Determinants of Minority Mental Health and Wellness

Sana Loue · Martha Sajatovic
Editors

Determinants of Minority Mental Health and Wellness

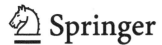 Springer

Editors

Sana Loue
Case Western Reserve
Cleveland, OH
sana.loue@case.edu

Martha Sajatovic
University of Cleveland
Cleveland, OH
martha.sajatovic@uhhs.com

ISBN 978-1-4419-2598-5   e-ISBN 978-0-387-75659-2
DOI 10.1007/978-0-387-75659-2

Printed on acid-free paper

springer.com

Preface

The United States is experiencing a dramatic shift in demographics, with minorities comprising a rapidly growing proportion of the population. It is anticipated that this will likely lead to substantial changes in previously established values, needs, and priorities of the population, including health and mental health for individuals, families, and society at large. This volume focuses on determinants of minority mental health and wellness. This emphasis necessarily raises the question of just who is a minority and how is minority to be defined.

The term has been defined in any number of ways. Wirth (1945, p. 347) offered one of the earliest definitions of minority:

> We may define a minority as a group of people who, because of their physical or cultural characteristics, are singled out from the others in the society in which they live for differential and unequal treatment, and who therefore regard themselves as objects of collective discrimination. The existence of a minority in a society implies the existence of a corresponding dominant group enjoying higher social status and greater privileges.

Numerous scholars have asserted that the central feature of a minority group is the power deficiency relative to that group (Blalock, 1960; Dworkin & Dworkin, 1982; Geschwender, 1978; Wilson, 1973) and the resulting oppression of one group by another. This imbalance of power may be manifested in the economic, political, and social domains of life (Ashmore, 1970; Barron, 1957; Howard, 1970; Kinloch, 1979; Ramaga, 1992; Wagley & Harris, 1958) through overt or more subtle forms of influence, exploitation, domination, oppression, and discrimination (Meyers, 1984; Ramaga, 1992). This power imbalance allows the establishment and maintenance of both control and dependency (Manderson, 1997).

Within this paradigm, it is the relative power or lack of it that is determinative of minority group status, rather than the numerical superiority or inferiority of a group (Meyers, 1984; Ramaga, 1992). The disempowerment and oppression of the black majority by a white minority in South Africa during the years of apartheid serves as such an example. Some writers, however, have refused to characterize a group as a minority if the group is larger in relative size within the population under discussion or if the group has no desire to preserve the characteristics which are believed to render it distinct (Anon, 2007; Schermerhorn, 1964).

Characteristics that have been linked to minority group identity include sex, sexual orientation, disability, ethnicity, nationality, race (without debating the validity of that concept), language, culture, and religion (Baron & Byrne, 1977; Barron, 1957; Hacker, 1951; Pap, 2003; Rose, 1964; Wagley & Harris, 1958), although religion has rarely been relied upon to define a minority in the United States (Minority, 2008). One scholar explained,

> Minorities are sub-groups within a culture which are distinguishable from the dominant group by reasons of differences in physiology, language, customs, or culture patterns (including any combination of these factors). Such sub-groups are regarded as inherently different and not belonging to the dominant groups; for this reason they are consciously or unconsciously excluded from full participation in the life of the culture .... Some minorities are physically different but culturally similar with respect to the majority ... others are culturally different but physically similar ... and still others are both culturally and physically different .... The cultural and/or physical differences between majority and minority actually may be so minute as to make it impossible to detect by simple observation who is a member of the minority and who is a member of the majority.
>
> (Schermerhorn, 1949, p. 5)

As such, an individual essentially inherits his or her status as a minority group member and cannot change that status unless the status of the group itself should change or he or she denies group membership, something that is not possible in the case of skin color or biological sex (Harris, 1959). The transformation of the Catholic population in New York from a despised and persecuted minority to a powerful force in the City's economic and political infrastructure serves as an example of how the status of a minority group may change over time (Collins, 2008).

Accordingly, each of the chapters within this volume addresses mental health and mental illness within the framework of one or more such groups. Sajatovic and colleagues lay the foundation for this exploration with their opening chapter that examines the meanings of mental health and wellness. The chapters that follow relating to urbanization, law, migration, media, health care systems, and systems of support examine the impact of these systems on minority health and wellness. Community-level and family-level and factors are discussed in the subsequent chapters that focus on religion, cultural perspectives of healing, racism, psychoeducation, and family dynamics. The importance of individual-level characteristics is addressed in the chapters relating to gender, socioeconomic status, genetics, substance use, cognitive functioning, and stress and resilience. The volume concludes with an examination of methodologic difficulties inherent in the conduct of research relating to mental health and wellness among minority groups and directions for future research.

Several themes emerge consistently throughout these chapters. Foremost among these is the discrimination encountered by members of minority groups defined on the basis of their skin color, ethnicity, biological sex, sexual orientation, gender, and language. It is equally apparent, however, that individuals face prejudice, hostility, and discrimination by virtue of their mental illness alone. Consequently, individuals who both are members of one or more defined minority groups and have a mental illness diagnosis may be multiply stigmatized (Capitanio & Herek, 1999; Herek, 1999; Herek & Capitanio, 1999; McBride, 1998; Reidpath & Chan, 2005).

Second, the discussion focusing on the larger environmental context of mental health and wellness underscores the complex nature of mental health and illness and the failure of many of our systems, including media, health care, housing, and law, to provide adequate support to individuals to enable them to function to their maximum ability within our society.

Finally, it is evident from these chapters that minority individuals, families, and communities often possess remarkable strengths that often remain unidentified or underutilized in their efforts to address life's challenges. Guarnaccia's final chapter highlighting directions for future research challenges us to identify mechanisms to address the deficiencies within our systems and to maximize the resources potentially available to individuals at the levels of the individual, family, and community.

Cleveland, OH   Sana Loue
                                                                                        Martha Sajatovic

References

Anon. (2007). Redefining minority undesirable controversy. *The Statesman (India)*, April 15. Retrieved May 21, 2008 from http://www.lexis.com/us/academic/delivery/PrintDoc.do?fromcart-false$dnldFilePath = %2F1-n%... [subscription required].

Ashmore, R. D. (1970). The problem of intergroup prejudice. In B. E. Collins (Ed.), *Social psychology* (pp. 246–296). Reading, Massachusetts: Addison-Wesley.

Baron, R. A., & Byrne, D. (1977). *Social psychology: Understanding human interaction* (2nd ed.). Boston, Massachusetts: Bacon and Allyn.

Barron, M. L. (Ed.). (1957). *American minorities: A textbook of readings in intergroup relations*. New York: Knopf.

Blalock, H. M. Jr. (1960). A power analysis of racial discrimination. *Social Forces, 39,* 53–59.

Capitanio, J. P., & Herek, G. M. (1999). AIDS-related stigma and attitudes towards injecting drug users among black and white Americans. *American Behavioral Scientist, 42*(7), 1148–1161.

Collins, G. (2008). Persecuted to powerful: Exhibiting a history of New York's Catholics. *New York Times, May 15,* sec. B, p. 2, col. 0.

Dworkin, A. G., & Dworkin, R. J. (Eds.). (1982). *The minority report: An introduction to racial, ethnic and gender relations* (2nd ed.). New York: Holt, Rinehart & Winston.

Geschwender, J. A. (1978). *Racial stratification in America*. Dubuque, Iowa: William C. Brown.

Hacker, H. M. (1951). Women as a minority group. *Social Forces*, 30(1), 60–69.

Harris, M. (1959). Caste, class, and minority. *Social Forces*, 37(3), 248–254.

Herek, G. M. (1999). AIDS and stigma. *American Behavioral Scientist, 42*(7), 1106–1116.

Herek, G. M., & Capitanio, J. P. (1999). AIDS stigma and sexual prejudice. *American Behavioral Scientist, 42*(7), 1130–1147.

Howard, J. R. (Ed.). (1970). *Awakening minorities: American Indians, Mexican Americans, Puerto Ricans.* Chicago: Aldine.

Kinloch, G. C. (1979). *The sociology of minority group relations.* Englewood Cliffs, New Jersey: Prentice-Hall.

Manderson, L. (1997). Migration, prostitution and medical surveillance in early twentieth-century Malaysia. In L. Marks & M. Worboys (Eds.). *Migrants, minorities, and health* (pp. 49–69). London: Routledge.

McBride, C. A. (1998). The discounting principle and attitudes towards victims of HIV infection. *Journal of Applied Social Psychology, 28*(7), 595–608.

Meyers, B. (1984). Minority group: An ideological formulation. *Social Problems, 32*(1), 1–15.

Minority. (2008). In *Encyclopedia Britannica.* Last accessed March 19, 2008; Available at *Encyclopedia Britannica Online,* http://www.britannica.com/eb/article-9052878

Pap, A. L. (2003). Ethnicization and European identity policies: Window-shopping with risks. *Dialectical Anthropology, 27,* 227–248.

Ramaga, P. V. (1992). Relativity of the minority concept. *Human Rights Quarterly, 14*(1), 104–119.

Reidpath, D. D., & Chan, K. Y. (2005). A method for the quantitative analysis of the layering of HIV-related stigma. *AIDS Care, 17*(4), 425–432.

Rose, A. M. (1964). Race and minority group relations. In J. Gould & W. L. Kolb (Eds.). *A dictionary of the social sciences* (pp. 570–571). New York: Free Press.

Schermerhorn, R. A. (1949). *These our people: Minorities in American culture.* Boston, Massachusetts: D.C. Heath.

Schermerhorn, R. A. (1964). Toward a general theory of minority groups. *Phylon, 25*(3), 238–246.

Wagley, C., & Harris, M. (1958). *Minorities in the New World.* New York: Columbia University Press.

Wilson, W. J. (1973). *Power, racism, and privilege: Race relations in theoretical and socio-historical perspective.* New York: Macmillan.

Wirth, L. (1945). The problem of minority groups. In R. Linton (Ed.). *The science of man in the world crisis* (pp. 347–372). New York: Columbia University Press.

Contents

Contributors

Ana F. Abraído-Lanza Mailman School of Public Health, Columbia University, New York, NY

AnnaMaria Aguirre McLaughlin Case Western Reserve University, Cleveland, Ohio

Stephanie Aldebot University of Miami, Coral Gables, Florida

Declan Barry, Ph.D. Yale University School of Medicine, New Haven, CT

Mark Beitel, Ph.D. Yale University School of Medicine, New Haven, CT

Kathryn A. Bottonari, M.A., M.S. Medical College of Georgia, Augusta, GA

Alice L. Costiuc Case Western Reserve University, Cleveland, OH

Radha Dunham, M.S. University of Miami, Coral Gables, Florida

Norah C. Feeney, Ph.D. Case Western Reserve University, Cleveland, OH

Susan Hatters Friedman, M.D. Case Western Reserve University, School of Medicine, Cleveland, OH

Prashant Gajwani, M.D. University Hospitals Case Medical Center, School of Medicine, Case Western Reserve University, Cleveland, OH

Sandro Galea, M.D., Dr.P.H. University of Michigan, School of Public Health, Ann Arbor, MI

Andres G. Gil, Ph.D. Florida International University, Office of Research and University Graduate School, Miami, FL

Deborah Goebert, Dr.P.H. University of Hawaii, John A. Burns School of Medicine, Honolulu, Hawaii

Emily Goldmann, M.P.H. University of Michigan, School of Public Health, Ann Arbor, MI

Peter Guarnaccia, Ph.D. Institute for Health, Health Care Policy, and Aging Research, Rutgers University, New Brunswick, NJ

Leslie J. Heinberg, Ph.D. Cleveland Clinic Lerner College of Medicine of Case Western Reserve University, Cleveland, OH

Franklin J. Hickman, J.D. Hickman & Lowder Co., L.P.A., Cleveland, OH

Siran M. Koroukian, Ph.D. Case Western Reserve University, School of Medicine, Cleveland, OH

Sana Loue, J.D., Ph.D., M.P.H. Case Western Reserve University, School of Medicine, Cleveland, OH

Andrea Maxwell University of Michigan, School of Public Health, Ann Arbor, MI

Lara Nochomovitz Hickman & Lowder Co., L.P.A., Cleveland, OH

Amir Poreh, Ph.D. Cleveland State University, Cleveland, OH

Martha Sajatovic, M.D. University Hospitals Case Medical Center, Case Western Reserve University, School of Medicine, Cleveland, OH

Saif Siddiqui, M.A. University of Illinois, College of Medicine, Chicago, IL

Laura Simonelli, Ph.D. Cleveland Clinic Foundation, Cleveland, OH

Joy Stankowski, M.D. Northcoast Behavioral Healthcare, Cleveland, OH

Lara M. Stepleman, Ph.D. Medical College of Georgia, Augusta, GA

Lisa Stines Doane Case Western Reserve University, Cleveland, OH

Alya Sultan, M.A. Cleveland State University, Cleveland, OH

Sandra S. Swantek, M.D. Northwestern University, Feinberg School of Medicine, Northwestern Memorial Hospital, Stone Institute of Psychiatry, Chicago, IL

Naomi Tuchman University of Miami, Coral Gables, Florida

William A. Vega, Ph.D. David Geffen School of Medicine, University of California Los Angeles, CA

Anahí Viladrich, Ph.D. The School of Health Sciences, The Schools of the Health Professions, Hunter College of the City of New York, School of Health Sciences, New York, NY

Stephanie Wasserman University of Miami, Coral Gables, Florida

Stevan Weine, M.D. University of Illinois, Psychiatric Institute, Chicago, IL

Amy Weisman de Mamani, Ph.D. University of Miami, Coral Gables FL

Dustin E. Wright, Ph.D. Medical College of Georgia, Augusta, GA

Chapter 1
Health and Wellness

Susan Hatters Friedman, Joy Stankowski, and Martha Sajatovic

Health: Definitions

Health is defined by the *Merriam-Webster Dictionary* as "the condition of being sound in body, mind, or spirit; *especially,* freedom from physical disease or pain" (*Merriam-Webster Dictionary*, 2007a). The emphasis is on the absence of disease or any condition that impairs normal functioning. For much of the last century, this impairment has been viewed mostly in biological terms, an approach known as the "medical model." Under this model, there have been significant advances in microbiology, genetics, and medication over the last half-century (McCulloch, 2005). Many nevertheless feel this model is too limiting, as it does not weigh psychological and social contributors to disease (Engel, 1977).

The World Health Organization, which coordinates health care for countries within the United Nations, emphasized a more broad definition of health in its 1946 Constitution: "Health is a state of complete physical, mental and social well-being and not merely the absence of disease or infirmity" (Yamey, 2002). In this definition, the emphasis is on complete well-being in many domains and contexts.

It can be argued that although this broader conceptualization of health is ideal, it is not practical (Saracci, 1997). First, it is likely that no human being ever achieves a complete state of well-being in all areas of life. Suffering is an intrinsic and, some argue, necessary component of human experience (Bhat, 2006). Second, a lack of disease can be defined objectively, but "complete well-being" is a subjective concept, especially as applied to one's mental and social health. One person may be depressed because he/she lives alone; another may be depressed because he/she lives with many people. Third, the variety of reasons that people lack well-being not only varies among individuals but changes frequently in the same individual. How is a nation, with limited resources and

M. Sajatovic (✉)
University Hospitals Case Medical Center, Case Western Reserve University, School of Medicine, Cleveland, OH
e-mail: Martha.Sajatovic@uhhs.com

S. Loue, M. Sajatovic (eds.), *Determinants of Minority Mental Health and Wellness*, DOI 10.1007/978-0-387-75659-2_1,
© Springer Science+Business Media, LLC 2009

health care dollars, to determine, measure, and realize the subjective and changing needs of all its citizens?

One author suggests a new definition of health: "a condition of well being free of disease or infirmity, and a basic and universal human right" (Saracci, 1997, pp. 1409–1410). The advantage of this definition is that it retains the idealistic goal of achieving well-being but describes this in practical terms of freedom from disease. Furthermore, this freedom is classified as a basic right. In following this guideline, nations are given a clear mandate to provide health for all citizens and can use the measuring sticks of disease or infirmity to track progress.

Health: In Practice

As discussed above, the medical model historically focuses on physical disease and treatment, a bias that is mirrored in the traditional medical school curriculum: first year, mastery of the normally functioning body; second year, exposure to the many ways the body can malfunction. By the time students begin to interact with patients, they have already learned to look for disease independent of the person suffering from the disease.

Although this model has been effective at finding and curing or controlling known diseases, it does not address how disease impacts the patient as a whole and complex person, and therefore does not necessarily improve or restore well-being. Research shows a positive correlation between the quality of doctor–patient communication and patient satisfaction with treatment (Hickson, 2002). Likewise, most patients who sue for medical malpractice do so because they perceive a lack of care and commitment, not necessarily because care was actually lacking (Teutsch, 2003). The fact that many medical schools are restructuring their curricula to include communication skills (Teutsch, 2003) indicates that restoring patient health clearly goes beyond removing physical disease.

As our understanding of health goes beyond the medical model, so does the breadth of treatments and providers. The prevalence of complementary alternative medicine in the last 30 years has steadily risen; many insurance providers now routinely accept treatment modalities such as chiropractic care, acupuncture, and massage. Health care is no longer provided just by doctors and nurses.

Wellness: Definition

Wellness has been described as "the quality or state of being in good health, especially as an actively sought goal" (*Merriam-Webster Dictionary*, 2007b). Health, therefore, is a state of being; wellness is the process of pursuing that state of being. This pursuit can center on treatment, for example, of an already contracted disease, or on prevention of a particular disease or diseases. The concept of wellness is thus a more inclusive construct than health and is also particularly relevant for groups within a larger population that may reflect ethnic, gender, religious, or other types of diversity and different ways of "being," including health, illness, and culturally or socially determines lifestyles and goals of living.

Wellness: Barriers

Barriers to wellness occur at both national and individual levels. First, a nation must identify which diseases plague their citizens. Public health officials assist by tracking the prevalence and course of disease in different locales. In the United States, heart disease is a primary cause of morbidity and mortality (Oyama et al., 2007), but in Africa malaria is of more concern.

Once common and preventable diseases are identified, the public must be educated, which can be difficult in the case of immigrants or persons without access to mass media. Finally, educated individuals must be motivated to change their behaviors. Lifestyle changes such as smoking cessation or weight loss are difficult, even when people are faced with life-threatening illness (Oyama et al., 2007). Furthermore, individuals must trust that the changes will cause benefit and not harm, as in the case of hormone replacement therapy for bone health causing increased cancer risk in post-menopausal women (Minelli, 2004).

Wellness: Facilitators

Most nations have pursued policies to prevent diseases that are endemic. In the United States, both public and privately funded organizations such as the American Heart Association help educate the public. In addition, as health care costs for employers rise, workplaces have become involved in prevention and control of common risk factors for heart disease, such as obesity and smoking (Oberlinner et al., 2007). In recent years, organizations supporting the education, treatment, and supports of mental health have also become prevalent. The most well-known is probably the National Alliance on Mental Illness (NAMI). Founded in 1979, NAMI now has offices in every state and over 1000 local communities, all "dedicated to the eradication of mental illnesses and to the improvement of the quality of life of all whose lives are affected by these diseases" (National Alliance for the Mentally Ill, 2008) (Table 1.1).

Table 1.1 Characteristics of health vs. wellness

Health	Wellness
• More disease/illness focused— specifically denotes *absence* of disease	• Broader, more holistic focus
• Often viewed in biological terms/ "medical model"	• Often viewed in social and cultural context
• A state of "being"	• A process of pursuing a state of being
• Has an industry (Health Care) devoted to primarily treating illness	• Has movements/advocacy groups that emphasize lifestyle, education, support

Mental Health: History

Throughout much of history, the mentally ill were feared and avoided. In medieval Europe, the mentally ill were thought to be witches, and 19 "witches" were burned at the stake in Salem, Massachusetts. Mentally ill persons in England were institutionalized or banished to the colonies in the United States or Australia.

Reform began in the 18th century with prominent speakers and educators. Cotton Mather proposed a physical cause for mental illness, and Benjamin Rush advocated for better treatment for mentally ill. Although treatment largely consisted of institutionalization, reformers such as Pinel argued for "moral treatment" of institutionalized patients (Bragg & Cohen, 2007). The discovery in 1952 that chlorpromazine could reduce psychosis revolutionalized our understanding and approach to mental illness. The success of psychopharmacology continued with lithium for mood stabilization and medication for depression. The effectiveness of this treatment helped spur the mass movement of psychiatric patients from institutions to the community in the 1970s (Miller, 1981).

Mental Health: Definitions

In psychiatry, mental illness is defined as subjective distress by a patient or impairment in functioning in one or more major life areas (Spitzer, Gibbon, Skodol, Williams, & First, 2001). Mental health is therefore the absence of any distress or impairment, and wellness is pursuing or maintaining this health. In mental health, consideration of factors beyond the physical is vital. Because distress is always subjective and unique to the individual, health care providers should consider how cultural, gender, religious, and age differences influence distress in a given individual.

In many ways, the definition and treatment of problems with mental health differs from that of physical health. As discussed above, in the United States mainstream health care is tied to the medical model, with a focus on finding and treating physical disease. This way of thinking about disease has spread beyond health care workers into the common culture. People most readily accept that someone is sick, or suffering, if the impairment is easily demonstrated, for example, a missing limb. In contrast, a person complaining of illness in the absence of any visible impairment—such as in the case of mental illness—is often viewed with suspicion (Johnston & Scholler-Jaquish, 2007). This stigma can make a person with mental illness reluctant to seek help.

This bias is also found in the business of medicine. Over time, salaries for physicians who perform procedures (such as surgeons, dermatologists, and radiologists) have increased significantly more than the salaries of non-procedure-oriented specialties (primary care, psychiatry) (American Medical Association, 2005).

For young doctors leaving medical school with debt that can reach several hundred thousand dollars, the incentive to choose a specialty that rewards finding and fixing physical disease is clear. Hospitals and institutions face similar incentives, since insurance reimburses physical illness more than mental. A new cardiology wing brings patients who require expensive monitoring and procedures; a new psychiatry wing brings patients who often require non-reimbursable social, financial, and medical assistance.

Mental Health in Minority Groups

Major mental illness is found worldwide, across all races and ethnicities. Are American minorities more likely to experience mental health problems? Data indicate that "the prevalence of mental disorder for racial and ethnic minorities in the United States is similar to that for whites" (United States Department of Health and Human Services, 2001). However, minorities may also be more likely to be poor or socially disadvantaged, which are known risk factors for mental illness. Additionally, the majority of those with mental illness do not get treatment, regardless of race or ethnicity. Unfortunately, minorities often receive less care and poorer quality care (United States Department of Health and Human Services, 2001).

Potential barriers to seeking mental health care include access difficulties, financial and transportation barriers, as well as stigma, cultural issues, and discrimination and mistrust (Aldrivez & Azocar, 1999; United States Department of Health and Human Services, 2001). Women with a mood or anxiety disorder and those with less education were more likely to anticipate stigma than other women (Aldrivez & Azocar, 1999). Stigma associated with getting mental health care varies across different subcultures. Cultural differences in social support and family involvement may play a role in mental health, acceptance of and adherence to treatment of mental illness (Snowden, 2007). For example, African American women may delay treatment for their own illnesses though they seek it for others (Loue, 1999).

Cultural differences between the health care practitioner and the patient should be considered. Potential obstacles between patients and care providers include difficulty understanding how a symptom is conceptualized in the culture (and whether it is pathological), language difficulty, and difficulty establishing rapport.

As the Group for Advancement of Psychiatry (GAP) aptly described, "cultural factors interact with and are molded by the specific historical experiences of the patient as well as by his or her race, gender, age, values and belief systems, country of origin, family migration events, language, and social and ethnic factors, with their resulting degrees of discrimination and disenfranchisement" (GAP Cultural, 2002). Individuals from various cultures may have different ways of experiencing and expressing distress. The meaning of being mentally ill within a specific culture and for that individual should be explored (Loue, 1999). Herbal medications or other remedies may be utilized within the community, which the mental health provider may need to ask about. Beliefs about disease causation, including disease as punishment for past offences or sins, disease related to ancestral spirits, or disease as externally generated (for example, voodoo or curse), may affect health practitioner choice—for example seeking care from traditional healers or clergy. Congruence in beliefs with healers is important, and by learning more about diverse cultures and culture-specific beliefs with regard to mental health and wellness, psychiatrists and other mental health providers can attempt to negotiate this often-complex issue.

Ethnic/Racial Minorities

In the United States, 75% of the population self-identify as Caucasian, while 12% self-identify as African American, 4% Asian American, and 1% Native American. Within these, 13% self-identify as Latino (United States Census Bureau, 2002). Though Caucasians may be in the majority, they too subsume or reflect many different cultures of origin. Minorities often face inequalities such as racism, violence, and poverty. Racism is stressful and could increase depression and anxiety. Poverty also increases the risk of mental illness (United States Department of Health and Human Services, 2001).

Regarding mental illness in the United States, African Americans "appear to have relatively low prevalence rates despite a history of prejudice, discrimination, and the resulting stress" (Sue & Chu, 2003, p. 447). They may have protective factors such as strong religious values and strong family support (Walker, 2007). African Americans, however, are overrepresented in groups vulnerable to mental illness, including the homeless, incarcerated, and children in foster care (United States Department of Health and Human Services, 2001). Additionally, African Americans may be more likely to be misdiagnosed with schizophrenia in cases where their true diagnosis is bipolar disorder or psychotic depression, leading to inappropriate treatments, and also to receive higher doses of antipsychotic medications, leading to increased propensity for medication-related adverse effects.

Members of the Asian community may report fatigue and pain, rather than sadness, in depression. Diversity of expression of mental illness occurs across various Asian subgroups as well. For example, Asians and Pacific Islanders include 43 ethnic groups and 100 languages or dialects (United States Department of Health and Human Services, 2001). They often delay care until symptoms are severe. They may have a different metabolism and require lower doses of medication.

There are over 500 federally recognized Native American tribes (United States Department of Health and Human Services, 2001). The Indian Health Service was established in 1955, the federal agency charged with providing physical and mental health care. One quarter of the Native American population lives in poverty. Native Americans have also been plagued with high rates of substance abuse and mood disorder. They are five times more likely to die of alcohol-related causes than Whites (United States Department of Health and Human Services, 2001). Their suicide rate is 50% higher than the U.S. national rate (United States Department of Health and Human Services, 2001).

Latinos are a quickly growing minority population in the United States. They are quite diverse, including immigrants and their descendents from Mexico, Puerto Rico, Central and South America, as well as Cuba. The average age of the Latino population is 26 years and educational levels often lower compared to non-Latinos (Galanti, 2003). Degree of acculturation varies depending on the time of immigration, residing community, and ethnic identity. There is a wide variation of mental health needs across different groups of Latinos. For example, Latinos born in the United States may suffer more mental illness than those born in Mexico or Puerto Rico. Latino youths are at higher risk of depression, anxiety, and suicide attempts. They may also experience poor access to ethnically similar health care providers (United States Department of Health and Human Services, 2001).

Among Latino groups, somatic complaints may be an "idiom of distress, nervousness." Headaches are "popular metaphors that connote specific sources of interpersonal stress rather than indicate somatization of psychological distress" (Koss-Chioino, 1999). Culture must be considered in assessing and diagnosing mental illness in minorities. For example, in some developing countries, hearing the voice of a deceased relative is not considered pathologic. Professionals must use caution rather than interpreting all voices as hallucinations indicative of illness. Various syndromes have been labeled by the *Diagnostic and Statistical Manual (DSM)* as psychiatric culture-bound phenomena such as "ataque de nervios" and "amok"; however, these likely represent only a small proportion of mental illnesses that are affected by culture. Finally, caution must be used to not perpetuate American ethnocentric ideas. For example, anorexia nervosa and dissociative identity disorder may be U.S. majority culture-bound syndromes (Simpson, 2007).

Gender Minorities

Men could be considered a minority in their seeking of mental health care, because women are the predominant care consumers. When depression is characterized as a weakness or lack of power, men may be hesitant to seek help (Emslie, Ridge, Ziebland, & Hunt, 2006). Men tend to have higher rates of substance abuse and antisocial personality disorder (Regier et al., 1998) compared to women. Mentally ill persons are overrepresented in the legal system, which has been known as "criminalization of the mentally ill" (Grekin, Jemelka, & Trupin, 1994, p. 411). Men (predominantly, and some women) may become involved in forensic mental health care due to involvement with criminal courts and incarceration.

Overall, women have an increased risk of developing major depression compared to men. Prenatal and postpartum depressions cause substantial burden and disability, including reduced functional status, increased risk of suicide, and increased risk of poor bonding with the infant. While there are multiple risk factors, mothers with socioeconomic disadvantage are at increased risk of postpartum depression. Some innovative clinics are able to combine obstetrics visits with psychiatric assessment and treatment so that one barrier to care is removed. Management of mental illness in pregnancy and lactation can be quite complex due to potential risks of malformations, infant toxicity, or medication withdrawal at birth and maternal side-effects. However, pregnant and postpartum women, as well as any woman of childbearing age in many cases, have been excluded from research studies traditionally, due to concerns about risk to the unborn or infant. Unfortunately, there is limited information regarding the best treatments of mental illness in pregnancy and the postpartum among minority women.

Religious Minorities

Religion and psychiatry have a complex relationship. In a 2001 survey in the United States, of those who responded regarding religion, 81% of individuals self-identified as Christian, 1% as Jewish, 1% Buddhist, 1% as Muslim, and 1% as agnostic/atheist (United States Census Bureau, 2001). Some religions (e.g., Scientology) eschew or openly protest against psychiatry. Alternatively, some religious institutions are quite effective partners in care with the traditional model mental health team. Approximately half of Americans with mental illness seek pastoral help (which is often free) rather than traditional model psychiatric help (Spangler, 2001).

For culturally informed mental health assessment and diagnosis, an understanding of the core beliefs of those in a specific religion is important. What may sound like a delusion initially may represent a normal religious belief. Consider, for example, if Christianity were not a widely accepted religion, how some of its core beliefs (immaculate conception, revival from the dead, visions and prophets) might be interpreted. In cases of less mainstream religions in the context of which a patient is seeking mental health care, it can be helpful to speak with others in the religion to ascertain the range of normative, culturally held beliefs. For example, belief in voodoo may be considered culturally appropriate in some religions or cultures and a paranoid delusion in others.

Therapists may be of the same or of different faith than their patients. A 2007 survey of physicians found that psychiatrists were more likely to be Jewish or without a religious affiliation and less likely to be Christian or even to be religious in general, than other physicians. Psychiatrists often considered themselves spiritual rather than religious (Curlin et al., 2007a). Individuals struggling with symptoms of mental illness may seek treatment by spiritual counselors or practitioners who can integrate components of traditional psychiatry and faith-based practices such as prayer. Mental health providers may not incorporate the patient's spiritual beliefs in their evaluation or treatment. While they are aware of the positive influence of spirituality on health, psychiatrists also note the potential for negative emotions related to increased suffering (Curlin et al., 2007b).

Sexual Orientation Minorities

Lesbian and gay mental health issues have a paucity of research devoted to them. Heterosexism is also believed to affect what is researched (Trettin, Moses-Kolko, & Wisner, 2006) and what trainees are taught. Homosexuality is a topic to which little attention is paid in medical school. Barriers to care exist for lesbian/gay, as well as other minority populations. Internalized homophobia, stigma, discrimination, and violence victimization may each play a role (Meyer, 1995). Further, the lack of benefits for same-sex partners in many cases may represent a barrier to care. If they are seeking psychiatric care, a gay therapist may be sought after for potentially better understanding of the issues (GAP Homosexuality, 2000). The U.S. military's policy on homosexuality could potentially affect access to psychiatric care, and having to hide one's sexuality could cause more stress, anxiety, and depression. Issues such as concern about acceptance are plentiful when the person faces "coming out" to friends and family as gay.

Rather embarrassingly, society's views about sexual issues have been paralleled by the psychiatric profession, apparently not based on research evidence. Freud himself described paranoia as a "defense against unconscious homosexual wishes" (GAP Homosexuality, 2000). Over a quarter-century ago, members of the American Psychiatric Association voted to remove homosexuality from the list of mental disorders (*Psychiatric News*, 2007). Since 1973 the APA has opposed discrimination against homosexuals, including in the Armed Services (American Psychiatric Association, 1990). The *DSM*'s bias is noted in that transsexualism is considered a gender identity disorder in mainstream U.S. society but may be considered culturally accepted behavior among some groups (Loue, 1999).

Immigrants

Immigrants, particularly refugees or those seeking asylum, may have been victims of torture or may have lost family members. While PTSD and depression are more common amongst those experiencing violence or trauma, the immigrant experience may be made difficult due to financial hardship, underemployment or unemployment, or language and cultural barriers. (For additional discussion of the effects of migration on mental health, see the chapter by Loue in this volume.) In addition to immigration stress, acculturation is another issue in mental health which may be different across immigration groups. For example, acculturation "is negatively related to mental health for Mexican Americans and positively related to mental health for Asian Americans" (Sue & Chu, 2003).

In some countries, such as China and Russia, it has been reported that psychiatric hospitalization has been used as a way of disposing of political dissidents. While this is not considered an ethical practice in the United States, previous life experience among immigrants experiencing political persecution could bias against individuals seeking psychiatric care in the new host country.

Military and Workforce Minorities

In the past, those returning from military service such as the Vietnam War, were often misunderstood and victims of prejudice. In addition, some soldiers may have suffered severe trauma during their service and are at risk for post-traumatic stress disorder (Engelhard et al., 2007). Services available to military veterans may be insufficient to meet their needs.

Lack of health insurance coverage among the working poor is an issue, and minorities are overrepresented in this group (United States Department of Health and Human Services, 2001). Minorities who are illegal immigrants typically have no or minimal access to any health care. Lack of mental health care seeking among these individuals is understandable as care seeking/use could lead to detection and subsequent deportation.

Individuals and Groups Who May Be Disproportionately Disadvantaged

Some groups may simultaneously represent multiple minorities. For example, women working in male male-dominated professions may experience bias against them and increased stress. Women physicians may be promoted more slowly than their male counterparts (Tesch, Wood, Helwig, & Nattinger, 1995). White female physicians (who may not traditionally be considered as "disadvantaged") have an elevated suicide rate, compared to the employed U.S. population (Petersen & Burnett, 2007). While suicide rates among male police officers in the New York Police Department were comparable to rates of male New York City residents, female police officers had a higher risk of suicide than female residents of New York City (Marzuk, Nock, Leon, Portera, & Tardiff, 2002).

Future Trends in the U.S. Population Anticipated to Affect Minority Mental Health

Demographic trends occurring in the United States that may be anticipated to affect minority populations and mental health among minority subgroups include increasing life span and a growing population of elderly, increasing ethnic and cultural diversity, and a "majority" culture that is shrinking in size and influence. Life expectancy in the United States has increased dramatically from 49 years in 1900 to 76.5 currently (Federal Interagency Forum on Aging-Related Statistics, 2000), and the elderly population is expected to continue to grow at a rapid pace. By the year 2030, one in three Americans will be aged 55 and older, and one in five will be at least aged 65. Individuals aged 85 and older are one of the fastest-growing subgroups in the United States (Federal Inter-agency Forum on Aging-Related Statistics, 2000). It is anticipated that the growing proportion of elderly will have increased need of medical services given the typical association of medical comorbidity and aging. Medical disability is known to be associated with depression and anxiety and is often underrecognized and undertreated in primary care settings (Young, Klapp, & Sherbourne, 2001). The number of individuals with dementing conditions such as Alzheimer's disease and the resultant neuropsychiatric syndromes that occur in these disorders is expected to increase. Health care costs for an expanding population of elderly will be increased for both individuals and society, and it can be anticipated that health care resources might require prioritization or rationing. It is not clear how minority populations will be affected by aging demographic trends, although one might anticipate that the problems of limited access and lower quality care will persist for minorities, especially elderly individuals with fewer resources, fewer supports, and less advocacy.

Currently minorities make up approximately 33% of the U.S. population, with 12.5% of those individuals being immigrants (United States Census Bureau, 2006). Latinos are currently the largest minority ethnic group, with expected continued robust growth in the Latino population. Latinos currently comprise 50% of the national population growth, and by 2050 are expected to number 102.6 million, or 24.4% of the U.S. population (Kramer, Resendez, & Ahmed, 2008; United States Census Bureau, 2004). Asian Americans make up more than 4% of the current U.S. population, a figure that is expected to double by 2025. Currently, approximately 71% of the U.S. Asian population is immigrants (Kramer, Kwong, Lee, & Chung, 2002). In contrast, U.S. African American population grew by only 1.3% during a 1-year period (2004–2005), with 18% of the increase being due to immigration (United States Census Bureau, 2004). Finally, in tandem with the rapid increase in ethnic subgroups within the United States it is anticipated that the Caucasian population will no longer be a majority, shrinking in both size and influence. This is likely to have substantial impact on health care resource use patterns and public policy.

Effects of Demographic Trends on Individuals and Communities

Minority subgroups have differing life experiences, prevalence, and presentation of mental illnesses. Experiences with war and trauma may be a particular focus of concern among some subgroups (Kramer et al., 2008). Acculturation for immigrants appears to be related to increasing rates of mental disorders, for example, the Mexican American Prevalence and Services Survey (MAPSS) demonstrated that lifetime mental disorder rate for immigrants who had lived in the United States for more than 13 years was nearly double that for newer immigrants (Dey & Lucas, 2006). The process of acculturation, however, may be modified for ethnic groups that have become so large that they may no longer be considered "minorities." For many non-American cultures the family is the focus of major decision making, including how, when, and where to seek health care. The process of health care seeking with respect to acculturation across the generations and individuals of differing age groups might be expected to change as minorities become "super minorities" or even a dominant subgroup. For example, elderly Latinos who have been living in the United States for decades may feel in some respects more culturally matched with their age-matched peers in the larger U.S. community compared to young adults who are recent immigrants from Mexico.

Growth in ethnic subgroups within the United States will eventually translate into more health care providers, including psychiatrists and other mental health care that are culturally matched to their patients with mental illness. This might decrease language and other barriers and lead to care that is more culturally informed. On the other hand, given the large number of subgroups within some of the major ethnic categories (for example, Latinos and Asian Americans), it is very likely that substantial barriers will persist. Finally, recent years have seen growth in minority public figures and policy makers such as Dr. Jocelyn Elders and Dr. Antonia Novello as the first African American and Latina U.S. Surgeon Generals, respectively. It is hoped that representation by minorities will result in legislation that mandates equity for minorities and leads to improved mental health outcomes and quality of life.

References

Aldrivez, J., & Azocar, F. (1999). Distressed women's clinic patients: preferences for mental health treatments and perceived obstacles. *General Hospital Psychiatry, 21*(5), 340–347.

American Medical Association. (2005). Last accessed January 16, 2008; Available at www.ama-assn.org/ama/pub/category/9922.html.

American Psychiatric Association. (1990). *Homosexuality and the armed services position statement*. APA Reference document 900013. Last accessed November 17, 2007; Available at www.psych.org/edu/other_res/lib_archives/archives/199013.pdf.

Bhat, S. K. (2006). The death of a Buddha. *Journal of Clinical Psychiatry, 67*, 1647–1648.

Bragg, T., & Cohen, B. (2007). From asylum to hospital to psychiatric health care system. *American Journal of Psychiatry, 164*(6), 883.

Curlin, F. A., Odell, S. V., Lawrence, R. E., Chin, M. H., Lantos, J. D., Meador, K. G., et al. (2007a). The relationship between psychiatry and religion among U.S. physicians. *Psychiatric Services, 58*(9), 1193–1198.

Curlin, F. A., Lawrence, R. E., Odell, S., Chin, M. H., Lantos, J. D., Koenig, H. G., et al. (2007b). Spirituality, and medicine: psychiatrists' and other physicians' differing observations, interpretations, and clinical approaches. *American Journal of Psychiatry, 164*(12), 1825–1831.

Dey, A. N., & Lucas, J. W. (2006). *Physical and mental health characteristics of U.S.- and foreign-born adults: United States, 1998–2003, Advance data from vital and health statistics, no. 369*. Hyattsville, Maryland: National Center for Health Statistics.

Emslie, C., Ridge, D., Ziebland, S., & Hunt, K. (2006). Men's accounts of depression: reconstructing or resisting hegemonic masculinity? *Social Science & Medicine, 62*(9), 2246–2257.

Engel, G. L. (1977). The need for a new medical model: a challenge for biomedicine. *Science, 196*(4286), 129–136.

Engelhard, I. M., Van Den Hout, M. A., Weerts, J., et al. (2007) Deployment-related stress and trauma in Dutch soldiers returning from Iraq. *British Journal of Psychiatry, 191*, 140–145.

Federal Interagency Forum on Aging-Related Statistics. (2000). *Older Americans 2000: Key indicators of well-being*. Washington, District of Columbia: U.S. Government Printing Office.

Galanti, G. A. (2003). The Hispanic family and male-female relationships: an overview. *Journal of Transcultural Nursing, 14*(3), 180–185.

Grekin, P. M., Jemelka, R., & Trupin, E. W. (1994). Racial differences in the criminalization of the mentally ill. *Bulletin of the American Academy of Psychiatry, 22*(3), 411–420.

Group for the Advancement of Psychiatry, Committee on Cultural Psychiatry. (2002). *Cultural assessment in psychiatry*. Washington, District of Columbia: American Psychiatric Publishing, Inc.

Group for the Advancement of Psychiatry, Committee on Human Sexuality. (2000). *Homosexuality and the mental health professions*. Hillsdale, New Jersey: Analytic Press.

Hickson, G. B. (2002). Patient complaints and malpractice risk. *Journal of the American Medical Association, 287*(22), 2951–2957.

Johnston, N. E., & Scholler-Jaquish, A. (2007). *Meaning in suffering: caring practices in the health professions*. Madison, Wisconsin: University of Wisconsin Press.

Koss-Chioino, J. D. (1999). Depression among Puerto Rican women: culture, etiology, and diagnosis. *Hispanic Journal of Behavioral Sciences, 21*(3), 330–350.

Kramer, E. J., Kwong, K., Lee, E., & Chung, H. (2002). Cultural factors influencing the mental health of Asian Americans. *Western Journal of Medicine, 176*(4), 227–231.

Kramer, E. J., Resendez, D. I., & Ahmed, I. (2008). Training the next generation of health care professionals. In S. Loue & M. Sajatovic (Eds.). *Diversity issues in the diagnosis, treatment, and research of mood disorders* (pp. 270–300). New York: Oxford University Press, Inc.

Loue, S. (1999). *Gender, ethnicity, and health research*. New York: Kluwer Academic/Plenum.

Marzuk, P. M., Nock, M. K., Leon, A. C., Portera, L., & Tardiff, K. (2002). Suicide among New York City police officers, 1977–1996. *American Journal of Psychiatry, 159*(12), 2069–2071.

McCulloch, A. (2005). Has the medical model a future? *The Mental Health Review, 10*, 7–15.

Merriam-Webster Dictionary (2007a). Last accessed January 16, 2008; Available at www.m-w.com/dictionary/health.

Merriam-Webster Dictionary (2007b). Last accessed January 16, 2008; Available at www.m-w.com/dictionary/wellness

Meyer, I. H. (1995). Minority stress and mental health in gay men. *Journal of Health & Social Behavior, 36*(1), 38–56.

Miller, R. D. (1981). Beyond the old state hospital: new opportunities ahead. *Hospital and Community Psychiatry, 32*(1), 27–31.

Minelli, C. (2004). Benefits and harms associated with hormone replacement therapy: clinical decision analysis. *British Medical Journal, 328*(7436), 371.

National Alliance for the Mentally Ill. (2008). About NAMI. Last accessed February 25, 2008; Available at www.nami.org/template.cfm?section = About_NAMI

Oberlinner, C., Lang, S., Germann, C., Trauth, B., Eberle, F., Pluto, R., et al. (2007). Prevention of overweight and obesity in the workplace. BASF-health promotion campaign "trim down the pounds – losing weight without losing your mind". *Gesundheitswesen, 69*(7), 385–392.

Oyama, N., Gona, P., Salton, C. J., Chuang, M. L., Jhaveri, R. R., Blease, S. J., et al. (2007). Differential impact of age, sex, and hypertension on aortic atherosclerosis. The Framingham Heart Study. *Arteriosclerosis, Thrombosis, & Vascular Biology, 28*(1), 155–159. [Epub ahead of print].

Petersen, M. R., & Burnett, C. A., (2007). The suicide mortality of working physicians and dentists. *Occupational Medicine (London)*, *58*(1), 25–29.

Psychiatric News (ref 35). (2007). *Panelists recount events leading to deleting homosexuality as a psychiatric disorder from DSM*. Last accessed October 29, 2007; Available at www.psych. org/pnews/98-07-17/dsm.html.

Regier, D. A., Boyd, J. H., Burke, J. D. Jr., Rae, D. S., Myers, J. K., Kramer, M., et al. (1988). One-month prevalence of mental disorders in the United States. Based on five Epidemiologic Catchment Area sites. *Archives of General Psychiatry*, *45*(11), 977–986.

Saracci, R. (1997). The World Health Organization needs to reconsider its definition of health. *British Medical Journal*, *314*, 1409.

Simpson, A. I. F. (2007). Responding to cultural difference: ethics, constitutionality or efficacy? Invited presentation at the American Academy of Psychiatry and the Law, Miami, Florida.

Snowden, L. R. (2007). Explaining mental health treatment disparities: ethnic and cultural differences in family involvement. *Culture, Medicine, and Psychiatry*, *31*(3), 389–402.

Spangler, P. R. (2001). The counseling role of Baptist ministers in rural and urban West Virginia counties. *West Virginia Medical Journal*, *97*(2), 115–117.

Spitzer, R. L., Gibbon, M., Skodol, A. E., Williams, J. B. W., & First, M. B. (2001). *DSM IV-TR case book*. Washington, District of Columbia: American Psychiatric Publishing.

Sue, S., & Chu, J.Y. (2003). The mental health of ethnic minority groups: challenges posed by the supplement to the surgeon general's report on mental health. *Culture, Medicine, & Psychiatry*, *27*(4), 447–465.

Tesch, B. J., Wood, H. M., Helwig, A. L., & Nattinger, A. B. (1995). Promotion of women physicians in academic medicine. Glass ceiling or sticky floor? *Journal of the American Medical Association*, *273*(13), 1022–1025.

Teutsch, C. (2003). Patient-doctor communication. *Medical Clinics of North America*, *87*(5), 1115–1145.

Trettin, S., Moses-Kolko, E. L., & Wisner, K. L. (2006). Lesbian perinatal depression and the heterosexism that affects knowledge about this minority population. *Archives of Women's Mental Health*, *9*(2), 67–73.

United States Census Bureau. (2001). *Self-described religious identification of adult population: 1990 and 2001*. Last accessed December 12, 2007; Available at www.census.gov/compen dia/statab/cats/population/religion.html.

United States Census Bureau. (2002). *United States Summary: Census 2000 Profile*. Last accessed November 17, 2007, Available at www.census.gov/prod/ 2002pubs/ c2kprof00-us.pdf.

United States Census Bureau. (2004). *U.S. Interim Projections by Age, Sex, Race and Hispanic Origin*. Last accessed October 26, 2006; Available at www.census.gov/ipc/www/usinter improj/natprojtab01a.pdf.

United States Census Bureau. (2006). *Nation's Population One-Third Minority*. Last accessed May 10, 2006; Available at www.census.gov/PressRelease/www/ releases/ archives/popu lation/006808.html.

United States Department of Health and Human Services. (2001). *Mental Health: Culture, Race, and Ethnicity—A Supplement to Mental Health: A Report of the Surgeon General*. Rockville, Maryland: United States Department of Health and Human Services, Substance Abuse and Mental Health Services Administration, and Center for Mental Health Services. Last accessed February 25, 2008; Available at http://download.ncadi.samhsa. gov/ken/pdf/SMA-01-3613/sma-01-3613A.pdf.

Walker, R. L. (2007). Acculturation and acculturative stress as indicators for suicide risk among African Americans. *American Journal of Orthopsychiatry*, *77*(3), 386–391.

Yamey, G. (2002). Have the latest reforms reversed WHO's decline? *British Medical Journal*, *325*, 1107–1112.

Young, A. S., Klapp, R., & Sherbourne, C. D. (2001). The quality of care for depressive and anxiety disorders in the United States. *Archives of General Psychiatry*, *58*, 55–61.

Chapter 2
City Living and Mental Health in History

Sandro Galea, Emily Goldmann, and Andrea Maxwell

Cities have long been the subject of literary and academic interest as a powerful force shaping the health of populations. Writers from several eras in Western European history considered cities as places that were detrimental to health, and in many ways, for much of history, cities were characterized by features that were unquestionably linked to poor health. Percy Bysshe Shelley (1819), an English romantic poet, observed that "Hell is a city much like London." Indeed, a full collection of the writings that have denounced cites or deplored living conditions in cities would fill several volumes (Marsella, 1995).

It is worth considering why historically so many leading thinkers have considered that cities could be detrimental to health. Most of the early thought about cities and how they might unfavorably influence human health arose from the growing role played by cities in European life over much of the past millennium. As cities grew—particularly as the Industrial Revolution accelerated—population density, marginalized populations, pollution, and crime frequently increased, resulting in health in cities being worse than it was outside of cities in many countries. Literary observers and social commentators, reflecting on these observations, ascribed to city living an etiologic role in shaping health (Dickens, 1850; Durant & Durant, 1967; Durkheim, 1897; Engels, 1887).

In many ways, it was the process of rapid urbanization itself during the eighteenth and nineteenth centuries that prompted developments in public health (Coleman, 1982; Glaab & Brown, 1976). For example, in France during the first half of the nineteenth century, rapidly changing demographics and the economic situation in urban areas contributed to *hygiene publique*, or public health, becoming formally constituted as a science (Coleman, 1982). Louis René Villermé and other *hygienistes* recognized the contribution that inadequate water supplies, overcrowding, and poor housing were making to poor health in France's burgeoning cities and implemented programs aimed at

S. Galea (✉)
University of Michigan, School of Public Health, Ann Arbor, MI
e-mail: sgalea@umich.edu

S. Loue, M. Sajatovic (eds.), *Determinants of Minority Mental Health and Wellness*, DOI 10.1007/978-0-387-75659-2_2,
© Springer Science+Business Media, LLC 2009

improving urban living conditions. Indeed, the urban environment in many Western cities improved dramatically at the turn of the twentieth century; coincident with this improvement, health of urban populations also improved (Vogele, 1994). In many parts of the world, however, the conditions that were prevalent in Western cities during the eighteenth and nineteenth century remain prevalent today.

Why should cities and city living affect the prevalence of disorders? More particularly, why should cities affect mental health overall and the mental health of minority populations in specific? Before addressing these questions, a couple of cautions are in order.

First, there is no "one way" in which city living may affect mental health. Although for the sake of explication we generally discuss mechanisms and mental health, the mechanisms that potentially explain the relations between urban living and mental disorders frequently depend on the specific type of mental disorder. As we discuss potential mechanisms, we consider "mental health" as one construct but make reference to specific theoretic distinctions and empiric examples that suggest how different factors may be differentially important for diverse mental disorders.

Second, cities are ultimately places. Although cities are not static—in fact the very dynamism of cities is one of their defining features—considering mental health in cities is ultimately the study of how a particular type of place may affect mental health. Explanations for these potential effects then rest primarily on how *characteristics* of places—in this case cities—may be important determinants of mental health.

In this book, we are primarily interested in the determinants of the mental health of minorities. Very little peer-reviewed literature exists that has shown that urban living, or urbanization, is differentially associated with the health of minorities compared to other racial/ethnic groups. It is the intent of this chapter first to highlight *why* city living may be associated with the mental health of minorities; second, to summarize the extant literature about the relation between city living and mental health in general, while drawing attention to the mental health of minorities where applicable; and third, to stimulate discussion about the topic at hand.

Why Would City Living Affect Mental Health?

Several characteristics of cities may be important determinants of mental health, each having multiple implications for urban dwellers in general and potentially for minority groups in particular. Building on the extant literature, we consider here five concepts that may be particularly relevant to mental health: social disorganization/strain, social resources, social contagion, spatial segregation, and the urban physical environment. Although there is overlap between each of these concepts, considering each in turn lends insight into the potential causal relations between urban living and mental health.

Social Disorganization/Strain

One of the primary explanations for the relation between urban living and health that has been posited in different guises in several disciplines can be conceptualized within the rubric of social disorganization/social strain theories. Social disorganization theory was first developed in studies of urban crime by sociologists in Chicago in the 1920s and 1930s. In brief, social order, stability, and integration are conducive to conformity, while disorder is conducive to crime and poor integration into social structures (Shaw & McKay, 1969). More recent theoretical and empirical refinements to social disorganization theory have held that social control is the hallmark of social disorganization theory and affects the likelihood of crime in cities (Sampson & Groves, 1989). A parallel theory, frequently referred to as anomie/strain theory, while arising from a separate disciplinary focus, similarly suggests explanations for the relations between social structure and behavior. Emile Durkheim (1897) used the term "anomie" to refer to the state of a lack of social regulation in modern society as one of the conditions that makes for higher rates of suicide. Drawing on this work, Robert Merton (1938) suggested that anomie is the lack of societal integration that arises from the tension between aspirations of industrialized persons and the means available to them to achieve those aspirations. In the U.S. context in particular, the exposure of persons of all social classes to high aspirations that are practically unachievable produces *strain* or pressure on these groups to take advantage of whatever effective means to income and success they can find, even if these means are illegitimate or illegal. Hence, Merton argued that social strain can be associated with crime.

Contemporary anomie/strain theories, such as general strain theory, expand on the connection between sources of strain, strain-induced negative emotion, and individual criminal behavior. Agnew (1992) suggests that there are other sources of strain in modern living, including confrontation with unpleasant stimuli. In a recent modification of general strain theory, Agnew (2001) more clearly specifies that the types of strain most likely to lead to criminal or delinquent coping are strains that are seen as unjust, high in magnitude, emanating from situations in which social control is undermined, and pressuring the individual into criminal or delinquent associations.

Social disorganization and social strain theories have important implications for mental disorders in cities. A substantial body of research has documented the role of stress in shaping health in general and mental health in particular (Pearlin, Lieberman, Menaghan, & Mullan, 1981). Although most of this work has considered stress processes at the individual level (Noh & Avison, 1996), there is a growing appreciation of the fact that environmental context may itself be an important determinant of health or may shape the impact of other stressors on individual mental health (Elliott, 2000). Urban areas are generally characterized by higher social disorganization, socioeconomic disparities, dense and diverse populations, higher crime rates, and migratory populations posing considerable stress on their residents.

It is worth noting the particular role that minority status may then play in generating substantial social strain in urban areas. Many cities worldwide are highly segregated with multiple historical, logistical, and practical barriers to mixing of social groups. In addition, minority groups often reside in parts of urban environments that are more disadvantaged than non-minority groups. Urban segregation also contributes to the strain faced by minority groups in urban areas. For example, a study assessing the relationships between perceptions of one's neighborhood and depressive symptoms found that perceptions of neighborhood characteristics (vandalism, litter or trash, vacant housing, teenagers loitering, burglary, drug selling, and robbery) predicted depressive symptoms at a 9-month follow-up interview. This suggests that social disorganization and social strain are determinants of depressive symptoms (Latkin & Curry, 2003).

Several studies have shown that social strain is associated with poorer overall mental health (e.g., Amick et al., 1998), depression (Beach, Schulz, Yee, & Jackson, 2000), and substance use (Velleman & Templeton, 2003), though few of these studies have specifically assessed the relations among the urban environment, social strain, and mental health. Urban areas characterized by greater deviant behavior also may have a higher likelihood of traumatic event experiences for their residents (e.g., rape, interpersonal violence), which are consistently linked to poorer mental health, including anxiety and mood disorders (Seedat, Nyamai, Njenga, Vythilingum, & Stein, 2004).

Social Resources

Further refinements on social strain theory in urban areas include an appreciation of the fact that in urban areas persons with different socioeconomic status both may be faced with different stressors and may have disparate access to resources that could help them cope with stressors. This is particularly an issue for minority group members who frequently have substantially lower socioeconomic status than majority group members. (Socioeconomic status and mental health and illness are addressed by Stepleman et al. in Chapter 15 of this volume.) However, the relation between urban stressors and mental disorders is likely buffered by salutary resources (e.g., health care, social services) that are frequently more prevalent in urban compared to non-urban areas. For disadvantaged urban populations, formal local resources can complement or substitute for individual or family resources. Although these resources may be available to urban residents, socioeconomic disparities in cities are linked to differential access to these resources; this suggests that persons at different ends of the socioeconomic spectrum—such as minorities—may have different opportunities to benefit from the resources available in cities. This discrepant exposure to stressors and access to resources has been called the "differential vulnerability" hypothesis, positing that persons with lower socioeconomic status are both exposed to more stressors and also have fewer resources to help cope with them (Pearlin, 1999). This hypothesis may be particularly important in urban areas characterized by socioeconomic disparities.

Individual social experiences also may be important determinants of mental disorders in cities. For example, limited social support may predispose persons to poorer coping and adverse health (McLeod & Kessler, 1990). In one national forensic autopsy of suicides, it was shown that urban suicides were more likely to be preceded by a recent separation from a partner than were rural suicides (Isometsa et al., 1997). This suggests that social connectedness may play a different role in determining mental disorders in urban versus rural areas. Importantly, there is scant evidence that social connectedness in cities is better or worse than in non-urban areas. It is more likely that the nature of individual connections vary in different contexts, and it is the interrelation between urban social and physical environmental stressors, availability and access to material resources, and psychosocial resources that ultimately would explain any relation between urban living and mental disorders.

Several other forms of social resources have been shown to affect health in cities. Informal social ties are an important feature of city living that affects social support, network, and cohesion (Fullilove, 1998). Social capital effects, including manifestations at the contextual level (e.g., at the level of the whole city or of urban neighborhoods) and the social network level, are thought to offer general economic and social support on an ongoing basis in addition to making specific resources available at times of stress (Kawachi & Berkman, 2001). Social capital is often defined in terms of social organization, and as such, it has been hypothesized that social capital is associated with lower levels of criminal activity through the enforcement of social norms as discussed earlier. However, the relation between social capital and crime is likely reciprocal: while social capital is associated with lower crime rates through the suppression of deviant behavior, high crime rates erode bonds in communities and weaken protective institutions, allowing for further criminal activity (Sampson, 2000). In the context of cities, the greater spatial proximity of one's immediate network may well accentuate the role of networks in shaping health. Social networks have been shown to be importantly associated with a range of health behaviors, including misuse of substances (Kafka & London, 1991). However, there is very little evidence about interracial/ethnic group differences in the relation between informal social resources and mental health in urban areas.

Social Contagion

Other theories that explain how urban living may affect mental disorder emphasize the role of group influence on individual health and behavior. Social learning theory emphasizes the importance of observing and modeling the behaviors and attitudes of others (Bandura, 1986). This is particularly the case in densely populated areas where there are several persons on whom behavior can be modeled. In diverse urban settings, social learning can both set social norms and set norms for social network behaviors. Similarly, theories of collective socialization emphasize the influence of group membership on the individual (Wilson, 1987; Coleman, 1988). These theories suggest that persons who are in positions of authority or influence in specific areas can affect norms and behavior of others in direct and indirect ways. Institutional socialization theory has been closely linked to the allocation of social resources within city neighborhoods (White, 2001), which in turn has implications for health in cities as discussed above. This issue is particularly relevant to minority groups in contexts of urban racial/ethnic segregation, which exists in many cities world-wide (and in most American cities) (White, 2001).

One of the concepts that is linked to social learning and may have substantial implications for public health is "contagiousness." Models of biological con-tagion, particularly in the context of infectious disease, are well established. However, newer theories include the possibility of contagiousness of ideas and social examples. Contagion theory is employed by sociologists as one explana-tion for crowd behavior. In epidemiology, it is understood that—all things being equal—urban populations, characterized by high population density, are at higher risk of transmission of biological organisms. Also, because con-centrated urban populations share common resources (e.g., water) the practices of one group can affect the health of others. These observations may be extended to behavior and to mental disorder. A classic example of this has been referred to as the Werther effect. The Werther effect suggests that media representations of suicide may have some influence on the actions of those exposed to them such that suicide becomes more likely. Several studies have provided both theoretical and empirical reasons to suggest that media repre-sentations of suicide could have some influence on a person's suicidality (Frei et al., 2003); other examples of media representation reinforcing unhealthy behavior include self-mutilation (Favazza, 1998).

In the urban context, the concentrated proximity of both persons and sources of information may be a "crucible" for the exacerbation of this effect (Eaton, 1986). One obvious such example would be the consequences of an urban disaster. A disaster in a densely populated urban area may well have substantial implications for mental health and behavior that would not be the case in a disaster in a less densely populated urban area. One example is the case of the September 11 terrorist attacks. The North Tower of the World Trade Center (WTC) in Manhattan, New York City (NYC), was hit by an American Airlines Boeing 767 passenger plane at 8:45 am on Tuesday, September 11, 2001. NYC residents learned of the crash in near real-time via the internet, all-news channels, or by looking up to see the WTC burning on the morning commute to work. New Yorkers were watching early reports of the first attack when a second plane struck the WTC South Tower. In the hours that followed, two other airplanes crashed elsewhere, the WTC towers collapsed, and thou-sands of persons were evacuated from lower Manhattan, while others searched for missing family and friends or assisted in the rescue efforts. In NYC, the days and weeks after September 11 were characterized by a growing awareness of the magnitude of the loss of life and fear of other potential terrorist attacks. Therefore, the attacks on the WTC were experienced by a substantial propor- tion of New Yorkers in real time, either via witnessing these events firsthand or hearing about them by word of mouth. Subsequent research after the attacks has shown that up to one-fifth of persons interviewed in a representative sample of residents of NYC reported seeing some of the events in person. A substantial proportion of the population *not directly affected by the attacks* reported symptoms consistent with posttraumatic stress disorder related to the Septem- ber 11 attacks (Galea et al., 2003). Intriguingly, the persons who were not directly affected by the attacks (those who did not see the attacks or lose possessions or relatives) would not be considered "exposed" to the traumatic event by classic DSM-IV criterion A definitions. It can be argued that the urban context in general was instrumental for the contagion of both exposure to the event in NYC and the subsequent development of mental health symptoms. Tying back to the notion of spatial racial/ethnic segregation introduced earlier, the concentration of persons of minority racial/ethnic groups into specific parts of the urban environment can further exacerbate the behavioral contagion discussed here.

The Urban Physical Environment

Urban areas typically feature a heavily built environment, reliance on human- made systems of water and food provision, and reliance on housing that is frequently substandard. It has been argued that the primary feature distinguish- ing the twentieth century from previous ones and cities from non-urban areas is the degree to which humans have become the primary influence on the physical environment (McNeill, 2000). The urban physical environment interacts with the other domains discussed above to shape health in cities. As cities grow, the ability of the physical environment to affect health can also grow. Highways and streets can destroy green space, influence motor vehicle use and accident rates, increase urban noise, and heighten the daily hassles of urban living. Green space has been associated with overall health and better mental health function- ing in several studies (Takano, Nakamura, & Watanabe, 2002). Automobile use of unleaded gasoline can increase lead levels in the environment. In turn, higher lead levels may be teratogenic in utero; prenatal exposure to teratogens has been associated with adult onset of mental illness, an example of environmental toxins contributing to the incidence of psychiatric disorders (Watson, Mednick, Huttunen, & Wang, 1999). Noise exposure in turn may contribute to hearing impairment, psychological distress, and hypertension (Evans, 2003). There is extensive environmental justice literature showing that adverse neighborhood conditions are much more prevalent in minority communities than in other urban communities, further contributing to poor mental health in these groups (Corburn, 2002; Maantay, 2007).

The urban infrastructure is also part of the physical environment. As the expensive urban infrastructure ages in a period of declining municipal resources, breakdowns may increase. This may not only cause physical health problems related to water, sewage, or disposal of waste but also limit municipalities' ability to adequately provide salutary resources. Ultimately, urban design may also influence crime and violence rates, demonstrating the close interactions between urban physical and social environments (Sampson, Raudenbush, & Earls, 1997). Recent empiric research that has assessed how characteristics of intraurban environments are associated with health has improved our understanding of the relation between the urban physical environment and mental health (Yang, 2000). Once again, differential exposure to adverse urban circumstances in many cities substantially disadvantages minority racial/ethnic groups, making these groups much more likely to be adversely influenced by the potential relation between urban characteristics and mental illness.

Spatial Segregation

Although mentioned throughout the discussion above, it is worth concluding this section with a recognition that much of the particular way in which the urban environment may influence mental health of minorities rests on the spatial segregation of different racial/ethnic and socioeconomic groups in cities. The role of spatial segregation in shaping mental health has long been recognized. In their seminal work of mental disorder in urban areas, Faris and Dunham (1939) described in detail a Chicago that had concentric circles wherein dwelled distinct groups whose social status was relatively unchanged even with migration of populations over time. Spatial segregation can have multiple effects, including the enforcement of homogeneity in resources and social network ties. Considering the role of spatial segregation in conjunction with concepts of social learning, spatial proximity to beneficial role models may be critical for socioeconomically disadvantaged persons to identify avenues to improve their social status. Perhaps more importantly, spatial proximity to persons of higher socioeconomic status could permit the formation of social networks that are critical for obtaining employment and opportunities for social mobility. Spatial heterogeneity also permits persons of higher socioeconomic status to appreciate the issues faced by others and to use their power, money, and prestige to influence the development of better distributed salutary resources.

Conversely, it is worth noting that spatial segregation may serve to minimize social strain by virtue of keeping persons who are different apart from one another. It has been shown in some studies that minorities living in highly segregated areas who only come into contact with other racial/ethnic groups infrequently experience less discrimination than minorities who regularly come into contact with persons of other racial/ethnic groups (Krieger, 2000). Discrimination in turn has been associated with poor mental health in minority groups (Cochran & Mays, 1994). However, it is important to note that segregation of minority groups into urban or peri-urban slum areas in many developing world countries represents a substantial threat to these populations' physical health and—as increasingly suggested by empiric research—mental health (Blue & Harpham, 1996).

Summary

In summary, several mechanisms exist that may explain how cities affect mental health, with different mechanisms being differentially important for different types of mental disorders and for different racial/ethnic groups. Indeed, a "big picture" perspective on the relation between characteristics of city living and mental health would suggest that any such relations are undoubtedly complicated. While specific features of cities may affect certain conditions adversely, other features may offer protection. Interrelationships between features of the urban environment (e.g., between spatial segregation and potential social strain) complicates attempts at generalization. However, in the context of concern with the mental health of racial/ethnic minorities, it is clear that the spatial segregation of racial/ethnic groups in many ways sets the stage for minority groups to be exposed to more concentrated disadvantage and more adverse social conditions than majority groups. As such, minority groups are more susceptible to the potential adverse health consequences of city living.

The empiric work that has explicitly assessed how urban living affects mental disorder has only begun to "scratch the surface" of the topic; there is very little research that has explicitly considered the interaction between city living and racial/ethnic minority group status. In the following section, we summarize the key research in the area in three distinct eras, drawing on seminal work that has established a link between city living and mental health and highlighting how this work may be extended to help us consider the role of city living in shaping the mental health of racial/ethnic minority populations.

The Evidence

Pre-1980: Before DSM-III

The past century has seen a flourishing of empiricism in health research, and in hand, a number of epidemiologic studies have sought to understand the potential relations between urban living and mental disorders. Empiric work produced conflicting results at the beginning of the twentieth century. For example, in a U.S. study, White (1902) found mental disorders to be higher in urban areas, while in a study of four regions of Scotland, Sutherland (1901) found higher rates of insanity in rural areas. Sorokin and Zimmerman (1929) reviewed data from a number of sources and concluded that psychiatric morbidity was higher in urban areas in the United States overall. These early studies were limited by a number of methodologic difficulties, primarily the use of crude definitions of outcomes and issues of sampling. Still, they acknowledged and established that place of residence and characteristics of the urban (and rural) environments may play a role in shaping individual mental health. In landmark research that laid the groundwork for much of the thinking behind the relation between urban living and mental health, Faris and Dunham (1939) conducted an ecological study in Chicago neighborhoods and found a high degree of association between different types of psychoses and certain conditions of communities. As we shall discuss further in subsequent sections, although recent work suggests that the association between urban living and psychotic disorders is likely complex, in many ways Faris and Dunham's work presaged thinking about characteristics of urban neighborhoods that may be associated with mental health.

During this period, a seminal study, the Midtown Manhattan (1962) study, provided a basis for comparison between urban and rural areas and had a marked influence on subsequent research (Srole et al., 1962). The fundamental postulate of this study was that *sociocultural conditions have measurable consequences reflected in mental health differences.* It built explicitly on some of the earlier theoretical work that suggested that sociocultural features of urban living (such as disorganization) may shape mental health. This study was a cross-sectional, in-person survey study, sampling residents (including hospitalized or institutionalized persons) of midtown Manhattan between 20 and 59 years old (n = 1,660). Among the principal findings from this study, it was shown that there was a particularly high prevalence of mental pathology among single men; additionally, low parental and adult socioeconomic status was associated with a greater likelihood of psychological impairment. The authors suggested that economic factors, potentially linked through pathways of discrimination, shape psychological factors that may affect adult mental health. Subsequently, other work compared the prevalence of psychiatric disorders in less urban areas to data obtained in the Midtown Manhattan study using comparable assessment methods. Using records from Minnesota, Laird (1973) estimated that the prevalence of severe psychiatric disorders in rural areas of Minnesota was one tenth of that reported by the Midtown Manhattan Study. In contrast, in a comparison of psychiatric morbidity from the Stirling County Study (a study of the prevalence of psychiatric morbidity in rural Nova Scotia, Canada), Srole (1977) concluded that the prevalence of psychiatric disorders was lower in Midtown Manhattan than it was in rural Nova Scotia.

Some of the most interesting research in this era that considered potential relations between urban living and mental disorders studied psychiatric disorders in children. In a small study of 175, 5- to 6-year-old pre-school children, Kalstrup (1977) did not find differences in the prevalence of psychiatric disorders between children recruited from the urban municipality of Århus and the rural municipality of Samsø in Åarhus County, Denmark. This study was limited by a relatively small sample size and by crude assessment of psychiatric disorders. In contrast, a contemporaneous study of adolescents that used personal psychiatric interviews, questionnaires, and school information to assess total psychiatric disorder among 483 adolescents in Norway found that the prevalence of psychiatric disorders was 16.9% in Oslo compared to 7.9% in a rural area in South-East Norway (1977).

In the mid-1970s, an influential series of studies, collectively referred to as the Isle of Wight Studies, rigorously and systematically assessed psychiatric disorders in 9- to 11-year-old children and provided some of the most compelling data relevant to questions of interest here (Rutter, Tizard, Yule, Graham, & Whitmore, 1976). In a comparison between 10-year-olds in the Isle of Wight and 10-year-olds attending school in an inner-city London district, it was shown that the prevalence of psychiatric disorder was twice as high in London as it was in the Isle of Wight. This discrepancy was more pronounced in girls (26.2% vs. 10.8% comparing London to the Isle of Wight) than it was in boys (18.3% vs. 13.0%) (Rutter, Cox, Tupling, Berger, & Yule, 1975). Reading retardation was nearly three times higher in London than in Isle of Wight children (9.9% vs. 3.9% respectively) (Berger, Yule, & Rutter, 1975). These studies were notable in their efforts to take into account the possible confounding effects of migration and social selection and in considering the principal reasons that might explain these differences in prevalence. The authors suggested that the higher proportion of children with psychiatric disorders in London was linked to a relatively higher proportion of family discord and social disadvantage in London than in the Isle of Wight (Rutter, Yule, et al., 1975). In some ways, these observations foreshadow more recent studies, some of which are discussed in the next section, that have begun to consider how characteristics of urban neighborhoods contribute to intraurban and interurban differences in the incidence and prevalence of both adult and child psychiatric disorders (Ford, Goodman, & Meltzer, 2004).

Clearly very little work during this era formally considered the specific role of urban living in influencing the health of different racial/ethnic groups. However, this early work was invaluable in establishing the framework for our understanding of the relation between city living and mental health. The principal epidemiologic work in the area during most of the twentieth century was summarized in a review by Dohrenwend and Dohrenwend (1974) that considered the best empiric evidence in an attempt to determine whether there was evidence that urban settings were associated with a greater prevalence of psychiatric disorders than rural settings. Limiting their observations to nine epidemiologic studies that reported prevalence of adult psychiatric disorders in both urban and rural sites conducted from 1942 to 1969 (in multiple cities including Tokyo, Japan, Reykjavik, Iceland, and Abeokuta, Nigeria), the authors suggested that a consistent pattern emerged from these disparate studies and stated that "there appears to be a tendency for total rates of psychiatric disorders to be higher in urban than in rural areas." A substantial portion of the difference in the urban-rural prevalence of mental disorders was influenced by higher prevalences of neurosis and personality disorders in urban communities. However, the authors noted that many of the studies they reviewed were limited by substantial methodologic difficulties, making comparisons across studies challenging. The Dohrenwends' conclusions have been challenged by authors who note that the samples that were the subject of this review were small and that the urban-rural differences reported were themselves also small (Fischer, 1976). In addition, a number of the "urban" areas in the studies reviewed by the Dohrenwends were atypically small urban communities and not usefully representative of modern urban areas.

1980s and 1990s: Community Prevalence Studies

The past two decades have witnessed a dramatic systematization of the study of psychiatric epidemiology in general, and more than a dozen community surveys have been published that have described the urban versus rural epidemiology of different mental disorders. In the United States, the Epidemiologic Catchment Area (ECA) project, a multi-stage probability sample of U.S. residents using in-person interviews, was the first community survey to assess psychiatric disorders using standardized instruments based on the DSM-III. Analysis using ECA data has specifically assessed urban-rural differences in the prevalence of psychiatric disorders in the United States, finding a twofold higher prevalence of major depression in persons living in urban areas vs. rural areas but no difference between small metropolitan areas and rural areas (Blazer, George, & Landerman, 1985). The prevalence of drug abuse/dependence was also higher in large metropolitan areas assessed in the ECA. The question of urban-rural differences was reconsidered using data from the National Comorbidity Survey (NCS), a community survey carried out in five sites across the United States. Using similar large and small metropolitan and rural area definitions as the ECA did, two NCS analyses found no difference in the prevalence of major depressive episodes, affective disorders, substance use disorders, antisocial personality disorder, or psychological disorders overall between persons living in different size metropolitan or rural areas (Blazer, Kessler, McGonagle, & Swartz, 1994; Kessler et al., 1994). A Canadian study using similar methodology also failed to find an urban-rural difference for a range of psychiatric disorders (Parikh, Wasylenki, Goering, & Wong, 1996). It is worth noting that all of these studies used lay administration of structured instruments, leaving open the possibility of non-differential misclassification.

In Europe, population-based surveys (two U.K. and one Dutch) have assessed the prevalence of mental disorders and examined urban-rural differences. In the first of these studies, the U.K. Health and Lifestyle Survey, an association was found between urban residence and the prevalence of psychiatric morbidity. This study used interviewers' subjective assessment of respondents' homes to determine urban versus rural living (Lewis & Booth, 1994). Subsequently, the Household Survey of National Morbidity of Great Britain, a multi-stage community sample using in-person interviews, also used interviewer ratings to determine urban versus rural residence and found that urban residents had a higher prevalence of alcohol and drug dependence and psychiatric morbidity in general (Paykel, Abbott, Jenkins, Brugha, & Meltzer, 2000). The Netherlands Mental Health Survey and Incidence Study (NEMESIS), a multi-stage, stratified, random study in the Netherlands, documented a higher likelihood of mood, substance use, and psychotic disorders in urban versus rural residents (Bijl, van Zessen, Ravelli, de Rijk, & Langendoen, 1998). The same study did not find urban-rural differences in anxiety disorders (Bijl, Ravelli, & van Zessen, 1998). Other European studies that have specifically focused on the relation between urban living and schizophrenia are discussed later in this chapter.

Four studies have assessed urban-rural differences using population-based surveys in Asian countries. The first of these was a multi-stage random sampling of households using in-person interviews (administered as part of the Clinical Interview Schedule) in Taiwan (Cheng, 1989). This study found no significant differences in the prevalence of total psychological morbidity, anxiety states, or depression between the urban and rural areas; additionally, no differences were observed in symptom profiles between the areas. A contemporaneous larger multi-stage random community sample, using in-person interviews based on the DSM-III, assessed persons in metropolitan Taipei, small towns, and rural villages in Taiwan (Hwu, Yeh, & Chang, 1989). In contrast to the Cheng et al. findings, this study found that the small town samples had a higher lifetime prevalence of eight disorders including major depressive disorders, dysthymic disorder, panic disorder, generalized anxiety disorder, alcohol abuse/dependence, and drug dependence. A comparative study, carried out in Korea, found a higher lifetime prevalence of many psychiatric disorders in less urban areas compared to Seoul, including alcohol abuse/dependence, agoraphobia, panic disorder, and cognitive impairment (Lee et al., 1990). This study found a higher prevalence of antisocial personality disorder in Seoul versus the rest of the country and no differences in schizophreniform disorders or affective disorders (including depression). A smaller study of persons over age 65 in Korea also failed to find urban-rural differences in depression (Kim, Shin, Yoon, & Stewart, 2002). One study in New Zealand that used a cross-sectional random community mail survey found no rural-urban differences in measures of psychiatric morbidity (Romans-Clarkson, Walton, Herbison, & Mullen, 1990).

In sum, the studies in the past 20 years that have documented urban-rural comparisons in the prevalence of psychiatric disorders do not suggest that there is a consistent urban-rural difference in mental morbidity in general or for specific mental disorders, with the possible exceptions of psychosis and child behavior disorders. These findings are consistent across different countries and different racial/ethnic groups, though none of these studies specifically assessed whether there were urban-rural differences between racial/ethnic minorities living in these two environments. The published data does hint that certain morbidities, particularly alcohol abuse/dependence, may be more likely in rural versus urban areas, although the inconsistency in the assessment of alcohol abuse/dependence across these studies suggests the need for further work to clarify this suggestion. It is important to note that none of these community surveys have been carried out in developing world countries.

Twenty-First Century: Studies that Consider Characteristics of Urban Areas and Mental Health

While the advent of community prevalence studies over the past 20 years provided rich opportunity for urban-rural comparisons, most of the relevant studies in the period were not predicated on the earlier theoretical work that, as summarized earlier, suggested specific mechanisms through which urban living may be associated with mental health. As such, these studies ultimately have limited usefulness in determining whether urban living is a determinant of mental health, what the features of urban living that may affect mental health are, and the mechanisms through which urban areas may affect the health of the residents within them. It is not surprising that different urban-rural comparisons have provided conflicting evidence about the relative burden of mental health in urban and non-urban areas. Changing conditions within cities over time and differences in living conditions (e.g., qualities of the built environment, exposure to environmental toxins) between cities suggest that these studies at best provide a snapshot of how the mass of urban living conditions at one point in time may be affecting population mental health.

More recently, several studies have assessed how particular characteristics of urban living are associated with mental disorders in individuals. This group of studies typically focused on spatial groupings of individuals (often conceived as "neighborhoods", although several studies assessed the contribution of administrative groupings that are not necessarily meaningful to residents as neighborhoods) and considered the role of one's community of residence within an urban area in shaping individual mental health. These studies come full circle, applying new empiric methods to earlier theories that describe how city living may affect health. The growing use of multilevel modeling techniques in epidemiology has made studies like these both more common and more methodologically robust, providing insight into how features of both the urban physical and social environment may influence health. However, most of the literature in the area has focused on physical health, with few published studies that consider mental health outcomes.

A systematic review of neighborhood characteristics and health outcomes, summarizing the literature before June 1998, only identified one study (out of twenty-five reviewed) that considered mental disorders (Pickett & Pearl, 2001). The study, which used a random sample of adult residents in Amsterdam, failed to observe a relation between living in socioeconomically disadvantaged urban neighborhoods and mental disorders (Reijneveld, 1998). In contrast, some more recent studies have observed a relation between disadvantaged neighborhoods and mental disorders in general. A study discussed earlier showed that neighborhood social disorganization was associated with depressive symptoms (Latkin & Curry, 2003). Another study looking at the association between features of the urban-built environment and mental health assessed the relation between the quality of one's living environment and the likelihood of depression using a cross-sectional survey (Weich et al., 2002). The study found that persons living in poor quality physical environments were more likely to report symptoms consistent with depression after accounting for individual characteristics. Other work has shown that living in more deprived neighborhoods is associated with a higher incidence of non-psychotic disorders (Driessen, Gunther, & Van Os, 1998). A recent study corroborating these observations made use of a randomized controlled trial in New York City in which families were moved from public housing in high poverty neighborhoods to private housing in non-poor neighborhoods (Leventhal & Brooks-Gunn, 2003). This experimental study showed that both parents and children who were moved to the better housing and better neighborhoods reported fewer psychological distress symptoms than did control families who were not moved (although the difference in mental health was noted in boys but not in girls).

Tremendous growth in work that has considered neighborhood influences on health has occurred in the past decade. A more recent review that summarized studies between January 1990 and August 2007 and considered urban neighborhood influences on depression found 24 studies with populations ranging from 200 to 56,428 adult subjects concerned with this issue (Mair, Diez Roux, & Galea, In press). Some of the studies restricted their populations to specific racial/ethnic groups or age categories, while others included a wide range of demographic characteristics. Of the 24 studies, only 7 studies specifically focused on the mental health of minorities, with 6 restricting their study population to African Americans (Fitzpatrick, Piko, Wright, & LaGory, 2005; Caughy, O'Campo, & Muntaner, 2003; Simons et al., 2002; Schulz et al., 2006; Cutrona, Russell, Hessling, Brown, & Murry, 2000; Cutrona et al., 2005) and one study examining Mexican Americans (Ostir, Eschbach, Markides, & Goodwin, 2003). The remaining studies enrolled a mixture of racial/ethnic groups, typically using random sampling of their study populations, although several sampled equal numbers of African Americans and whites (Henderson et al., 2005; Schieman & Meersman, 2004).

The small number of studies that compared different race/ethnic groups found some evidence of heterogeneity of neighborhood effects by race/ethnicity (Aneshensel & Sucoff, 1996; Ostir et al., 2003; Weich, Lewis, & Jenkins, 2001). In a Baltimore study, community cohesion was associated with less depression amongst whites but was not associated with depression amongst African Americans (Gary, Stark, & Laveist, 2007). One study found Mexican Americans had better mental health in areas with high concentrations of Mexican Americans, whereas another study found that African Americans had worse mental health in areas with higher concentrations of African Americans (Ostir et al., 2003; Henderson et al. 2005).

Thus, while a relatively nascent area of research, multilevel analyses assessing relations between characteristics of urban environments and individual mental health promise to advance our understanding of the question well beyond the insights possible from the comparative descriptive studies of the 1980s and 1990s. However, the implications of such multilevel analyses may be difficult to generalize to other cities or urban areas more broadly. For example, the observation in one study that the quality of residences in London is associated with the likelihood of depression among urban residents may not necessarily be relevant in another urban context where the social environment plays an equally important role in shaping individual mental health. This example reflects both the complexity of the factors that may shape mental health in cities and the limitations of extant methods in fully assessing how urban living conditions may affect health.

A Research Agenda—What Are the Features of Urban Living that Affect Mental Health of Minorities?

In 1991, the World Health Organization identified mental illness as one of the diseases that deserved special attention in light of trends (including urbanization) that could have an impact on mental health (Harpham & Blue, 1995). However, mental health continues to be an underfunded area of research given its importance in the global burden of disease and given that significant questions concerning the impact of trends such as urbanicity and urbanization on mental health remain unanswered. The growing realization of persistent, and in some cases expanding racial/ethnic disparities in mental health, and the recent resurgence of interest in urban health (Vlahov & Galea, 2003) provide an opportunity to frame and consider questions concerning mental health and urbanicity.

We suggest that there are three primary areas of research that urgently need exploration as we seek to improve our understanding of the relation between cities and health in general and the role of urbanicity and urbanization in shaping the mental health of minorities in particular.

First, as we hope the discussion here has shown, both the theoretical considerations that explain why cities may affect mental health and the conflicting evidence on the relation between city living and mental health suggest that research needs to move beyond thinking about cities as a whole and start considering specific features of cities that may contribute to poor mental health or improve mental health. In particular, much more research is needed that specifically focuses on the mental health of minority populations and how urban living contributes to the mental health of these groups. The cross-sectional surveys that highlighted the potential differences in the prevalence of mental health problems between urban and rural areas unfortunately raise more questions than they answer. It is likely that the primary reason for the conflicting results documented by these surveys is the complexity of urban factors that may affect mental health. Prevalence studies cannot differentiate between the determinants of incidence of psychiatric disorders and the determinants of prevalence of these disorders, which may include factors that affect disease duration and severity that may be different from those associated with disease onset. Also, it is difficult to adequately control for factors such as selective migration or socioeconomic factors that may introduce bias or unmeasured confounding, particularly in cross-sectional surveys (Neff, 1983).

Although there is growing evidence of the role that characteristics of neighborhoods may play in determining physical health, relatively little of this work has concentrated on mental health and even less on the mental health of minorities. Recent work, discussed above, has provided early experimental evidence that living in poor neighborhoods is associated with psychological distress, anxiety/depressive symptoms, and dependency (Leventhal & Brooks-Gunn, 2003), suggesting avenues for future research and intervention. Better study designs, particularly the use of longitudinal or experimental studies, will obviate some of the concerns about most of the extant research. More importantly, it will be helpful to appreciate that a diverse set of risk factors determine mental health and that the complexity of urban circumstance and urban living frequently results in these factors manifesting differently in different contexts. This points to the importance of future research focused on understanding specific characteristics of urban living that shape mental health and how these characteristics interrelate.

Second, while assessing the urban determinants of mental health—in particular the role of urban living in shaping minority mental health—is an important first step, elucidating the mechanisms through which risk factors are associated with mental health is equally important and particularly germane to the development of effective interventions. As discussed in this chapter, a diverse set of mechanisms including stress processes, the availability of resources, varying degrees of social connectedness, and exposure to infectious agents and environmental toxins may explain how characteristics of cities affect urban health. Clearer elucidation of the pathways between urban determinants and mental health involving empiric tests to determine which mechanisms may be more important in particular contexts can guide interventions and the development of city policies that promote health. For example, if the relation between the urban-built environment and depression (Weich et al., 2002) is mediated by how the built environment facilitates (or discourages) social ties, different solutions are indicated than if the relation between the built environment and mental health is mediated by stress processes. If the former pathway is correct, one could easily conceive of efforts to promote social connectedness as a way of minimizing depression in lieu of ambitious and expensive renovation of dilapidated built environments. However, if the latter pathway is correct, successful interventions must improve the quality of the built environment itself in order to plausibly affect depression in the urban context.

It is likely, of course, that multiple mechanisms are responsible for the relations between different urban characteristics and mental health and that observed epidemiologic relations are mediated through multiple etiologic pathways. In addition, different mechanisms may be important for the etiology of different racial/ethnic groups. Improved understanding of associations, effect modifiers, and mediators can provide insight into how mental health interventions in cities can best be designed and tailored to maximize effectiveness. As a corollary to this direction, future work that considers how the urban environment jointly affects poor physical and mental health may provide insight into the role of the urban context in shaping overall population disability and function.

Third, as the pace of urbanization in less wealthy countries far exceeds urbanization in wealthier countries, consideration of the urban determinants of mental health in different countries acquires increasing importance. Although mental health in developing countries has historically received less attention than other causes of morbidity, particularly communicable disease, mental health is an increasingly important issue in developing countries. For example, for women in less wealthy countries, neuropsychiatric diseases account for the second largest burden of disease after cardiovascular disease among all non-communicable diseases (Harpham & Blue, 1995). However, most of the research in the area has been conducted in wealthier countries, to the detriment of our understanding of how urban living in other contexts may shape mental health. A research agenda for urban mental health must include work that identifies the unique urban determinants of mental health in different national contexts and how urbanization, a process that is much more prevalent in developing countries than it is in developed countries, is itself a determinant of mental health. It is likely that differences in baseline vulnerability, social resources, the physical environment, social connectedness, and conceptions of health and illness all may contribute to differences in the role that cities play in shaping mental health in different parts of the world. Research in developing countries and comparative multisite research can help elucidate these differences and direct creative solutions to improving population mental health.

Acknowledgments The authors are grateful to Robin Konkle Mays for editorial assistance. Work on this chapter was funded in part by grants DA 02270, DA 017642, and MH078152 from the National Institutes of Health. This chapter is in part adapted from Galea, S., Bresnahan, M., & Susser, S. (2006). Mental health in the city. In N. Freudenberg, S. Galea, & D. N. Vlahov (Eds.), *Cities and the health of the public* (pp. 247–276). TN: Vanderbilt University Press.

References

Agnew, R. (1992). Foundation for a general strain theory of crime and delinquency. *Criminology, 30*, 47–87.

Agnew, R. (2001). Building on the foundation of general strain theory: Specifying the types of strain most likely to lead to crime and delinquency. *Journal of Research in Crime and Delinquency, 38*, 319–361.

Amick, B. C. III, Kawachi, I., Coakley, E. H., Lerner, D., Levine, S., & Colditz, G. A. (1998). Relationship of job strain and iso-strain to health status in a cohort of women in the United States. *Scandinavian Journal of Work, Environment, & Health, 24*(1), 54–61.

Aneshensel, C. S., & Sucoff, C. A. (1996). The neighborhood context of adolescent mental health. *Journal of Health & Social Behavior, 37* 293–310.

Bandura, A. (1986). *Social foundations of thought and action: A social cognitive theory.* Engelwood Hills, NJ: Prentice-Hall.

Beach, S. R., Schulz, R., Yee, J. L., & Jackson, S. (2000). Negative and positive health effects of caring for a disabled spouse: Longitudinal findings from the caregiver health effects study. *Psychology & Aging, 15*(2), 259–271.

Berger, M., Yule, W., & Rutter, M. (1975). Attainment and adjustment in two geographical areas. II: The prevalence of specific reading retardation. *British Journal of Psychiatry, 126,* 510–519.

Bijl, R. V., Ravelli, A., & van Zessen, G. (1998). Prevalence of psychiatric disorders in the general population: Results of the Netherlands mental health survey and incidence study (nemesis). *Social Psychiatry & Psychiatric Epidemiology, 33,* 587–595.

Bijl, R. V., van Zessen, G., Ravelli, A., de Rijk, C., & Langendoen, Y. (1998). The Netherlands mental health survey and incidence study (nemesis): Objectives and design. *Social Psychiatry & Psychiatric Epidemiology, 33,* 581–586.

Blazer, D., George, L. K., Landerman, R., Pennybacker, M., Melville, M. L., Woodbury, M., et al. (1985). Psychiatric disorders: A rural/urban comparison. *Archives of General Psychiatry, 42,* 651–656.

Blazer, D. G., Kessler, R. C., McGonagle, K. A., & Swartz, M. S. (1994). The prevalence and distribution of major depression in a national comorbidity sample: The national comorbidity survey. *American Journal of Psychiatry, 151,* 979–996.

Blue, L., & Harpham, T. (1996). Urbanization and mental health in developing countries. *Current Issues in Public Health, 2,* 181–185.

Caughy, M.O., O'Campo, P.J., & Muntaner, C. (2003). When being alone might be better: Neighborhood poverty, social capital, and child mental health. *Social Science & Medicine, 57,* 227–237.

Cheng, T. A. (1989). Urbanization and minor psychiatric morbidity: A community study in Taiwan. *Social Psychiatry & Psychiatric Epidemiology, 24,* 309–316.

Cochran, S.D., & Mays, V.M. (1994). Depressive distress among homosexually active African American men and women. *American Journal of Psychiatry, 151,* 524–529.

Coleman, C. (1982). *Death is a social disease: Public health and political economy in early industrial France.* Madison, WI: The University of Wisconsin Press.

Coleman, J. S. (1988). Social capital in the creation of human capital. *American Journal of Sociology, 94,* S95–120.

Corburn, J. (2002). Environmental justice, local knowledge, and risk: The discourse of a community-based cumulative exposure assessment. *Environmental Management, 29,* 451–456.

Cutrona, C. E., Russell, D. W., Hessling, R. M, Brown, P. A., & Murry, V. (2000). Direct and moderating effects of community context on the psychological well-being of African American women. *Journal of Personality & Social Psychology, 79,* 1088–1101.

Cutrona, C. E., Russell, D. W., Brown, P. A., Clark, L. A., Hessling, R. M., & Gardner, K. A. (2005). Neighborhood context, personality, and stressful life events as predictors of depression among African American women. *Journal of Abnormal Psychology, 114,* 3–15.

Dickens, C. (1850). *The personal history and experience of David Copperfield the younger* Harvard Classics Shelf of Fiction. New York, NY: PF Collier & Son.

Driessen, G., Gunther, N., & Van Os, J. (1998). Share social environment and psychiatric disorder: A multilevel analysis of individual and ecological effects. *Social Psychiatry & Psychiatric Epidemiology, 33,* 606–612.

Dohrenwend, B. P., & Dohrenwend, B. S. (1974). Psychiatric disorders in urban settings. In S. Arieti (Ed.), *American handbook of psychiatry* (Vol. 11). New York, NY: Basic Books.

Durant, W., & Durant, A. (1967). *The story of civilization: Volume X: The age of Rousseau.* New York, NY: Simon and Schuster.

Durkheim, E. (1897). *Suicide.* (J. A. Spaulding & G. Simpson, Trans.). Reissue: Glencoe, IL: The Free Press.

Eaton, W. W. (1986). *The sociology of mental disorders* (2nd ed.). New York, NY: Praeger.

Elliott, M. (2000). The stress process in neighborhood context. *Health Place, 6,* 287–299.

Engels, F. (1887). *The condition of the working class in England.* New York, NY: John W. Lovell Company.

Evans, G. M. (2003). The built environment and mental health. *Journal of Urban Health, 80,* 536–555.

Faris, R. E. L., & Dunham, H. W. (1939). *Mental disorders in urban areas: An ecological study of schizophrenia and other psychoses.* Chicago, IL: The University of Chicago Press.

Favazza, R. (1998). The coming age of self-mutilation. *Journal of Nervous & Mental Disease, 186,* 259–266.

Fischer, C. S. (1976). *The urban experience.* New York, NY: Harcourt Brace Jovanovich.

Fitzpatrick, K. M., Piko, B. F., Wright, D. R., &, LaGory, M. (2005). Depressive symptomatology, exposure to violence, and the role of social capital among African American adolescents. *American Journal of Orthopsychiatry, 75,* 262–274.

Ford, T, Goodman, R. & Meltzer, H. (2004). *Social Psychiatry and Psychiatric Epidemiology, 39,* 87–96.

Frei, A., Schenker, T., Finzen, A., Dittmann, V., Kraeuchi, K., & Hoffmann-Richter, U. (2003). The Werther effect and assisted suicide. *Suicide & Life Threatening Behavior, 33,* 192–200.

Fullilove, M. T. (1998). Promoting social cohesion to improve health. *Journal of the American Medical Women's Association, 53,* 72–76.

Galea, S., Vlahov, D., Resnick, H., Ahern, J., Susser, E., Gold, J., et al. (2003). Trends in probable posttraumatic stress disorder in New York City after the September 11 terrorist attacks. *American Journal of Epidemiology, 158*(6), 514–524.

Gary, T. L., Stark, S. A., & Laveist, T. A. (2007). Neighborhood characteristics and mental health among African Americans and whites living in a racially integrated urban community. *Health & Place, 13,* 569–575.

Glaab, C. N., & Brown, A. T. (1976). *A history of urban America.* Toronto, ON: Macmillan Company.

Harpham, T., & Blue, I. (1995). Urbanization and mental health in developing countries: An introduction. In T. Harpham & I. Blue (Eds.), *Urbanization and mental health in developing countries* (pp. 3–14). Aldershot, UK: Avebury.

Henderson, C., Diez Roux, A. V., Jacobs, D. R. Jr., Kiefe, C. I., West, D., & Williams, D. R. (2005). Neighbourhood characteristics, individual level socioeconomic factors, and depressive symptoms in young adults: The CARDIA study. *Journal of Epidemiology & Community Health, 59,* 322–328.

Hwu, H.-G., Yeh, E.-K., & Chang, L.-Y. (1989). Prevalence of psychiatric disorders in Taiwan defined by the Chinese diagnostic interview schedule. *Acta Psychiatrica Scandinavia, 79,* 136–147.

Isometsa, E., Heikkinen, M., Henriksson, M., Marttunen, M., Aro, H., & Lonnqvist, J. (1997). Differences between urban and rural suicides. *Acta Psychiatrica Scandinavia, 95,* 297–305.

Kafka, R. R., & London, P. (1991). Communication in relationships and adolescent substance use: The influence of parents and friends. *Adolescence, 26,* 587–598.

Kalstrup, M. (1977). Urban-rural differences in 6 year olds. In P. J. Graham (Ed.).*Epidemiological approaches in child psychiatry* (pp. 165–180). New York, NY: Academic Press.

Kawachi, I., & Berkman, L. F. (2001). Social ties and mental health. *Journal of Urban Health, 78,* 458–467.

Kessler, R. C., McGonagle, K. A., Zhao, S., Nelson, C. B., Hughes, M., Eshleman, S., et al. (1994). Lifetime and 12-month prevalence of DSM-III-R psychiatric disorders in the United States. *Archives of General Psychiatry, 41,* 8–19.

Kim, J.-M., Shin, I.-S., Yoon, J.-S., & Stewart, R. (2002). Prevalence and correlates of late-life depression compared between urban and rural populations in Korea. *International Journal of Geriatric Psychiatry, 17,* 409–415.

Krieger, N. (2000). Discrimination and health. In L. Berkman & I. Kawachi (Eds.), *Social epidemiology* (pp. 36–75). Oxford, UK: Oxford University Press.

Laird, J. T. (1973). Mental health and population density. *Journal of Psychology, 85,* 171–177.

Latkin, C. A., & Curry, A. D. (2003). Stressful neighborhoods and depression: A prospective study of the impact of neighborhood disorder. *Journal of Health & Social Behavior, 44,* 34–44.

Lee, C. K., Kwak, Y. S., Yamamoto, J., Rhee, H., Kim, Y. S., Han, J. H., et al. (1990). Psychiatric epidemiology in Korea. Part II: Urban and rural differences. *Journal of Nervous & Mental Disease, 178,* 247–252.

Leventhal, T., & Brooks-Gunn, J. (2003). Moving to opportunity: An experimental study of neighborhood effects on mental health. *American Journal of Public Health, 93,* 1576–1582.

Lewis, G., & Booth, M. (1994). Are cities bad for your mental health? *Psychological Medicine, 24,* 913–915.

Maantay, J. (2007). Asthma and air pollution in the Bronx: Methodological and data considerations in using GIS for environmental justice and health research. *Health & Place, 13,* 32–56.

Mair, C.L.F., Diez Roux, A. V., & Galea, S. (2008, Epub ahead of print). Are neighborhood characteristics associated with depressive symptoms? A critical review.*Journal of Epidemiology and Community Health.*

Marsella, A. J. (1995). Urbanization, mental health and psychosocial well-being: Some historical perspectives and considerations. In T. Harpham & I. Blue (Eds.), *Urbanization and mental health in developing countries* (pp. 3–14). Aldershot, UK: Avebury.

McLeod, L., & Kessler, R. (1990). Socioeconomic status differences in vulnerability to undesirable life events. *Journal of Health & Social Behavior, 31,* 162–172.

McNeill, J. R. (2000). *Something new under the sun: An environmental history of the twentieth century.* New York, NY: Norton.

Merton, R. K. (1938). Social structure and anomie. *American Sociology Review, 3,* 672–682.

Neff, J. A. (1983). Urbanicity and depression reconsidered: The evidence regarding depressive symptomatology. *Journal of Nervous & Mental Disease, 171,* 546–552.

Noh, S., & Avison, W. R. (1996), Asian immigrants and the stress process: A study of Koreans in Canada. *Journal of Health & Social Behavior, 37,* 192–206.

Ostir, G. V., Eschbach, K., Markides, K. S., & Goodwin, J. S. (2003). Neighbourhood composition and depressive symptoms among older Mexican Americans. *Journal of Epidemiology & Community Health, 57,* 987–992.

Parikh, S. V., Wasylenki, D., Goering, P., & Wong, J. (1996). Mood disorders: Rural/urban differences in prevalence, health care utilization and disability in Ontario. *Journal of Affective Disorders,, 38,* 57–65.

Paykel, E. S., Abbott, R., Jenkins, R., Brugha, T. S., & Meltzer, H. (2000). Urban-rural mental health differences in Great Britain: Findings from the national morbidity survey. *Psychological Medicine, 30,* 269–280.

Pearlin, L. (1999). Stress and mental health: A conceptual overview. In A. Horwitz & T. Scheid (Eds.), *A handbook for the study of mental health* (pp. 161–175). Cambridge, UK: Cambridge University Press.

Pearlin, L., Lieberman, M., Menaghan, E., & Mullan, J. (1981). The stress process. *Journal of Health & Social Behavior, 22,* 337–356.

Pickett, K. E., & Pearl, M. (2001). Multilevel analyses of neighborhood socioeconomic context and health outcomes: A critical review. *Journal of Epidemiology & Community Health, 55,* 111–122.

Reijneveld, S. (1998). The impact of individual and area characteristics on urban socioeconomic differences in health and smoking. *International Journal of Epidemiology, 27,* 33–40.

Romans-Clarkson, S. E., Walton, V. A., Herbison, P. G., & Mullen, P. E. (1990). Psychiatric morbidity among women in urban and rural New Zealand: Psycho-social correlates. *British Journal of Psychiatry, 156*, 84–91.

Rutter, M., Tizard, J., Yule, W., Graham, P., & Whitmore, K. (1974). The Isle of wight studies, 1964–1974. *Psychological Medicine, 6*, 313–332.

Rutter, M., Cox, A., Tupling, C., Berger, M., & Yule, W. (1975). Attainment and adjustment in two geographical areas. I: The prevalence of psychiatric disorder. *British Journal of Psychiatry, 126*, 493–509.

Rutter, M., Yule, B., Quinton, D., Rowlands, O., Yule, W., & Berger, M. (1975). Attainment and adjustment in two geographical areas. III: Some factors accounting for area differences. *British Journal of Psychiatry, 125*, 520–533.

Sampson, R. J. (2000). Public health and safety in context: Lessons from community-level theory on social capital. In: B. D. Smedly & S. L. Syme (Eds.),*Promoting health: Intervention strategies from social and behavioral research* (pp. 366–390). Washington, DC: National Academy Press, Washington.

Sampson, R. J., & Groves, W. B. (1989). Community structure and crime: Testing social-disorganization theory. *American Journal of Sociology, 94*, 774–802.

Sampson, R. J., Raudenbush, S. W., & Earls, F. (1997). Neighborhoods and violent crime: A multilevel study of collective efficacy. *Science, 277*, 918–924.

Schieman, S., & Meersman, S. C. (2004). Neighborhood problems and health among older adults: Received and donated social support and the sense of mastery as effect modifiers. *Journal of Gerontology B: Psychological Science & Social Science, 59*, S89–97.

Schulz, A. J., Israel, B. A., Zenk, S. N., Parker, E. A., Lichtenstein, R., Shellman-Weir, S.,et al. (2006). Psychosocial stress and social support as mediators of relationships between income, length of residence and depressive symptoms among African American women on Detroit's eastside. *Social Science & Medicine, 62*, 510–522.

Seedat, S., Nyamai, C., Njenga, F., Vythilingum, B., & Stein, D. J. (2004). Trauma exposure and post-traumatic stress symptoms in urban African schools: Survey in CapeTown and Nairobi. *British Journal of Psychiatry, 184*, 169–175.

Shaw, C. R., & McKay, H. D. (1969). *Juvenile delinquency and urban areas*. Chicago, IL: The University of Chicago Press.

Shelley, P. B. (1819). *Peter Bell the Third*, "Hell", stanza 1.

Simons, R. L., Murry, V., McLoyd, V., Lin, K. H., Cutrona, C., & Conger, R. D. (2002). Discrimination, crime, ethnic identity, and parenting as correlates of depressive symptoms among African American children: A multilevel analysis. *Developmental Psychopathology, 14*, 371–393.

Sorokin, P., & Zimmerman, C. C. (1929). *Principles of urban-rural sociology*. New York, NY: Henry Holt.

Srole, L. (1977). The city vs. town and country: New evidence on an ancient bias. *Mental health in the metropolis*. Revised ed. New York, NY: Harper.

Srole, L., Langner, T. S., Michael, S. T., Kirkpatrick, P., Opler, M., & Rennie, T. A. (1962). *Mental health in the metropolis*. New York, NY: Harper & Row.

Sutherland J. (1901). *The growth and geographical distribution of lunacy in Scotland*. London, UK: British Association for the Advancement of Science.

Takano, T., Nakamura, K., & Watanabe, M. (2002). Urban residential environments and senior citizens' longevity in megacity areas: The importance of walkable green spaces. *Journal of Epidemiology & Community Health, 56*, 913–918.

Velleman, R., & Templeton, L. (2003). UK alcohol, drugs and the family research group. Alcohol, drugs and the family: Results from a long-running research programme within the UK. *European Addiction Research, 9*, 103–112.

Vlahov, D., & Galea, S. (2003). Urban health: A new discipline. *Lancet, 362*, 1091–1092.

Vogele, J. P. (1994). Urban infant mortality in Imperial Germany. *Social History of Medicine, 7*(3), 401–425.

Watson, J. B., Mednick, S. A., Huttunen, M., & Wang, X. (1999). Prenatal teratogens and the development of adult mental illness. *Developmental Psychopathology, 11*, 457–466.

Weich, S., Blanchard, M., Prince, M., Burton, E., Erens, B., & Sproston, K. (2002). Mental health and the built environment: Cross-sectional survey of individual and contextual risk factors for depression. *British Journal of Psychiatry, 180*, 428–433.

Weich, S., Lewis, G., & Jenkins, S.P. (2001). Income inequality and the prevalence of common mental disorders in Britain. *The British Journal of Psychiatry, 178*, 222–227.

White, M. J. (2001). Demographic effects of segregation. *Encyclopedia of social sciences* (pp. 13250–13254). Elseviear Science.

White, W. (1902). The geographical distribution of insanity in the United States. *Journal of Nervous & Mental Disease, 30*, 257–279.

Wilson, W. J. (1987). *The truly disadvantaged: The inner city, the underclass and public policy.* Chicago, IL: University of Chicago Press.

World Health Organization. (1991). *Health trends and emerging issues in the 1990s and the 21st century.* Geneva, Switzerland: Monitoring, Evaluation, and Projection Methodology Unit, World Health Organization.

Yang, M. J. (2000). Neighborhood experience and mental health. *Chang Gung Medical Journal, 23*, 747–754.

Chapter 3
Mental Health, Mental Health Courts, and Minorities

Lara Nochomovitz and Franklin J. Hickman

Introduction

Racial and ethnic minorities are less likely than their white counterparts to receive mental health services. Experts agree that, regardless of race or ethnicity, the majority of people with diagnosable disorders do not receive needed treatment (Office of the Surgeon General, 1999), while membership in a racial or ethnic minority[1] exacerbates the barriers to receiving mental health treatment. A report completed by the Surgeon General found that mental health services are less available to minorities, minorities have less access to mental health services, and the quality of mental health services that minorities receive is likely to be of comparatively poor quality. The disparities in the availability of services are attributable to cost, fragmentation of services, stigma associated with mental illness, mistrust and fear of treatment, racism and discrimination, and differences in language and communication (U.S. Department of Health and Human Services, 1999).

Lack of treatment increases the likelihood that a person with active mental illness will struggle with housing, employment and other common activities, and become involved in criminal activity. Available statistics confirm that, like racial minorities, individuals with mental illness are disproportionately represented in the criminal justice system. Though 2006 statistics are not available, in 2005, 45% of federal inmates, 56% of state inmates, and 64% of persons in local jails nationwide suffered from a mental health problem (James & Glaze, 2006). By comparison, 12.9% of adults in the general population received some sort of treatment for a mental health problem (James & Glaze, 2006). Based on such

---

[1] The terms "racial and ethnic minority" and "minorities" refer to Blacks, Hispanics, Native Americans, Asian Americans and Pacific Islanders.

F.J. Hickman (✉)
Hickman & Lowder Co., L.P.A., Penton Building, 1300 East Ninth Street, Suite 1020, Cleveland, OH 44114
e-mail: FHickman@hickman-lowder.com

S. Loue, M. Sajatovic (eds.), *Determinants of Minority Mental Health and Wellness*, DOI 10.1007/978-0-387-75659-2_3,
© Springer Science+Business Media, LLC 2009

statistics, one author asserted, "prisons may now be the largest mental health provider in the Unites States" (Fellner, 2006, p. 391).

Attempting to explain the disparity in incarceration of the mentally ill, a commission organized by President George W. Bush contended that "the mental health delivery system is fragmented and in disarray ... lead[ing] to unnecessary and costly disability, homelessness, school failure and incarceration" (President's New Freedom Commission on Mental Health, 2007, p. 3). Police officers have been found to be almost twice as likely to arrest someone who appears to have a mental illness in comparison with an individual engaging in the same behavior who does not appear to be mentally ill (Bernstein & Seltzer, 2003). Such practices—even if subconscious—further contribute to the overrepresentation of mentally ill individuals involved with the criminal justice system. Despite the disproportionate representation of the mentally ill in the criminal justice system, and the unique needs of such individuals, legal professionals, including lawyers and judges, are inadequately trained to deal with mental illnesses (Bernstein & Seltzer, 2003).

Mental Health Courts as an Intervention Model

To ameliorate the justice system's ability to address needs of overly represented mentally ill persons, the federal government began promulgating the development of "mental health courts." Mental Health Courts provide a model for effective intervention for persons with mental illness who are involved in the criminal justice system. The principles which make these courts effective can be applied to some, but not all, types of civil proceedings involving persons with mental illness. This chapter will define the essential characteristics of a mental health court and apply those characteristics to two common civil proceedings which affect persons with mental illness living in the community: evictions and employment discrimination claims. The structure of mental health courts can be more readily applied in eviction cases where there is a predictable forum for most proceedings and claims which can be readily remedied at the court level. Employment claims are less amenable to a mental health court model under current structures because, by the time persons with mental illness gain access to administrative or judicial review, there is little potential for correcting the procedural and substantive problems which led to the claims. The chapter will suggest alternative approaches which can enhance access to effective civil remedies in situations more similar to employment disputes.

Characteristics of Mental Health Courts

Currently, there are more than 100 mental health courts nationwide (Bureau of Justice Assistance, 2005). While each of these courts operates uniquely, the courts have one significant commonality: a dedicated mental health docket. The overarching objectives of these dockets include: creating alternatives to hospitalization and incarceration; providing more appropriate sanctions and long-term treatment for mentally ill defendants; alleviating the burden on the criminal justice system; and, reducing recidivism. Mental health dockets generally employ a team comprising court staff and mental health professionals to identify and assess participants and to achieve the aforementioned goals (Council of State Governments, 2005a). The success of mental health courts is often measured in subjective terms based on the sanctions that participants receive and how individual mentally ill defendants perceive that they are being treated during criminal proceedings.

Common Problems Associated with Mental Health Courts

While mental health courts are typically viewed as an asset to the criminal justice system, the courts are often underinclusive. For example, 60% of mental health courts accept only individuals with "serious and persistent mental illness" (Council of State Governments, 2005b, p. 3). Not all mental health courts accept felony cases, and many require that participants plead guilty (Council of State Governments, 2005b). Even the federal government recognizes that a mental health court should be viewed as only one component in a larger systematic strategy to improve the response to individuals with mental illness (Council of State Governments, 2005a).

Many mental health courts, such as the court in Cuyahoga County, Ohio, have implemented strategies in an attempt to remedy underinclusiveness and benefit as many participants as possible. Cuyahoga County requires that a mental health court participant receive a mental illness diagnosis within six months prior to arraignment. Recognizing that some beneficiaries may not have a confirmed diagnosis due to limited access to mental health services, the Court collaborates with community organizations and provides pretrial services to identify individuals who would benefit from mental health court (Cuyahoga County Common Pleas Court Local Rule 30.1). Even if a diagnosis occurs after arraignment, an Administrative Judge has the discretion to assign a case to a mental health docket.

Some mental health courts do not implement such proactive services to identify individuals who qualify for mental health court. Racial and ethnic minorities with mental illness are the least likely to have previously received mental health services. Consequently, this population is the most likely to suffer from a mental illness, yet not receive the benefits of a mental health court.

Even in a county such as Cuyahoga, where there are safeguards in place to identify indigent and other previously undiagnosed individuals with mental illnesses, the benefits of mental health court are limited. If an individual is convicted of a crime and is transferred to a state penal institution, the most that the mental health court can do is transfer that individual's treatment history, diagnoses, and medication to the state institution; no mechanism exists to ensure that individuals with mental illness continue to receive appropriate services or treatment. Once an individual is transferred to the state penal system that individual once again becomes subject to the rules and procedures of individuals who are not necessarily knowledgeable about mental illnesses.

The criminal justice system's ability to accommodate offenders with mental illness remains imperfect. Nevertheless, Mental Health Courts render the criminal justice system better equipped than the civil law system to meet the needs of individuals with mental illness who are involved in a lawsuit. Except in limited cases, such as those related to guardianship or civil commitment, civil courts lack a uniform procedural mechanism to ascertain whether a party has a mental illness and to intervene with solutions to the problems arising from the mental illness. Individuals with mental illness might benefit from special accommodations in the civil court system based on the mental health court model.

The Mental Health Court Model, Eviction Proceedings, and Mental Health

Stress related to the inability to secure and maintain housing may exacerbate the negative symptoms of mental illness, including anxiety and depression. The inability to secure permanent housing also decreases the likelihood that an individual will achieve independence or self-sufficiency (Pearson, Locke, Montgomery, & Buron, 2007). Consequently, individuals with mental illness who are unable to secure permanent housing experience increased feelings of marginalization, decreased self-worth, and an increased risk of homelessness.

Despite the importance of permanent housing, stabilized housing often evades individuals with mental illness. Individuals with mental illness often face financial barriers to securing stable housing due to the disparity between the cost of adequate housing and the sum provided to individuals by Supplemental Security Income (SSI) benefits.[2] It has been found that "not one housing market in the United States exists in which an individual receiving SSI benefits can afford to rent a modest efficiency or one-bedroom unit" (Substance Abuse and Mental Health Services Administration, 2004, p. 23). In 2000, people with disabilities receiving SSI needed to pay, on average, 98% of their SSI benefits to rent a modest, one-bedroom unit at fair market rent, as determined by the U.S. department of Housing and Urban Development (O'Hara & Miller, 2003; Substance Abuse and Mental Health Services Administration, 2004). Behavioral problems also put individuals with mental illness at higher risk of losing housing due to eviction actions. For example, individuals with untreated mental illness may disturb their neighbors, be a threat to themselves or others, miss rent or utility payments, or neglect their housekeeping and, as a consequence, be evicted.

---

[2] SSI benefits consist of a monthly federal stipend which is available to disabled individuals, including mentally ill persons, who cannot work.

Some remedies already exist to protect individuals with mental illness from eviction. This chapter will focus on remedies that are available nationally – (1) the Fair Housing Act Amendments of 1988 (FHAA) and (2) the Americans Disabilities Act (ADA). A survey of state-by-state protections is beyond the scope of this chapter, but advocates and attorneys should be aware that each state likely has unique provisions to protect individuals who are mentally ill or otherwise disabled from discriminatory housing practices. This paper limits its examination of state based anti-discrimination procedures to those available in Ohio because the authors' primary experiences have been in Ohio.

Current Remedies

Fair Housing Act Amendments

The FHAA prohibits rental practices which are discriminatory toward individuals with disability, including mental illness (Fair Housing Act Amendments, 1988). Discriminatory practices include failures to make "reasonable" accommodations or modifications to prevent a disabled renter from receiving treatment that is unequal to that received by other tenants (Fair Housing Act, 1988). Whereas a reasonable modification typically requires a structural change to a building, a reasonable accommodation "is a change, exception, or adjustment to a rule, policy, practice, or service" (U.S. Department of Housing and Urban Development, 2008). It is more likely that an individual with mental illness will require a reasonable accommodation than a reasonable modification.

Prevailing on a claim that a landlord failed to make reasonable accommodations, requires establishing that:

> [The individual] suffered from a "handicap" (or "disability"), (2) the landlord knew or should have known of the disability, (3) an accommodation of the disability may be necessary to afford the tenant an equal opportunity to use and enjoy her apartment, (4) the tenant requested a reasonable accommodation, and (5) the landlord refused to grant a reasonable accommodation.
>
> (*Douglas v. Kriegsfeld Corp.*, 2004, p. 1129).

While FHAA protections and reasonable accommodations can prevent individuals who are facing eviction from losing their housing, the FHAA guarantees are not foolproof safeguards to ensure stable housing. The FHAA protections are particularly likely to fail individuals who have not sought mental health treatment. An individual who does not know, or is unwilling to acknowledge, that he suffers from a mental illness is unlikely to request an accommodation or otherwise try to seek FHAA protections. The policy allowing tenants to request reasonable accommodations at *any time* during tenancy eases the burden of qualifying for a reasonable accommodation (U.S. Department of Housing and Urban Development, 2008). A tenant who learns or accepts his mental illness after initially moving into rental housing could still qualify to receive an accommodation. This provision also protects individuals whose mental illnesses may not preclude the function of a major life activity when the individual moves into the housing, but whose mental illnesses deteriorate and begin to preclude major life functions.

However, individuals who do not know of or do not accept their mental illness diagnosis would struggle to establish the first, second, and fourth prongs of the prima facie case to show that a housing provider failed to make reasonable accommodations. As discussed above, individuals who are part of a racial minority are particularly susceptible to suffering from undiagnosed mental illness. Minorities with mental illness are the least likely population to receive FHAA benefits, including the reasonable accommodation guarantee.

The Americans with Disabilities Act (ADA) and the Ohio Civil Rights Commission (OCRC)

The Americans with Disabilities Act (ADA) provides alternative remedies for individuals suffering from mental illness who are subjected to discriminatory housing practices to assert a discrimination claim. The scope of the ADA protections is narrower than that under FHAA in that the ADA only extends to public housing and accommodations (42 U.S.C.S. § 12132).

Individual states may also have remedies for individuals with mental illnesses to assert discrimination claims. In Ohio, an individual who believes that he was the victim of a discriminatory housing practice may file a complaint with the Ohio Civil Rights Commission (OCRC) (http://crc.ohio.gov/about_us.htm). Under this scenario, the OCRC will spearhead an investigation of the charges and pursue mediation if feasible. The OCRC will make a determination of whether there is probable cause of discrimination.

Challenges to Providing Reasonable Accommodations

Meeting the prima facie standard to receive a reasonable accommodation does not entitle an individual to receive housing accommodations. For individuals whose disabilities prevent reasonable accommodations, there may not be adequate remedies. Case studies of compulsive hoarders, an individual's whose mental illnesses cause violent behavior, and tenants requiring service animals illustrate the ways that an individual's disability may preclude the implementation of a reasonable accommodation.

Exceptions to the Reasonable Accommodations Requirement

Compulsive Hoarding. A landlord has no obligation to lease to a tenant where the lease "would constitute a direct threat to the health or safety of other individuals or whose tenancy would result in substantial physical damage to the property of others" (Fair Housing Act, 2008). This provision is potentially prohibitive to individuals who are compulsive hoarders.

Approximately one-quarter of individuals diagnosed with obsessive-compulsive disorder are compulsive hoarders (Cobb et al., 2007). The endless acquisition of useless possessions by these individuals may result in such significant cluttering that their living spaces become essentially uninhabitable and may result in increased risk of fire, falling, poor sanitation, and health problems. A tenant who hoards compulsively cannot conceivably comply with health and safety requirements, which may exempt the landlord from accommodating this tenant who compulsively hoards, and the tenant would be at risk of eviction (Cobb et al., 2007).

Assuming that the tenant successfully overcomes these barriers and secures the accommodation, there are no existing protections if the tenant condition worsens and the tenant again becomes unable to comply with the lease agreement. These individuals will likely fail to establish that a housing provider refused to make a reasonable accommodation.

Violent and Criminal Behavior. Because mental illnesses can cause an individual to behave erratically, violently, or otherwise engage in unhealthy behavior, individuals with mental illness may be perceived as a threat to themselves or their neighbors. Whether accurate or not, such perceptions often result in the individuals' inability to secure and maintain housing.

In the case of *Boston Housing Authority v. Bridgewaters* (2007), the appellant, Emmett Bridgewater – a man suffering from bipolar disorder – assaulted his partially paralyzed brother during a physical altercation. The court rejected Bridgewaters' argument that, because he had started taking medication to stabilize his mental illness, the housing authority should allow him to retain his housing. The court held that "an individual who engages in conduct that is significantly inimical to an authority's obligation to provide a physically safe environment for its tenants is not ... entitled to ... [a] reasonable accommodations for ... handicapped tenants" (*Boston Housing Authority v. Bridgewaters*, 2007, p. 768).

It is unlikely that the FHAA will shield an individual with mental illness from eviction based on any criminal behavior, violent or not. Various Massachusetts courts have recently upheld this principle stating, "a ... housing authority must have the discretion to seek to terminate a lease based on criminal activity, occurring on the premises, or off, that constitutes a threat to public safety" (*Lowell Housing Authority v. Melendez*, 2007, p. 40).

Other Barriers to Creating Reasonable Accommodations

Even individuals with mental illness who do not face obstacles in establishing their entitlement to a reasonable accommodation may struggle to fashion an appropriate reasonable accommodation. Such obstacles are usually surmountable, but only after tenants have participated in litigation or court mediation. Mentally ill individuals who use service animals for emotional support are particularly susceptible to such barriers.

Many residential housing units do not allow pets. To maintain a service animal, an individual with mental illness will have to seek a reasonable accommodation to keep the animal. A disabled individual may reasonably maintain a service animal if the disability-based problems will be effectively resolved through the use of the requested service animal. Such determinations are fact specific and must be evaluated on a case-by-case basis (*Auburn Woods I Homeowners Association v. Fair Employment & Housing*, 2004; *Janush v. Charities Housing Development Corporation*, 2000; *Oras v. Housing Authority of City of Bayonne*, 2004; *State ex rel. Henderson v. Des Moines Municipal Housing Agency*, 2007). Though an individual will likely prevail in establishing that a service animal qualifies as an appropriate "reasonable accommodation," that individual may first be a party to a legal action to make the factual determination about reasonableness.

Applying the Mental Health Court Models to Eviction Cases

Suits where a tenant asserts a housing discrimination claim are most likely to be heard in a municipal court. Many municipal courts have a housing subdivision with a judge dedicated to covering a narrowly defined set of issues. This structure lends itself to having a specialized magistrate or other staff consultants who can focus on issues particular to housing and mental illness.

The development of specialized dockets in housing courts for individuals with mental illness would improve efforts to secure stable housing for individuals who are otherwise prone to eviction and homelessness. When an individual with mental illness has a dispute with a landlord, the specialized docket could help to prevent eviction. The magistrate could review that individual's mental health history, community supports, psychiatric treatment, and any reasonable accommodations. Based on the findings of this review and in consultation with mental health experts—much like in existing mental health courts in the criminal system—the magistrate could fashion a solution to prevent eviction, address a landlord's concerns, and prevent future recurrences of the event which led to the dispute. The magistrate could appoint a social service agency to construct adequate reasonable accommodations and assist the landlord in implementing these accommodations. The agency could also ensure that a tenant complies with his medication regimen and receives adequate community support.

The magistrate could also set up an intervention plan and identify a trained person for the landlord to contact in the event that the individual was struggling to comply with the lease agreement or had an acute mental health crisis. The involvement of a trained individual would reduce the incidents of futile efforts by the landlord—who is most likely not trained to address mental illness—to prompt a mentally ill tenant to comply with lease requirements. The landlord could implement the intervention plan as soon as he notices the tenant's behavior changes and, in so doing, avert an impending crisis.

A specialized mental health docket in housing court would hear a proportionately higher number of reasonable accommodations cases than other courts. The magistrate would residually develop specific experience in developing and knowledge about the relative success of various reasonable accommodations. This experience and knowledge would improve the efficacy of the specialized docket relative to other courts hearing housing discrimination claims. For particularly challenging or novel cases, the magistrate would have the flexibility to devote more time to fashioning an appropriate accommodation because his time would be dedicated to the specialized docket. Even for individuals for whom eviction is inevitable, a mental health docket at housing court could provide referrals and linkages to secure alternative housing and prevent the repetition of the original scenario under which that mentally ill individual lost his or her housing.

In the case of a compulsive hoarder, a court could provide the tenant with an opportunity to remove the clutter upon receiving an eviction notice (Cobb et al., 2007). The hoarder could agree to a contract whereby he completes specific chores to ensure that a home which has been "cured" of its clutter remains clean (Cobb et al., 2007). Contracting with a social service agency to monitor the hoarder would help to ensure compliance with the accommodation. The agency could also provide support to the landlord who owns the property where the compulsive hoarder resides.

In the case of an individual who exhibits violent and aggressive behaviors, the specialized court could work with a landlord to identify and remove "triggers." The court could order the tenant to attend individual or group counseling and take medication to control violent behavior. As with the compulsive hoarder, the court could provide the landlord with a community contact who would have the tools, training, and authority to monitor, evaluate, and modify the accommodation and respond in an emergency if the accommodation failed.

Encouraging Participaties in a Specialized Docket

Though the benefits of a specialized docket seem apparent, the court would have to strategize to promote the utilization of the specialized docket; the court cannot compel either individuals with mental illness or landlords to participate in the specialized docket. For tenants, the prospect of secured housing would likely serve as a great incentive to utilize the services of a mental health docket in housing court; the alternatives – including homelessness, institutionalization, or frequent relocation – are sufficiently unattractive.

For landlords, the incentives are less compelling; evicting and replacing a problematic tenant, or even providing minimal reasonable accommodations, are less time and resource consuming than participating in a program dedicated to creating holistic, comprehensive accommodations. Although participation in the specialized docket may reduce a landlord's potential civil liability for housing discrimination, due to underenforcement of the FHAA and the low burden to establish a good faith effort to create a reasonable accommodation, fear of civil liability is unlikely to incentivize landlord's utilization of the specialized docket. To encourage landlord participation, the court should create new incentives such as vouchers or tax rebates for landlords who work with the court and implement *comprehensive* reasonable accommodations for tenants.

Existing Model: The Tenancy Preservation Project

Massachusetts has already developed a program geared toward the prevention of homelessness among individuals with mental problems who become involved in housing court. The Tenancy Preservation Project (TPP) prevented homelessness in 297 of 371 cases throughout Massachusetts in 2007. While some of TPP's clients suffer from mental problems other than mental illness, such as substance abuse or mental retardation, mentally ill individuals comprise the majority of TPP's caseload.

TPP program participants are primarily low-income individuals who receive case management referrals from a judge, legal service provider, or social service agency. (Anderson, 2005). Individuals may also refer themselves to the program. TPP typically achieves one of three potential outcomes for program participants: (1) the preservation of the individual's tenancy, (2) the development of a plan for alternative housing when tenancy preservation is not feasible, and (3) referral of the individual to a homeless outreach program if he or she is unable or unwilling to work toward the first two alternatives (Anderson, 2005).

While officially a housing court initiative, TPP relies on the collaboration of various agencies and housing providers, including the Department of Mental Health, the Department of Public Health Bureau of Substance Abuse Services, MassHousing, the Department of Housing and Community Development, and Legal Services (Anderson, 2005). TPP has also successfully engaged private landlords, because TPP is viewed as a credible and responsive agency (The Better Homes Fund And The Massachusetts Housing Finance Agency, 1999; Burt, 2007). The comprehensive partnership has streamlined the process for individuals with mental illness and housing problems to secure services and, in doing so, made working with TPP more attractive.

TPP's success is also attributable to its holistic approach to resolving housing problems for individuals with mental illness. Case managers both provide needed services, such as mental health treatment or house cleaning services to clients, and also facilitate communication between provider agencies. TPP staff also develop lease compliance and clinical plans and recommendations to facilitate the housing Court's efforts to form an effective plan for participants in the program (The Better Homes Fund and The Massachusetts Housing Finance Agency, 1999; Burt, 2007).

Other jurisdictions considering developing a mental health docket for housing could refer to TPP as an appropriate model. The proposed housing court mental health docket should begin as a pilot project, preferably in an urban area. The jurisdiction should have a well-established housing court, as well as social service agencies that have the capacity and training to provide the recommended supports to both landlords and mentally ill tenants. The docket will require funding to cover the salary of a dedicated magistrate and to contract with the social service agencies. Apart from helping to secure housing for individuals with mental illness, the proposed docket will ameliorate the perceived disparities in access to legal services amongst mentally ill individuals.

The Mental Health Court Model, Employment, and Mental Health

According to Congressional findings, more than 43 million people suffer from some physical or mental disability (42 U.S.C.S. § 12101). Disability is a barrier to securing stabilized employment. "Individuals with disabilities continually encounter . . . discrimination, including outright intentional exclusion . . . failure to make modifications to existing facilities and practices, exclusionary qualification standards and criteria, segregation, and relegation to lesser . . . jobs" (42 U.S.C.S. § 12101). The ADA, the Family Medical Leave Act (FMLA), and state law provide employment discrimination protection for all disabled individuals. Typically, employment discrimination cases, whether brought under the ADA or FMLA, are heard by the Equal Employment Opportunities Commission (EEOC) (U.S. Equal Employment Opportunity Commission, 2008). According to statistics from EEOC, more than 15% of the cases that it resolved in 2007 stemmed from discrimination based on some form of mental illness (U.S. Equal Employment Opportunity Commission, 2008).

From a social and policy perspective, promoting stable employment amongst individuals with mental illness serves multiple functions. Stabilized employment increases an individual's self-sufficiency and presumably decreases that individual's reliance on SSI and other social welfare systems. Research shows that economic self-sufficiency is directly correlated to positive self-esteem and self-worth (Hubbard, 2004). The ability to maintain stabilized employment also decreases the likelihood that individuals with mental illness will face societal marginalization; the ability to work affords an individual with mental illness increased opportunities to participate socially and economically.

Existing Remedies

Americans with Disabilities Act (ADA)

The ADA may provide remedies to individuals with mental illness who are subject to employment discrimination. Whereas the ADA's protections against

housing discrimination only apply to public entities, protections against employment-based discrimination are broader. The ADA precludes any "employer,
employment agency, labor organization, or joint labor-management committee"
from discriminating against any individuals with a disability, in the workplace
(42 U.S.C.S. § 12111). The ADA requires an employer to provide "reasonable
accommodations" to ensure workplace accessibility for disabled individuals.

The Family Medical Leave Act (FMLA)

The FMLA precludes employers from terminating employees who require a
leave of absence due to, amongst other situations, a serious health condition
(29 U.S.C.S. § 2612). A "serious Health Condition" includes "a … mental
condition that involves – (A) inpatient care in a hospital, hospice, or residential
medical care facility; or (B) continuing treatment by a health care provider" (29
U.S.C.S. § 2611). An employee who can establish that he or she suffers from a
serious health condition qualifies for up to 12 weeks of employment leave (29
U.S.C.S. § 2612).

The FMLA has limited application. The FMLA will not protect workers
from hiring discrimination. To qualify for leave under the FMLA, an individual
must already have permanent employment from which to take leave. The anti-
discrimination act provides for up to 12 weeks of consecutive leave; the leave
cannot be utilized on an intermittent basis. However, an individual with mental
illness would likely receive a greater benefit from intermittent leave because it is
unlikely that a mental illness would afflict an employee for 12 consecutive weeks
but no other period of time over the course of employment (29 U.S.C.S. § 2612).
The FMLA will not protect employees from discriminatory termination unless
the termination is directly related to an employee's leave.

Even for those individuals who would benefit from FMLA coverage, the
certification requirements may pose an obstacle to enjoyment of benefits.
Certification must include the following: "(1) the date on which the serious
health condition commenced; (2) the probable duration of the condition; (3) the
appropriate medical facts within the knowledge of the health care provider
regarding the condition; (4) … a statement that the employee is unable to
perform the functions of the position of the employee" (29 U.S.C.S. § 2613).
Minorities with mental illness who, as previously established, are less likely than
non-minority counterparts to receive adequate mental health treatment are the
most likely to fail to provide the requisite certification from a medical provider
(29 U.S.C.S. § 2613).

State Remedies

State agencies and regulations may provide additional protections against
disability-based employment discrimination. In Ohio, the OCRC investigates
discrimination claims based on state law (Ohio Revised Code § 4112.04). In
addition to establishing that discrimination occurred – an almost identical

burden as that required under Federal law – to prevail on a discrimination claim under Ohio law, an individual must have a record of impairment (http://crc.ohio.gov/disc_em ployment.htm). Individuals who have not received a diagnosis or treatment because of cultural and socioeconomic biases would struggle to establish a record.

The EEOC interprets and enforces the ADA's provisions related to disability and employment. The ADA does not unequivocally recognize all problems caused by mental illness as bases for asserting discrimination claims; there is currently a disagreement among courts as to whether individuals who struggle to interact with others due to a mental disability are entitled to ADA protections (Mortlock, 2007).

Under the EEOC's narrow interpretation of "disabled," the ADA only protects individuals whose mental or physical impairments preclude the "form[ance of] a major life activity that the average person in the general population can perform" (Goldstein, 2001, p. 933). If an individual is able to "perform a major life activity while using a mitigating measure," such as medication, that individual is not considered disabled within the scope of the ADA (Goldstein, 2001; Paetzold, 2005).

This provision is particularly dangerous to individuals with mental illness who may struggle with medication compliance but are not able to qualify for ADA protection because of their ability to perform major life activities while medicated. Even individuals who do comply with their treatment may not qualify for reasonable accommodations under this provision of the ADA; oftentimes, medication will have side effects which require constant monitoring and may inhibit individuals' job performance. Individuals without adequate community supports to assist with medication compliance and monitoring are most susceptible to such obstacles under the ADA.

Reasonable accommodations may take various forms depending on an individual's disability. Under the ADA, accommodations may include job restructuring, modified work schedules, reassignment to an alternative position, modified equipment or devices, adjustment of examinations, training materials or policies, and/or the provision of readers or interpreters to support an individual in the performance of his or her employment responsibilities (42 U.S.C.S. § 12111). Modifications that may be of particular benefit to an individual with mental illness include reassignment to an environment with minimal stressful triggers (*Bultemeyer v. Fort Wayne Community Schools*, 1996), a reduction in workload (*Suppi v. Nicholson*, 2007), and allowing an employee to take a leave of absence to seek mental health treatment (*Suppi v. Nicholson*, 2007).

Unfortunately, most "reasonable accommodations" are geared toward individuals with physical rather than mental disabilities, limiting the potential benefit that the ADA can provide to an employee with mental illness. While employers are required to cooperate with mentally ill employees to try to fashion reasonable accommodations in the workplace, "the ADA ... is not intended to punish employers for behaving callously if, in fact, no accommodation for the employee's disability could reasonably have been made" (*Taylor v. Phoenixville School District*, 1999, p. 318). If an individual fails to request a reasonable accommodation, he or she cannot later claim that an employer's failure to make an accommodation equated to a violation of the ADA.

The ADA requires that individuals with mental illness provide their employers with notice of need for an accommodation (*Taylor v. Phoenixville School District*, 1999). There are few instances where an employee's symptoms alone are so severe as to put the employer on notice. (Rogers, 1998). If an individual has not sought mental health treatment, that individual may lack the requisite awareness of his disability to put the employer on notice. Because minorities with mental illness are prone to receiving inadequate mental health services and support, the reasonable notice requirement of the ADA is likely to impose a unique barrier to this population's receipt of employment discrimination protection. The pervasive stigma associated with mental illness is a further disincentive to disclosures necessary to establish the need for reasonable accommodations.

Applying the Mental Health Court Models to Employment Issues

The mental health court model would not be effective to prevent employment-based discrimination claims; the unique rules and restrictions of the ADA and FMLA limit the prospective utility of these protections for mentally ill employees. Both the ADA and FMLA are better suited to protect physically disabled individuals.

A docket dedicated to hearing discrimination claims of mentally ill employees would *not* improve the ability of individuals with mental illness to benefit from anti-discrimination laws. If an employee fails to give an employer adequate notice about his need for reasonable accommodations then the employee cannot later claim that the employer violated the ADA. By the time a discrimination case arrives in court, the employee has already failed to fulfill this burden; short of adapting the language of the ADA, a specialized court for mentally ill individuals cannot remedy the lack of notice.

A specialized court would not offer any remedies to an individual with mental illness who is able to perform major life functions with the assistance of mitigating measures. Even if that person were unable to comply with his or her treatment regimen, precedent implies that such an individual would not qualify to receive discrimination protection under the ADA. While employees who struggle to follow their treatment regimen may benefit from compliance assistance, a social worker is better suited to provide such assistance than a court.

Since the typical cases are filed in either the state's court of general jurisdiction or federal court, there is no forum that is identified as exclusively devoted to employment issues at the trial level. The EEOC and a state's review body may offer more of a focus on discrimination issues, but their offices are not widely distributed and lack the ability to gain access to local resources.

Eliminating Barriers

Rather than establishing a specialized court or docket to ensure that mentally ill individuals receive the same benefits from the ADA as physically disabled persons, advocates must lobby for changes to the statutory language and application. Three specific amendments would be particularly beneficial to individuals with mental illness. Congress should (1) ease the burden on employees to establish that they qualify for reasonable accommodations, (2) amend the provision that excludes from ADA protections mentally ill employees who are able to perform major life activities with the assistance of mitigating measures, and (3) amend notice requirements to prevent the automatic preclusion of individuals who do not request reasonable accommodations from ADA protections.

Compared to the population at large, minorities with mental illness are less likely to receive adequate mental health care or have stable community supports. These circumstances increase the barriers which minorities with mental illness face when navigating the notice and mitigating measures provisions of the ADA. Amending the federal law would eliminate some of the existing barriers to the receipt of ADA protections by mentally ill minorities.

Conclusion

The criminal justice system has provided a model which can effectively manage the unique problems posed by persons with mental illness who are accused of crimes. Major features of the mental health courts can be applied to some, but not all, types of civil cases. A specialized docket, modeled after the criminal justice system's mental health courts, could help to address root causes of mental illness which contribute to the involvement of individuals with mental illness in legal disputes.

Of the two particular types of cases evaluated—housing and employment— the housing courts appear to be most likely to benefit from a specialized mental health docket. Housing disputes have a predictable forum, housing courts, which are separate from the general civil dockets. Because housing courts exist in most large cities, such courts are more likely to be accessible to tenants with mental illness. In addition, the housing court is more likely to be able to develop the network of connections and referrals which would make a separate housing docket more effective.

The investment of resources to develop a specialized mental health docket in housing courts would benefit both tenants with mental illness in securing stabilized housing and landlords who may rent to such individuals. The specialized docket would reduce the burden that individuals with mental illness pose on the civil law system by creating comprehensive solutions to housing disputes. The specialized docket would ensure that any resolution to a housing dispute included provisions to safeguard against a repetition of the scenario that gave raise to the initial claim. Assuming that the implementation of specialized mental health docket in housing court was successful, the model could be replicated in other areas of civil law – such as bankruptcy courts – where there are centralized venues to hear cases, and individuals with mental health are likely to be a party to lawsuits. Specialized housing dockets would be of particular benefit to minorities with mental illness, who are the least likely to receive adequate mental health treatment or benefit from community supports.

Employment-related claims lack a similar venue which is widely available and designated to focus only on employment issues. Housing discrimination laws are also better suited to benefiting individuals with mental illness than employment discrimination law; the reasonable accommodations are more readily available in housing contexts than in employment.

References

Anderson, A. (2005). *The Tenancy Preservation Program Operations Manual.* Boston: MassHousing. (Sept. 2005). Last revised September, 2005; Last accessed April 30, 2008; Available at: https://www.masshousing.com/portal/server.pt/gateway/ PTARGS_0_2_1358_0_0_18/TPP_Manual.pdf.

Auburn Woods I Homeowners Association v. Fair Employment & Housing, 2004 121 Cal. App. 4th 1578 (Cal. App. 2004).

Bernstein, R., & Seltzer, T. (2003). Criminalization of people with mental illnesses: The role of mental health courts in system reform. *D.C. Law Review, 7*, 143–162.

Boston Housing Authority v. Bridgewaters, 2007 871 N.E.2d 1107 (Mass. App. 2007).

Bultemeyer v. Fort Wayne Community Schools, 1996 100 F.3d 1281 (7th Cir. 1996).

Burt, M. R. (2007). *History, principles, context, and approach: The special homelessness initiative of the Massachusetts Department of Mental Health.* Washington, D.C.: Urban Institute. Last accessed April 28, 2008; Available at http://www.urban.org/uploadedpdf/411500_special_homeless_initiaitve.pdf.

Cobb, T., Dunn, E., Torres Hernandez, V., Okleberry, J. M., Pfefferkorn, R., & Spector, C. E. (2007). Advocacy strategies to fight eviction in cases of compulsive hoarding and cluttering. *Clearinghouse Review: Journal of Poverty Law & Policy, 41*, 427–441.

Council of State Governments. (2005a). A guide to mental health court design and implementation. Last accessed April 28, 2008; Available at http://consensusproject.org/mhcp/Guide-MHC-Design.pdf.

Council of State Governments. (2005b). Mental health courts: A national snapshot. Last accessed April 28, 2008; Available at http://consensusproject.org/mhcp/national-snapshot.pdf.

Cuyahoga County Common Pleas Court Local Rule 30.1.

Douglas v. Kriegsfeld Corp., 2004 884 A.2d 1109, 1129 (D.C. App. 2004).

Fair Housing Act Amendments, 42 U.S.C.S. §§ 3601 et seq.

Fellner, J. (2006). A corrections quandary: Mental illness and prison rules. *Harvard Civil Rights-Civil Liberties Law Review*, 41, 391–412.

Goldstein, R. I. (2001). Mental illness in the workplace after *Sutton v. United Air Lines*. *Cornell Law Review, 86*, 927–973.

Hubbard, A. (2004). Meaningful lives and major life activities. *Alabama Law Review, 55*, 997–1042.

James, D. J., & Glaze, L. E. (2006). *Bureau of Justice Statistics special report: Mental health problems of prison and jail inmates.* Washington, D.C.: United States Department of Justice. Last accessed April 28, 2008; Available at http://www.ojp.usdoj.gov/bjs/mhppji. htm.

Janush v. Charities Housing Development Corporation, 2000 169 F. Supp. 2d 1133 (N.D. Cal. 2000).

Lowell Housing Authority v. Melendez, 2007 449 Mass. 34 (Mass. 2007).

Mortlock, S. (2007). Customer service rules: When a company cannot hire or retain a mentally ill employee with severely limited interpersonal skills. *Drake Law Review, 56,* 59–81.

Office of the Surgeon General. (1999). *Main findings: Mental illnesses are real, disabling conditions affecting all populations, regardless of race or ethnicity.* Washington, D.C.: United States Department of Health and Human Services, Substance Abuse and Mental Health Services Administration. Last accessed April 28, 2008; Available at http:// mentalhealth.samhsa.gov/cre/execsummary-2.asp.

O'Hara, A., & Miller, E. (2003). Priced out in 2002: The crisis continues. Boston: Technical Assistance Collaborative, Inc. Last accessed April 28, 2008; Available at http://www. tacinc.ord/Docs/HH/PricedOutIn2002.pdf.

Ohio Revised Code § 4112.04 (2008).

Oras v. Housing Authority of City of Bayonne, 2004 861 A.2d 194 (N.J. App. 2004).

Paetzold, R. L. (2005). Mental illness and reasonable accommodations at work: Definition of a disability under the ADA. *Psychiatric Services, 56,* 1188–1190.

Pearson, C., Locke, G., Montgomery, A., & Buron, L. (2007). *The applicability of housing first models to homeless persons with serious mental illness.* Cambridge, M.A.: United States Department of Housing and Urban Development.

President's New Freedom Commission on Mental Health. (2007). *Executive summary,* July 22. Last accessed April 28, 2008; Available at http://www.mentalhealthcommission.gov/ reports/FinalReport/FullReport.htm).

Rogers v. CH2M Hill, 18 F. Supp. 2d 1328, 1337 (N.D.A.L 1998).

Sabol, W. J., Couture, H., & Harrison, P. (2007). Prisoners in 2006. *Bureau of Justice Statistics Bulletin.* Washington, D.C.: United States Department of Justice. Last revised December 2007; Last accessed April 28, 2008; Available at http://www.ojp.usdoj.gov/bjs/pub/pdf/ p06.pdf.

State ex rel. Henderson v. Des Moines Municipal Housing Agency, 2007 Iowa App. LEXIS 1328, 18 (2007).

Substance Abuse and Mental Health Services Administration. (2004). *Blueprint for Change: Ending Chronic Homelessness for Persons with Serious Mental Illnesses and Co-Occurring Substance Use Disorders,* ch. 2. Last revised January 2004; Last accessed April 28, 2008; Available at http://mentalhealth.samhsa.gov/publications/allpubs/SMA04-3870/).

Suppi v. Nicholson, 2007 EEOPUB LEXIS 4238 (USEEOP 2007).

Taylor v. Phoenixville School District, 1999 184 F.3d 296, 318 (3d Cir. 1999).

The Better Homes Fund, & The Massachusetts Housing Finance Agency. (1999). *Tenancy preservation project: The first year in review: An evaluation report.* (Copy on file with author.).

The Sentencing Project. (2007). United States Sentencing Commission approves crack reform for federal prisoners. Last accessed April 28, 2008; Available at http://www. sentencingproject.org/NewsDetails.aspx?NewsID=530).

U.S. Census Bureau. (2001). *Overview of race and Hispanic origin 2000: Census 2000 brief.* Last accessed April 28, 2008; Available at: http://www.census.gov/prod/2001pubs/cenbr01-1.pdf.

U.S. Department of Health and Human Services. *Mental Health: A Report of the Surgeon General-Executive Summary.* Rockville, M.D.: U.S. Department of Health and Human Services, Substance Abuse and Mental Health Services Administration, Center for Mental Health Services, National Institutes of Health, National Institute of Mental Health, 1999.

U.S. Department of Housing and Urban Development. (2008). Joint Statement of the Department of Housing and Urban Development and the Department of Justice:

Reasonable Modifications Under the Fair Housing Act. Last accessed April 28, 2008; Available at http://www.hudgov/offices/fheo/disabilities/reasonable_modifications_-mar08.pdf.

U.S. Equal Employment Opportunity Commission. (2008). ADA Charge Data by Impairments/Bases – Merit Factor Resolutions FY 1997 – FY 2007 (February 2008). Last accessed April 30, 2008; Available at http://www.eeoc.gov/stats/ada-merit.html.

29 U.S.C.S. § 2611.

29 U.S.C.S. § 2612.

42 U.S.C.S. § 12101.

42 U.S.C.S. § 12111.

Chapter 4
Migration and Mental Health

Sana Loue

The Migration Experience

Migration has been defined as:

> the physical transition of an individual or a group from one society to another. This transition usually involves abandoning one social setting and entering a different one
>
> (Eisenstadt, 1955, p. 1).
>
> a relatively permanent moving away of . . . migrants, from one geographical location to another, preceded by decision-making on the part of the migrants on the basis of a hierarchically ordered set of values or valued ends and resulting in changes in the interactional set of migrants
>
> (Mangalam, 1968, p. 8).
>
> a permanent or semipermanent change of residence
>
> (Lee, 1966, p. 49).
>
> the process of social change whereby an individual moves from one cultural setting to another for the purpose of settling down either permanently or for a prolonged period
>
> (Bhugra & Jones, 2001, p. 216).

Accordingly, migration refers to both movement within and across national borders. It encompasses internal migrants, such as agricultural workers and immigrants, regardless of the manner or legality of their entry into a country. It is not only the movement of populations that affects health but also the context in which that movement occurs. Importantly, it occurs as the result of a decision-making process undertaken by an individual that is premised on a set of values that may or may not be explicit. This chapter focuses on the relationship between migration across international borders and the mental health of the individuals who so migrate.

Estimates suggest that currently 175 million people, or 2.9% of the world's population, live either permanently or temporarily outside of their countries of origin (International Organisation for Migration, 2003). In 1990 migrants accounted for 15% of the population of 52 countries (Council of Europe & Parliamentary Assembly, 2000). The International Organisation for Migration

S. Loue (✉)
Case Western Reserve University, School of Medicine, Cleveland, OH
e-mail: Sana.Loue@case.edu

S. Loue, M. Sajatovic (eds.), *Determinants of Minority Mental Health and Wellness*, DOI 10.1007/978-0-387-75659-2_4,
© Springer Science+Business Media, LLC 2009

has estimated that currently one in every 35 people in the world is an international migrant (Scott, 2004) and that by the year 2050, the number of international migrants will approach 250 million (International Labour Office, International Organisation for Migration, and the Office of the United Nations High Commissioner for Human Rights [ILO, IOM, OHCHR], 2001). These figures include migrant workers, permanent immigrants, and those who are seeking asylum or refugee status; it does not include individuals who migrate across borders illegally, who are known variously as "illegal," "undocumented," or "irregular" (World Health Organization, 2003). These individuals may migrate themselves; may be trafficked, a process that involves coercion or deception; or may be smuggled, meaning that their entry has been facilitated by others for profit (ILO, IOM, OHCHR, 2001). Consequently, these figures represent underestimates of the magnitude of migration and its demographic impact in various regions of the world (Council of Europe & Parliamentary Assembly, 2000).

Individuals may migrate from one area to another for any number of reasons. Circumstances at the point of origin that may "push" individuals to leave include poverty, unemployment, persecution, internal civil strife, a change in government or regime, and/or natural disasters, such as a hurricane. Refugees, in particular, migrate due to "push" factors. The 1951 United Nations Convention on Refugees, as modified by the 1967 Protocol Relating to the Status of Refugees, describes a refugee as a person who:

> owing to well-founded fear of being persecuted for reasons of race, religion, nationality, membership of a particular social group or political opinion, is outside the country of his nationality and is unable or, owing to such fear, is unwilling to avail himself of the protection of that country; or who, not having a nationality and being outside of his former habitual residence as a result of such events, is unable, or owing to such fear, is unwilling to return to it.

Individuals may also migrate because they feel a "pull" toward the intended destination as a result of perceived employment prospects, the ability to reunify with other family members, expectations of a better economic and/or political situation, freedom from persecution, and/or a safe haven from the ravages of man-made or natural disasters. Distinctions have accordingly been made between those immigrants who are "voluntary," such as students, tourists, and migrant workers, and those who are "forced" to migrate as the result of displacement due to internal conflict, environmental disaster, famine, or development projects (Loughna, n.d.).

The health of migrating individuals and groups, whether documented/regular or undocumented/irregular, voluntary or forced, and internal or international, may be shaped by each stage of the migration process. During the period preceding migration ("pre-migration stage"), that is, before individuals have physically left their place of origin/residence, individuals have formed beliefs about health, illness, disease, treatment, and expectations of care that they will carry with them to their intended destinations. They may also have developed mental illness or vulnerability for mental illness that they will bring with them.

During the process of migration itself ("peri-migration"), and following their arrival at their destination ("post-migration"), individuals will be affected by the conditions that they confront and the experiences that they undergo during this process. Accordingly, it is critical that migration not be treated as a unitary concept but, instead, that clinicians and researchers be cognizant of critical factors that differentiate immigration experiences, including relevant individual and group characteristics, the conditions of the emigration-immigration process, and the conditions that are encountered in the destination country. Table 4.1, below,

Table 4.1 Factors impacting immigrant mental health during phases of migration process

Premigration	Peri-migration	Post-migration
Economic conditions	Travel conditions	Level of acceptance in destination country
Political conditions	(Il)legality of immigration process	Extent of congruence between country of origin and country of destination (extent of "culture shock")
Social status	Exposure or witnessing of violence	Length of detention
Economic standing	Number and nature of traumatic events witnessed	Conditions of detention
Educational level	Experience of torture	Existence of ethnic enclave to provide support
Extent of social support	Lack of access to food and water	Extent of isolation
Family network		Existence of family network ("chain migration")
Preexisting mental illness		Extent of loss or bereavement
Experience of torture		Role change
Experiencing or witnessing of violence		Knowledge of language in destination country
Number and nature of traumatic events witnessed		Availability of employment and economic opportunities
Starvation and lack of water		Availability of mental health services
Lack of secure shelter		Availability of insurance or other payment mechanism for mental health services
Stigma associated with mental illness		
Availability of mental health services		
Availability of payment mechanism for mental health services		
Quality of mental health services		

illustrates the various factors that have been noted in the literature as possibly impacting an individual's mental health during each such phase of migration.

The effect of varied immigration experiences on immigrants' mental health is further evident in the following two examples. Consider first a situation in which the individual seeking entry into another country is doing so because of the persecution and torture that he has suffered in his country of origin. He is one of the world's 8.7 million refugees and 20.8 million "people of concern" (Craig, Jajua, & Warfa, 2006), seeking safe haven from the persecution he has experienced in his home country because of his race, religion, gender, or political beliefs. He has witnessed the slaughter of family members and neighbors and the torture of men, women, and children. He has endured pain of an intensity so great that it can never be conveyed in words.

Upon arrival at the border of his country of destination, he is immediately arrested for attempting to enter illegally and is detained for an indefinite period of time in a facility that resembles a prison but is called a detention center. Some of those with whom he is confined are there for similar reasons, awaiting a decision as to their fate. Others have been transferred to the detention facility to await their deportation after serving prison sentences for crimes ranging from burglary to murder. He is not screened for mental or emotional problems, and no services are offered to him.

Contrast this situation with that of a middle-class woman who was trained as an engineer in her country of origin. Because of her skill level, she was able to obtain employment in her country of destination and, as the result of her prospective employer's efforts, was granted permission to reside permanently in the country of her destination. She processes for her visa through the established procedures for her new home country. Upon arrival in her new country, she secures an apartment in a desirable area of her new hometown and is immediately welcomed by her new colleagues.

Prevalence and Risk of Mental Illness Among Immigrants

Schizophrenia

In one of the first studies to examine the relationship between migration and mental illness, Ödegaard (1932) reported that hospital admission rates for schizophrenia were significantly higher among immigrant Norwegians to the United States than among Norwegians who had remained in their native country. Later, studies from the U.K. found higher rates of hospital admission for schizophrenia among Irish, Indian, Pakistani, and Caribbean immigrants in comparison with native British whites (Cochrane & Bal, 1989). Studies from Jamaica (Hickling & Rodgers-Johnson, 1995), Trinidad (Bhugra et al., 2000b), and Barbados (Mahy, Mallett, Leff, & Bhugra, 1999) suggest that the rates of schizophrenia in these countries are lower than that found among African-Caribbean migrants to the U.K.

Increased rates of schizophrenia have been noted among other immigrant groups as well. A Netherlands-based study found an increased risk of schizophrenia among those born in Morocco, Surinam, and the Dutch Antilles but not among those originating from Turkey or Western nations (Selten et al., 2001; Schrier, van de Weterin, Mulder, & Selten, 2001). An increased risk of schizophrenia-like psychosis has been reported among East African immigrants to Sweden (Zolkowska, Cantor-Graae, & McNeil, 2001) and among first- and second-generation immigrants to Denmark (Cantor-Graae, Pedersen, McNeil, & Mortensen, 2003).

Several hypotheses have been advanced in an attempt to explain the seemingly increased rates of schizophrenia among immigrants, which are as follows:

1. Rates of schizophrenia are high in the sending countries.
2. Individuals with schizophrenia are more likely to migrate.
3. The process of migration is stressful and, consequently, particularly vulnerable individuals may develop schizophrenia.
4. The apparently increased rates observed among immigrants are attributable to misdiagnosis.
5. Schizophrenia is manifested differently within different populations.
6. Rates of schizophrenia appear higher among immigrant communities because of ethnic density.
7. Conditions within the receiving country, including the extent of disparity between expected achievement and actual achievement and the level of acceptance or discrimination encountered, may result in elevated rates (Bhugra, 2004; Cochrane & Bal, 1987).

Increasing evidence suggests that the apparent increased risk of schizophrenia that has been noted among immigrant populations may be attributable to a constellation of co-occurring circumstances that include social disadvantage, language differences, and the stresses of an urban environment (Hutchinson & Haasen, 2004). (Galea, Goldmann, and Maxwell discuss the relationship between urbanization and mental health and illness of minority populations in Chapter 3 of this volume.) Rates of schizophrenia in Caribbean countries are similar to those among the native-born in the U.K., while immigrants, many of whom are socially disadvantaged, display an increased risk (Cooper, 2005). A review of 17 studies reported an increased incidence of schizophrenia in individuals who were socially disadvantaged in comparison with native-born members of the population majority (Eaton & Harrison, 2000).

Nonpsychotic Disorders

Findings from studies of immigrant mental health have been inconsistent, with some researchers reporting lower rates of mental illness among immigrant populations compared to the native-born populations of the receiving countries and others reporting elevated rates. Two national studies (Grant et al., 2004; Ortega, Rosencheck, Alegria, & Desai, 2000) and two smaller regional studies (Burnam, Hough, Karno, Escobar, & Telles, 1987; Vega et al., 1998) conducted in the United States found that Mexican immigrants had lower rates of anxiety and mood disorders than did U.S.-born individuals of Mexican ethnicity. And, in a survey of Mexican Americans in Fresno County, California and Mexicans resident in Mexico City, it was found that the lifetime prevalence of mental disorders was lowest among recent immigrants to the United States and highest among Mexican immigrants to the United States who had resided in the United States for 13 years or more (Vega et al., 1998). The rates of mental illness among the Mexico City residents fell between that of the recent U.S. immigrants and the longer-term immigrants. Taken together, it has been suggested that these studies support both the healthy migrant theory, that is, that healthier individuals self-select for migration (Breslau et al., 2007) and the hardy person theory, which asserts that hardy persons—those who believe they can influence life events, have a sense of purpose, and view change as an exciting challenge— remain healthier under stress (Kuo & Tsai, 1986).

However, at least one other research group has reported that preexisting anxiety disorders among Mexican residents of Mexico predicted migration to the United States, thereby casting doubt on the healthy migrant hypothesis (Breslau et al., 2007). They found, additionally, that immigration predicted the later onset of anxiety and mood disorders, lending support to the acculturation stress hypothesis, that is, the idea that the stresses of living in one's newly adopted country and exposures associated with residence in the new country may increase the risk of a mental disorder (cf. Rogler, Cortes, & Malgady, 1991).

A number of studies may lend additional support to the acculturation stress hypothesis. A study conducted in Rotterdam found the children of Turkish immigrants five times as likely to commit suicide compared to Dutch children; Moroccan children were three times as likely to do so (Carballo & Nerukar, 2001). A U.K. study that examined symptoms of depression and anxiety among white British and Somali and Bengali first-generation immigrants found the prevalence of depression to be 25% among the Somalis, 77% among the Bengalis, and 25% among the east London whites (Silveira & Ebrahim, 1998). Social factors, including poor housing conditions, low family support, and inadequate community services were associated with depression in both Somalis and Bengalis, suggesting that post-migration factors played a critical role in the development of depression.

Consistent with these findings, an interview-based study of 40 Irish-born immigrants to England found that the majority of the 25 participants who suffered from depression attributed their depression to life events and circumstances unrelated to migration itself, including chronic physical illness, partner violence, and sexual identity conflict (Leavey, Rozmovits, Ryan, & King, 2007). Heavy alcohol use, however, was found to be associated with bereavement and loneliness, as well as chronic pain. Similarly, a study designed to investigate risk factors for psychiatric disorders among Latinos who were U.S.-born and those who arrived in the United States before and after the age of six concluded that nativity was a less important risk factor for psychiatric morbidity that had been hypothesized (Alegria et al., 2007). However, family conflict and burden were found to be related to the risk of mood disorders.

A study of native-born Swedes and immigrants to Sweden from Poland, the former Soviet Union, and other Eastern European countries found that Polish and other Eastern European immigrants experienced twice the rate of reported psychiatric illness and psychosomatic symptoms, while immigrants from the former Soviet Union experienced rates of mental illness similar to the native-born Swedes (Blomstedt, Johansson, & Sundquist, 2007). The authors specu-lated that the observed differences may have resulted from greater stigmatiza-tion of mental illness in the former Soviet Union, thereby impeding the report-ing of symptoms; lower levels of social support in Poland and other Eastern European countries, thereby increasing the likelihood of presentation for men-tal illness symptoms; or better mental health among individuals born in the former Soviet Union.

Numerous studies have reported that refugees and asylum seekers, in particular, may suffer from posttraumatic stress disorder and other mental illness. It has been estimated that in the European Union, two out of every three asylum seekers (the equivalent of a pending application for refugee status) have experienced some mental problems (Burnett & Peel, 2001). It has been estimated that up to 40% of refugees have experienced torture (Steel, Frommer, & Silove, 2004). In a study of 10 detained asylum seekers in the U.K., it was found that 6 had suffered torture, all 10 were suffering from depression, 4 were suicidal, and 2 had attempted suicide while in detention (Bracken & Gorst-Unsworth, 1991). Over one-half of a sample of 33 asylum seekers in Sydney, Australia reported having been subjected to physical torture (Sultan & O'Sullivan, 2001). A review of 20 studies providing results for 6,743 adults from 7 countries and 5 surveys of 260 refugee children from 3 countries reported that among the adults, 9% suffered from PTSD, 4% had generalized anxiety disorder, and 5% had major depression, while 11% of the children were diagnosed with PTSD (Fazel, Wheeler, & Danesh, 2005). The authors concluded that refugees are 10 times as likely to have PTSD compared to age-matched individuals in the native populations of the countries surveyed.

Other studies have also reported high rates of PTSD among refugee children. Almost all of the children in a sample of internally displaced Bosnian children were found to have PTSD (Goldstein, Wampler, & Wise, 1997). The prevalence of PTSD was almost 50% among children who had experienced war in Cam-bodia and the former Yugoslavia and had migrated to the United States (Mollica, Poole, Son, Murray, & Tor, 1997; Sack, Clarke, & Seeley, 1996; Weine et al., 1995). A study of refugee children aged 8–16 in London found that greater severity of PTSD was associated with premigration experiences of the violent death of family members and an unstable or insecure status following migration (Heptinstall, Sethna, & Taylor, 2004). Similar findings were reported from a study involving 87 children and adolescents who sought refuge in the United States from Cuba and had been held in refugee camps for up to 8 months prior to arrival in the United States (Rothe et al., 2002). More than half of the children (57%) evidenced symptoms of PTSD. Age and having witnessed violence in the camps were associated with PTSD. Consistent with findings from other studies (Chung, 1994; Chung & Kagawa-Singer, 1993; Steel, Silove, Phan, & Bauman, 2002), a dose-effect relationship was noted between the number of stressors and the severity of self-reported symptoms.

Research findings suggest that exposure to war and/or political unrest may heighten the risk of PTSD. A study comparing 258 immigrants from Central America and Mexico to the United States and 329 U.S-born Mexican Americans and Anglo-Americans found that 52% of the Central Americans who had migrated because of war and political violence experienced symptoms of PTSD, compared with 49% of Central Americans who had migrated for other reasons and 25% of Mexican immigrants (Cervantes, Salgado de Snyder, & Padilla, 1989).

Refugees who were subjected to torture appear to be at increased risk of developing not only PTSD but other psychiatric disorders as well. A study of ethnically Nepalese, religiously Hindu refugees from Bhutan who sought refuge in refugee camps in Nepal found that individuals who had been tortured were 5 times as likely to develop PTSD as those who had not been tortured, and 1.6 times as likely to have any psychiatric disorder (Van Ommerren et al., 2001). Researchers conducting the study estimated the 12-month prevalence of any psychiatric disorder at 74.4% among those refugees who had been tortured and 48% among those who had not been tortured. The impact of torture on mental health may be alleviated by the presence of family and social support from the immigrant community after arrival in the receiving country (Başoğlu & Paker, 1995; Schweitzer, Melville, Steel, & Lacherez, 2006).

Research suggests that individuals who are placed in detention facilities upon arrival at their destination country are often re-traumatized by this experience and suffer a worsening of their mental health in comparison with those who are not detained (Becker & Silove, 1993; Bracken & Gorst-Unsworth, 1991; Steel & Silove, 2001; Thompson & McGorry, 1998). In the previously mentioned study of 33 asylum seekers in Sydney, Australia, researchers noted a progressive deterioration in the mental health of the asylum seekers, who had been held in detention for an average period of 2 years (Sultan & O'Sullivan, 2001). The research team observed that, ultimately, many of these individuals were

> dominated by paranoid tendencies, leaving them in a chronic state of fear and apprehension and a feeling that no one, including other detainees, can be trusted. Long periods of time are spent alone and some develop frankly psychotic symptoms, such as delusions, ideas of reference and auditory hallucinations

> (Sultan & O'Sullivan, 2001, p. 595).

This is also true of refugee children in detention, whose distress may be exacerbated as a result of observing parental distress and suffering, separation from their parents with or without warning, suffering through repeated interviewing by immigration officials, witnessing violence and self-harm, and instability due to lengthy delays in the processing of their claims for refugee status (Zwi, Herzberg, Dossetor, & Field, 2003).

Diagnosis and Assessment of Mental Illness

Published studies suggest that the experience and expression of various disorders vary across cultures. This results in increased difficulty in diagnosing mental illness among immigrants, particularly where there exists a difference in language in addition to variations in the expression of a mental illness (Jackson, Zatzick, Harris, & Gardiner, 2008).

As an example, in a study conducted by Bughra and colleagues (2000a) in the U.K., it was found that almost one-third of Asians, Trinidadians, and British whites suffering from schizophrenia reported visual hallucinations, whereas none of the African-Caribbean participants reported such symptoms. However, the African-Caribbean individuals were more likely to experience delusions of reference and paranoia.

One study of 134 patients under the age of 55 from three ethnic groups living in the U.K., all of whom were on lithium prophylaxis, found that of the individuals who had been diagnosed with bipolar I disorder, African-origin patients were significantly more likely than the British white patients to display symptoms of mania, while the Afro-Caribbean patients were more likely to experience mood-incongruent delusions (Kirov & Murray, 1999). The investigators were unable to explain the underlying reasons for this difference in the expression of the disorder. Other researchers have similarly reported a greater tendency for African-Caribbean immigrants in the U.K. to present with manic symptoms compared with similarly diagnosed whites (van Os et al., 1996).

An investigation of bipolar I disorder first manic episode among African-Caribbean, African, and white European individuals in the U.K. found that the African-Caribbean and African individuals were significantly less likely to have experienced a depressive episode prior to the onset of the first episode of mania (Kennedy, Boydell, van Os, & Murray, 2004). This finding persisted even after controlling for differences across the groups in sex, occupational category, or educational level, and use of substances. The investigators hypothesized that this finding could be related to decreased access to care for depression among the African-Caribbean and African patients and a resulting absence of depression in the patient's history and/or cultural beliefs about the unacceptability of depression or treatment of depression.

Both the African-Caribbean and African groups in this study had experienced an earlier onset of mania and bipolar disorder compared with the group of European whites, which the authors attributed to differences in population distribution (Kennedy et al., 2004). These two groups were more likely to display symptoms of psychosis at the occurrence of first mania; these included persecutory delusions, delusions of influence, and auditory hallucinations. The authors were unable to account for this finding, but surmised that this severe clinical presentation might explain the overdiagnosis of schizophrenia that has been noted among African-American patients (Strakowski et al., 2003).

A study of individuals with bipolar disorder in Israel noted the predominance of manic episodes over time (Osher, Yaroslavsky, el-Rom, & Belmaker, 2000), in contrast to the pattern of predominantly depressive episodes noted among European patients with bipolar disorder (Angst, 1986; Judd et al., 2002). Two studies of the presentation and course of bipolar disorder in Nigeria also found that a unipolar manic course was most common (Makanjuola, 1982, 1985). All of these studies taken together suggest that the clinical presentation of bipolar disorder may vary across cultures due to a variety of possible factors.

Diagnosis of mental illness among immigrants may be further impeded by the complexities of interpretation and translation. In a case series of four individuals who migrated within Europe and were hospitalized in the U.K. for a manic episode, the clinicians reported significant problems due to the immigrants' inability to communicate in English and difficulties locating appropriate professionals (Gledhill, Warner, & Wakeling, 1996). The authors were unable to determine whether the mania had been precipitated by the stresses associated with travel or whether migration represented a manifestation of manic illness.

A lack of understanding of the immigrants' culture and immigration experience may also lead to misdiagnosis (Gonzalez, Natale, Pimentel, & Lane, 1999). Guardedness and suspiciousness may be misinterpreted as evidence of psychopathology, rather than an adaptive response to one's circumstances (Adebimpe, 1981). Jenkins (1991), for instance, noted that the women participating in her study of Salvadorean refugees to North America were suffering from nervios, a cultural category that encompasses such symptoms as dysphoria and nonspecific body aches. Jenkins argued that rather than reflecting underlying psychopathology, these symptoms constituted a culturally created normative response to abnormal stressors.

Help-Seeking and Utilization of Mental Health Services

Although research suggests that a large proportion of refugees may be in need of mental health services, relatively few are assessed for that need upon arrival in the United States. A survey of geographically dispersed large metropolitan refugee programs that received approximately 40% of all refugees during the study period revealed that only one-third of the sites performed mental status examinations (Vergara, Miller, Martin, & Cookson, 2003). Slightly more than three-quarters (78%), however, offered mental health care.

Portes, Kyle, and Eaton (1992) found in their study of mental health service utilization by Haitian refugees and Mariel Cubans that Cuban and Haitian refugees had lower rates of use but that Mariel Cuban refugees utilized mental health services to a far greater degree than did native-born persons. The researchers concluded that the different contexts of exit constituted the primary determinants of the mental health profile of each refugee group and that the mental health assistance received in the country of origin has a significant effect on knowledge of facilities in the receiving country. Additionally, they identified a series of variables relevant to help-seeking for mental health among refugee minorities in the United States. These include the context of their exit from their home country; the context of their reception by their receiving country; predisposing factors, such as age, sex, marital status, educational level, and knowledge of English; and enabling factors, including knowledge of the availability of services, the affordability of treatment, the availability of insurance or another payment mechanism. Factors such as the extent of resettlement assistance received, the existence of a family network in the receiving country, and the ethnicity of coworkers will also impact the decision to seek care.

Various factors have been found to impede refugees' ability and/or willingness to seek mental health care. These include a belief that the problem will resolve of its own accord, a lack of information about potential resources, and/ or shame, embarrassment, and concern about others' reactions to their help-seeking (Beiser, Simich, & Pandalangat, 2003).

Unlike refugees who may be able to access mental health care specifically because they hold legal status as refugees, temporary immigrants, undocumented immigrants, individuals awaiting a determination of their asylum claims, and many permanent residents may encounter significant obstacles in their attempts to access mental health care. In the United States, for instance, publicly funded mental health care is generally unavailable for temporary visitors, undocumented persons, and even permanent residents ("green card" holders) who are within the first 5 years of having received their permanent resident status (Personal Responsibility and Work Opportunity Reconciliation Act, 1996). A large proportion of immigrants to the United States do not have either employer-sponsored health insurance or sufficient funds to afford private health care insurance (Buchmueller, Lo Sasso, Lurie, & Dolfin, 2007; Grieco, 2004), further limiting their ability to obtain needed mental health treatment.

This situation is not peculiar to the United States. To provide another example, a study of 102 undocumented individuals (*gömda*) in Sweden revealed a relatively high prevalence of depression, anxiety disorders, and suicidal ideation (Médecins sans Frontières, n.d.). The immigrants reported a significant deterioration of their mental health status since their arrival in Sweden. However, the majority of the individuals in need of mental health care did not seek care out of fear that they would be returned to their home country and the lack of funding for such treatment.

When mental health care is sought, the type of help sought may vary across immigrant groups. A study of Turkish refugees resident in London found that they resorted simultaneously to a variety of treatments for their psychoses, including Turkish-speaking general practitioners and psychiatrists and traditional healers (Leavey, Guvenir, Haase-Casanovas, & Dein, 2007). Similarly, Tamil refugees in Toronto rarely sought help for their mental illness from a psychiatrist, and preferred instead to rely on rituals, traditional herbal remedies, religious stones and bracelets, and the services of an astrologer (Beiser, Simich, & Pandalangat, 2003).

Clinical and Research Implications

A number of key points are evident from this review. First, the diagnosis of mental illness in immigrant populations is complex due to variations in disease and illness definition, explanatory models of illness, symptom presentation, and language. Second, the context of individuals' exit and entry experiences may have a significant impact on individuals' willingness and ability to seek needed mental health services and their receptivity to the treatments offered. Finally, the passage of time may or may not alleviate the effects of immigrants' entry exit and entry experiences, and mental health care may be needed even years after they have apparently resettled in their new country. The clinician must be cognizant of these issues in his or her efforts to evaluate the genesis of behaviors and formulate potentially ameliorating interventions.

Research is needed in numerous areas so as to better inform clinical practice. These include the following: (1) the development of improved screening tools to identify those immigrants most in need of immediate mental health care; (2) the development and implementation of efficacious and effective interventions for the treatment of mental illness among immigrants; (3) the development in collaboration with legal systems of mechanisms to reduce the risk of mental status deterioration among detained immigrants; and (4) the identification of additional mechanisms for the provision of mental health care to all immigrants, as well as potential sources of revenue for such care.

References

Adebimpe, V. (1981). Overview: White norms and psychiatric diagnosis of black patients. *American Journal of Psychiatry, 138*, 279–285.

Alegria, M., Shrout, P. E., Woo, M., Guarnaccia, P., Sribney, W., Vila, D., et al. (2007). Understanding differences in past year psychiatric disorders for Latinos living in the US. *Social Science & Medicine, 65*, 214–230.

Angst, J. (1986). The course of affective disorders. *Psychopathology, 19*(2), 47–52.

Başoğlu, M., & Paker, M. (1995). Severity of trauma as a predictor of long-term psychological status in survivors of torture. *Journal of Anxiety Disorders, 9*, 339–350.

Becker, R., & Silove, D. (1993). Psychiatric and psychosocial effects of prolonged detention in asylum-seekers. In M. Crock (Ed.), *Protection or punishment: The detention of asylum-seekers in Australia* (pp. 46–63). Sydney, Australia: The Federation Press.

Beiser, M., Simich, L., & Pandalangat, N. (2003). Community in distress: Mental health needs and help-seeking in the Tamil community in Toronto. *International Migration, 41*(5), 233–245.

Bhugra, D. (2004). Migration and mental health. *Acta Psychiatrica Scandinavia, 109*, 243–258.

Bhugra, D., Hilwig, M., Corridan, B., Neehall, J., Rudge, S., Mallett, R., et al. (2000a). A comparison of symptoms in cases with first onset of schizophrenia across four groups. *European Journal of Psychiatry, 14*, 241–249.

Bhugra, D., Hilwig, M., Mallett, R., Corridan, J., Leff, J., Neehall, J., et al. (2000b). Factors in the onset of schizophrenia: A comparison between London and Trinidad samples. *Acta Psychiatrica Scandinavia, 101*, 135–141.

Bhugra, D., & Jones, P. (2001). Migration and mental illness. *Advances in Psychiatric Treatment, 7*, 216–223.

Blomstedt, Y., Johansson, S.-E., & Sundquist, J. (2007). Mental health of immigrants from the former Soviet Bloc: A future problem for primary health care in the enlarged European Union? A cross-sectional study. *BMC Public Health, 7*, 27. Last accessed February 18, 2007; Available at http://www.biomedcentral.com/ 1471-2458/7/27

Bracken, P., & Gorst-Unsworth, C. (1991). The mental state of detained asylum seekers. *Psychiatric Bulletin, 15*, 657–659.

Breslau, J., Aguilar-Gaxiola, S., Borges, G., Casilla-Puentes, R. C., Kendler, K. S., Medina-Mora, M.-E., et al. (2007). Mental disorders among English-speaking Mexican immigrants to the US compared to a national sample of Mexicans. *Psychiatry Research, 121*, 115–122.

Buchmueller, T. C., Lo Sasso, A. T., Lurie, I., & Dolfin, S. (2007). Immigrants and employer-sponsored health insurance. *Health Services Research, 42*, 286–310.

Burnam, M. A., Hough, R. L., Karno, M. Escobar, J. I., & Telles, C. A. (1987). Acculturation and lifetime prevalence of psychiatric disorders among Mexican-Americans in Los Angeles. *Journal of Health and Social Behavior, 28*, 89–102.

Burnett, A., & Peel, M. (2001). The health of survivors of torture and organized violence. *British Medical Journal, 322*, 606–609.

Cantor-Graae, E., Pedersen, C.B., McNeil, T.F., & Mortensen, P.B. (2003). Migration as a risk factor for schizophrenia: A Danish poulation-based cohort study. *British Journal of Psychiatry, 182*, 117–122.

Carballo, M., & Nerukar, A. (2001). Migration, refugees, and health risks. *Emerging Infectious Diseases, 7*, 556–560.

Cervantes, R. C., Salgado de Snyder, V. N., & Padilla, A. M. (1989). Posttraumatic stress in immigrants from Central American and Mexico. *Hospital and Community Psychiatry, 40*, 615–619.

Chung, P. (1994). Post-traumatic stress disorder among Cambodian refugees in New Zealand. *International Journal of Social Psychiatry, 40*, 17–26.

Chung, P., & Kagawa-Singer, M. (1993). Predictors of psychological distress among Southeast Asian refugees. *Social Science & Medicine, 36*, 631–639.

Cochrane, R., & Bal, S. S. (1987). Migration and schizophrenia: An examination of five hypotheses. *Social Psychiatry, 22*, 181–191.

Cochrane, R., & Bal, S. S. (1989). Mental hospital admission rates of migrants to England: A comparison of 1971 and 1981. *Social Psychiatry and Psychiatric Epidemiology, 24*, 2–12.

Convention Relating to the Status of Refugees, 189 U.N.T.S. 150 (1951), entered into force April 22, 1954.

Cooper, B. (2005). Immigration and schizophrenia: The social causation hypothesis revisited. *British Journal of Psychiatry, 186*, 361–363.

Council of Europe, Parliamentary Assembly. (2000). Health conditions of migrants and refugees in Europe: Report of the Committee on Migration, Refugees and Demography.

Last accessed June 14, 2006; Available at http://assemply.coe.int/Documents/Working Docs/ doc00/EDOC8650.htm

Craig, T., Jajua, P., & Warfa, N. (2006). Mental healthcare needs of refugees. *Psychiatry*, *5*, 405–408.

Eaton, W., & Harrison, G. (2000). Ethnic disadvantage and schizophrenia. *Acta Psychiatrica Scandinavica*, *407*(Suppl. 1), 38–43.

Eisenstadt, S. N. (1955). *The absorption of immigrants*. Glencoe, Illinois: Free Press.

Fazel, M., Wheeler, J., & Danesh, J. (2005). Prevalence of serious mental disorder in 7000 refugees settled in Western countries: A systematic review. *Lancet*, *365*, 1309–1314.

Gledhill, J., Warner, J., & Wakeling, A. (1996). Mania in European immigrants. *European Psychiatry*, *11*(Supp. 4), 341s–341s(1).

Goldstein, R., Wampler, N., & Wise, P. (1997). War experiences and distress symptoms of Bosnian children. *Pediatrics*, *100*, 873–878.

Gonzalez, E. A., Natale, R. A., Pimentel, C., & Lane, R. C. (1999). The narcissistic injury and psychopathology of migration: The case of a Nicaraguan man. *Journal of Contemporary Psychotherapy*, *29*(3), 185–194.

Grant, B. F., Stinson, F. S., Hasin, D. S., Dawson, D. A., Chou, S. P., & Anderson, K. (2004). Immigration and lifetime prevalence of DSM-IV psychiatric disorders among Mexican Americans and non-Hispanic whites in the United States: Results from the National Epidemiologic Survey on Alcohol and Related Conditions. *Archives of General Psychiatry*, *61*, 1226–1233.

Grieco, E. (2004). *Fact sheet #8: Health insurance coverage of the foreign born in the United States: Numbers and trends*. Washington, DC: Migration Policy Institute. Last accessed February 25, 2008; Available at http://www.migrationpolicy.org/ pubs/ eight_health.pdf

Heptinstall, E., Sethna, V., & Taylor, E. (2004). PTSD and depression in refugee children: Associations with pre-migration trauma and post-migration stress. *European Child & Adolescent Psychiatry*, *13*, 373–380.

Hickling, F., & Rodgers-Johnson, P. (1995). The incidence of first contact schizophrenia in Jamaica. *British Journal of Psychiatry*, *167*, 193–196.

Hutchinson, G., & Haasen, C. (2004). Migration and schizophrenia: The challenges for European psychiatry and implications for the future. *Social Psychiatry and Psychiatric Epidemiology*, *39*, 350–357.

International Labour Office, International Organization for Migration, Office of the United Nations High Commissioner for Human Rights. (2001). *International migration, racism, discrimination, and xenophobia*. Geneva, Switzerland: Authors.

International Organisation for Migration. (2003). *World migration report*. Geneva, Switzerland: Author.

Jackson, C., Zatzick, D., Harris, R., & Gardiner, L. Loss in translation: Considering the role of interpreters and language in the psychiatric evaluation of non-English speaking patients. In S. Loue & M. Sajatovic (Eds.), *Diversity issues in the diagnosis, treatment, and research of mood disorders* (pp. 135–163). New York: Oxford University Press.

Jenkins, J. H. (1991). A state construction of affect: Political ethos and mental health among Salvadorean refugees. *Culture, Medicine, and Psychiatry*, *15*, 139–165.

Judd, L. L., Akiskal, H. S., Schettler, P. J., Endicott, J., Maser, J., Solomon, D. A., et al. (2002). The long-term natural history of the weekly symptomatic status of bipolar I disorder. *Archives of General Psychiatry*, *59*, 530–537.

Kennedy, N., Boydell, J., van Os, J., & Murray, R. M. (2004). Ethnic differences in first clinical presentation of bipolar disorder: Results from an epidemiological study. *Journal of Affective Disorders*, *83*, 161–168.

Kirov, G., & Murray, R. M. (1999). Ethnic differences in the presentation of bipolar affective disorder. *European Psychiatry*, *14*(4), 199–204.

Kuo, W. H. & Tsai, Y.-M. (1986). Social networking, hardiness, and immigrant's mental health. *Journal of Health and Social Behavior*, *27*, 133–149.

Leavey, G., Guvenir, T., Haase-Casanovas, S., & Dein, S. (2007). Finding help: Turkish-speaking refugees and migrants with a history of psychosis. *Transcultural Psychiatry*, *44*(2), 258–274.

Leavey, G., Rozmovits, L., Ryan, L., & King, M. (2007). Explanations of depression among Irish migrants in Britain. *Social Science & Medicine*, *65*, 231–244.

Lee, E. (1966). A theory of migration. *Demography*, *3*, 47–57.

Loughna S. (n.d.). What is forced migration? Forced migration online. Last accessed June 21, 2006; Available at http://www.forcedmigration.org/whatisfm.htm

Mahy, G., Mallett, R., Leff, J., & Bhugra, D. (1999). First contact of incidence of schizophrenia in Barbados. *British Journal of Psychiatry*, *175*, 28–33.

Makanjuola, R. O. A. (1982). Manic disorder in Nigerians. *British Journal of Psychiatry*, *141*, 459–463.

Makanjuola, R. O. A. (1985). Recurrent unipolar manic disorder in the Yoruba Nigerian: Further evidence. *British Journal of Psychiatry*, *147*, 434–437.

Mangalam, J. J. (1968). *Human migration: A guide to migration literature in English 1955–1962*. Lexington, Kentucky: University of Kentucky.

Médecins sans Frontières. (n.d.). Experiences of gömda in Sweden: Exclusion from health care for immigrants living without legal status. Stockholm, Sweden: Author. Last accessed February 25, 2008; Available at http://lakareutangranser.org/ files/ReportGomdaSweden En.pdf

Mollica, R., Poole, C., Son, L., Murray, C., & Tor, S. (1997). Effects of war trauma on Cambodian refugee adolescents functional health and mental health status. *Journal of the American Academy of Child and Adolescent Psychiatry*, *36*, 1098–1106.

Ödegaard, O. (1932). Emigration and insanity. *Acta Psychiatrica et Neirologica Supplementum*, *4*, 1–206.

Ortega, A. N., Rosencheck, R., Alegria, M., & Desai, R. A. (2000). Acculturation and the lifetime risk of psychiatric and substance use disorders among Hispanics. *Journal of Nervous and Mental Disease*, *188*, 728–735.

Osher, Y., Yaroslavsky, Y., el-Rom, R., & Belmaker, R. H. (2000). Predominant polarity of bipolar patients in Israel. *World Journal of Biological Psychiatry*, *1*(4), 187–189.

Personal Responsibility and Work Opportunity Reconciliation Act. Pub. L. 104-193, 110 Stat. 2105 (August 22, 1996).

Portes, A., Kyle, D., & Eaton, W. W. (1992). Mental illness and help-seeking behavior among Mariel Cuban and Haitian refugees in South Florida. *Journal of Health and Social Behavior*, *33*, 283–298.

Protocol Relating to the Status of Refugees, 606 U.N.T.S. 267 (1967), entered into force October 4, 1967.

Rogler, L. H., Cortes, D. E., & Malgady, R. G. (1991). Acculturation and mental status among Hispanics: Convergence and new directions for research. *American Psychologist*, *46*, 585–597.

Rothe, E. M., Lewis, J., Castilo-Matos, H., Martinez, O., Busquets, R., & Martinez, I. (2002). Posttraumatic stress disorder among Cuban children and adolescents after release from a refugee camp. *Psychiatric Services*, *53*(8), 970–976.

Sack, W. H., Clarke, G., & Seeley, J. (1996). Multiple forms of stress in Cambodian adolescent refugees. *Child Development*, *67*, 107–116.

Schrier, A. C., van de Weterin, B. J., Mulder, P. G., & Selten, J. P. (2001). Point prevalence of schizophrenia in immigrant groups in Rotterdam: Data from outpatient facilities. *European Psychiatry*, *16*, 162–166.

Schweitzer, R., Melville, F., Steel, Z., & Lacherez, P. (2006). Trauma, post-migration living difficulties, and social support as predictors of psychological adjustment in resettled Sudanese refugees. *Australian and New Zealand Journal of Psychiatry 40*, 179–187.

Scott, P. (2004). Undocumented migrants in Germany and Britain: The human "rights" and "wrongs" regarding access to health care. *Electronic Journal of Sociology*, ISSN 1198 3655.

Last accessed June 14, 2006; Available at http://www.sociology.org/content/2004/tier2/scott.html

Selten, J. P., Veen, N., Feller, W., Blom, J. D., Schols, D., Camoenie, W., et al. (2001). Incidence of psychotic disorders in immigrant groups to the Netherlands. *British Journal of Psychiatry, 178*, 367–372.

Silveira, E. R., & Ebrahim, S. (1998). Social determinants of psychiatric morbidity and well-being in immigrant elders and whites in East London. *International Journal of Geriatric Psychiatry, 13*, 801–812.

Steel, Z., Frommer, N., & Silove, D. (2004). Part 1–The mental health effects of migration: the law and its effects; Failing to understand: Refugee determination and the traumatized applicant. *International Journal of Law and Psychiatry, 27*, 511–528.

Steel, Z., Silove, D., Phan, T., & Bauman, A. (2002). Long-term effect of psychological trauma on the mental health of Vietnamese refugees resettled in Australia: A population-based study. *Lancet, 360*, 1056–1062.

Strakowski, S. M., Keck, P. E., Arnold, L. M., Collins, J., Wilson, R. M., Fleck, D. E., et al. (2003). Ethnicity and diagnosis in patients with affective disorders. *Journal of Clinical Psychiatry, 64*, 747–754.

Sultan, A., & O'Sullivan, K. (2001). Psychological disturbances in asylum seekers held in long term detention: A participant-observer account. *Medical Journal of Australia, 175*, 593–596.

Thompson, M., & McGorry, P. (1998). Maribyrnong detention centre Tamil survey. In D. Silove & Z. Steel (Eds.), *The mental health and well-being of on-shore asylum seekers in Australia* (pp. 27–31). Sydney, Australia: University of New South Wales.

Van Ommerren, M., de Jong, J. T. V. M., Sharma, B., Komproe, I., Thapa, S., & Cardena, E. (2001). Psychiatric disorders among tortured Bhutanese refugees in Nepal. *Archives of General Psychiatry, 58*(5), 475–482.

Van Os, J., Takei, N., Castle, D. J., Wessely, S., Der, G., MacDonald, A. M., et al. (1996). The incidence of mania: Time trends in relation to gender and ethnicity. *Social Psychiatry and Psychiatric Epidemiology, 31*(3–4), 129–136.

Vega, W. A., Kolody, B., Aguilar-Gaxiola, S., Alderete, E., Catalano, R., & Caraveo-Anduaga, J. (1998). Lifetime prevalence of DSM-III-R psychiatric disorders among urban and rural Mexican Americans in California. *Archives of General Psychiatry, 55*, 771–778.

Vergara, A. E., Miller, J. H., Martin, D. R., & Cookson, S. T. (2003). A survey of refugee health assessments in the United States. *Journal of Immigrant Health, 5*(2), 67–73.

Weine, S., Becker, D., McGlashan, T., Vojvoda, D., Hartman, S., & Robbins, J. (1995). Adolescent survivors of "ethnic cleansing": Observations on the first year in America. *Journal of the American Academy of Child and Adolescent Psychiatry, 34*, 1153–1159.

World Health Organization. (2003). *International migration, health, & human rights*. Geneva, Switzerland: Author.

Zolkowska, K., Cantor-Graae, E., & McNeil, T. F. (2001). Increased rates of psychosis among immigrants to Sweden: Is migration a risk factor for psychosis? *Psychological Medicine, 31*, 669–678.

Zwi, K. J., Herzberg, B., Dossetor, D., & Field, J. (2003). A child in detention: Dilemmas faced by health professionals. *Medical Journal of Australia, 179*, 319–322.

Chapter 5
Media, Minorities, and the Stigma of Mental Illness

Sandra S. Swantek

The media is all brainstem, hot buttons, happy endings, ultimate evil, heroes, miracle cures. Not a lot of shading here.
                    Commentator John Hockenberry, The Infinite Mind, 2003.

Media is everywhere. Television, cable, radio, internet, newspapers, magazines, film—all vie daily for your attention. If you are like the majority of Americans, your primary source of information about mental illness is from the media (Tu & Cohen, 2008). This information is often inaccurate and perpetuates harmful misconceptions about people with mental illness (Corrigan, 1998; Wahl, 1992). The mainstream media's coverage of persons of color is frequently biased and misinformed (Biagi & Kern-Foxworth, 1997). The minority person with mental illness faces the challenge of succeeding in an unwelcoming culture, while also carrying a diagnosis that marks him or her as different even within the minority community. That mark is stigma (Goffman, 1963). Many researchers agree that it is one of the most debilitating handicaps faced by persons with mental illness (Corrigan, 2005; Hinshaw 2005, 2006, 2007; Otey & Fenton, 2004; U.S. Department of Health and Human Services, 1999, 2001). Stigma refers to a cluster of negative attitudes and beliefs that motivate the public to fear, reject, avoid, and discriminate against people with mental illnesses. The President's New Freedom Commission identified stigma as the number one obstacle preventing Americans from receiving excellent mental health care (Hogan, 2003).

Negative stereotypes result in a cascade of problems for a person with mental illness, including difficulty completing educational goals, finding employment and securing housing. Even making and keeping friends may become a challenge for the person with mental illness (Corrigan, 1998).

This chapter serves as a brief introduction to a dynamic, abundantly documented, and complex topic—the depiction of mental illness in the media (Morris, 2006; Wahl, 1995; Wahl, Wood & Richards, 2002). Less copiously

S.S. Swantek (✉)
Northwestern University, Feinberg School of Medicine, Northwestern Memorial Hospital, Stone Institute of Psychiatry, Chicago, IL
e-mail: sswantek@nmh.org

S. Loue, M. Sajatovic (eds.), *Determinants of Minority Mental Health and Wellness*, DOI 10.1007/978-0-387-75659-2_5,
© Springer Science+Business Media, LLC 2009

documented is the media image of the minority person with mental illness. This chapter begins with a limited review of studies examining the portrayal of mental illness and minority persons in fictional media. We discuss the depiction of the minority person with mental illness in the news media and the efforts of advocacy groups to encourage the fair portrayal of the mentally ill person in the media. The chapter concludes with recommendations regarding future research and efforts.

For the purposes of this chapter, the term media includes any means of communication that reaches or influences people widely whether via newspaper, magazine, radio, television, film, or internet (McQuail, 2005). The subject of mental illness in literature is so broad that it is not possible to address the subject in this chapter.

Media Images of Mentally Ill Persons

Images of the mentally ill abound in the media. The rebellious free spirit, violent seductress, narcissistic parasite, mad scientist, sly manipulator, helpless and depressed female, substance abusing starlet (or star), or the odd character used for comedic relief are the media-portrayed images of mental illness.

The implication that television perpetuates the stigma attached to mental illness first emerged in 1978 with the publication of the U.S. President's Commission on Mental Health (Chu & Falkson, 1978). Media depictions of mental illness emphasizing dangerousness, criminality, and unpredictability are often vivid and anxiety provoking for the viewer. Because of this, they are memorable and likely to contribute to stigma by providing inaccurate information that reinforces cultural stereotypes of the mentally ill. One event or series of events may overshadow many positive stories and solidifies culturally held negative stereotypes (Anderson, 2003; Haghighat, 2001).

The media focus on reactions to the mentally ill emphasizes fear, rejection, and ridicule, which then seeps malignantly into the cultural consciousness and affects both mentally ill and non-mentally ill members of society. Stigma emerges, affecting the lives of both the mentally ill and their families, by causing impaired self-esteem, reduced help-seeking behaviors, decreased medication adherence, and reduced chance of recovery for persons with mental illness.

Fictional Portrayals

Dramatic fictional images of the mentally ill provide potent reinforcement of stereotypes and stigma. In the United States, one-fifth of prime time television programs depict some aspect of mental illness and portray 2–3% of the adult characters as having mental health problems (Stuart, 2003). Williams examined broadcast and print depictions of mental illness and found that characters with mental illness looked different from "normal" people (Williams & Taylor, 1995). Nunnally (1957) tested this perception by comparing psychiatrists' perceptions of the appearance and behaviors of mentally ill people with media representations. In Nunally's study, psychiatrists shown a series of photos could not distinguish mentally ill from normal individuals, suggesting that potent stereotypes do not necessarily hold true. Regardless of this finding, media often portrays mentally ill persons as acting wildly, with bizarre behaviors including mumbling, drooling, and odd body movements (Nunnally, 1957; Wahl, 1995).

In an analysis of television roles in prime time television in the United States between 1969 and 1985, Signorielli (1989) found that 72% of characters depicted as mentally ill were violent, compared to 42% of normal characters. In reality, estimates of the percentage of mentally ill persons who are violent ranges from 3% to 10% (Monahan, 1992).

Movies such as *One Flew Over the Cuckoos Nest* portrayed the oppressive nature of early psychiatric treatment and created images of treatment that, while untrue, remain ingrained in the popular consciousness even today (Anderson, 2003; Freeman, 2001). Stigmatizing portrayals of mental illness are also found in children's television and films (Lawson & Fouts, 2004; Wilson, Nairn, Coverdale, & Panapa, 2000). Whether evil or comic, animated characters stereotypically and blatantly portray mentally ill characters negatively as objects of amusement, derision, or fear (Wilson et al., 2000). Thus, early exposure to negative depictions of mental illness encourages children to incorporate stigma into their understanding of people who are "different" (Wahl, 2003).

Alternatively, television drama can be a source of inspiration and support for the mentally ill. Actor Maurice Benard was 22 when he suffered his first episode of bipolar mood disorder (manic-depressive illness). Doctors prescribed Lithium to help control his illness. Benard felt that the medication hindered his acting and so he stopped taking it. Benard says he then plunged into a dark period, rapidly started losing control, and could not distinguish what was real from what was on TV. He realized that Lithium would be an integral part of his life. Shortly after signing on to play Sonny Corinthos on "General Hospital," he suffered his third episode of mood disorder. Benard is very open about his bipolar disorder. In magazine articles, television interviews and personal appearances, he describes the difficulties he endured. He is one of the first Hollywood and Hispanic celebrities to talk publicly about his experience with bipolar disorder.

Few studies assess the potential for the media positively impacting attitudes toward mental illness and treatment. A study by Ritterfeld and Jin (2006) suggested that viewing an accurate and empathetic movie portrayal increased knowledge acquisition and viewing an educational trailer influenced stigma reduction (Ritterfeld & Jin, 2006). Russell Crowe's portrayal of Nobel Laureate

John Nash's struggle with schizophrenia in the film *A Beautiful Mind* realistically depicted schizophrenia and increased public understanding of an illness that affects 1 in 10 Americans. While there is hope that such positive media depictions of mental illness would diminish the stigma associated with mental illness, there is little evidence demonstrating long lasting change as a result (Stout, Villegas, & Jennings, 2004; Wahl, 1992).

The Internet

Increasingly, people use the internet as a source of health information. It is an ideal resource for information that offers immediacy, privacy, and convenience. An enormous amount of health information is only a mouse click away. Chat rooms allow users to ask sensitive detailed questions while maintaining anonymity and avoiding the risk of judgment or stigma. Cotten and Gupta (2004) examined the characteristics of online information seekers and discovered that minority persons are much less likely than whites to use the internet for health information. Blacks may be more concerned compared to whites regarding the trustworthiness of information on the internet. They also described greater concern about unauthorized persons gaining access to their personal data (Brodie et al., 2000).

The News Media

Much of the news content distributed via television, radio, newspapers, and the internet is about events that take place today or within the past 24 hours and is typified by a "headline" followed by a report of the newsworthy event. In television or radio, the average news report lasts 33 seconds (Pribble et al., 2006). Print media operate under less strict time constraints that allow for a somewhat lengthier examination of an event. Regardless of format, all news media have deadlines to meet and a product cycle that requires daily renewal for broadcast and newspapers and weekly renewal for newsmagazines.

Stories involving fires, natural disasters, sex, and bloody violence attract news media attention because both print and electronic news organizations are primarily profit-making businesses. Pictures sell. Stories that stir the emotions sell. In Western culture, the media uses sex to sell everything from toothpaste to automobiles. Reporters emphasize the violent, delusional, and irrational behavior of persons with mental illness while sensationalizing the story in order to attract and maintain audience attention (Corrigan et al., 2005; Coverdale, Nairn, & Claasen, 2000; Olstead, 2002; Thornton & Wahl, 1996).

Fairness, Media, and Mental Illness

In a free society, we expect the media to act in the public interest and honor basic values of accuracy, objectivity, fairness, and balance. In doing this, the media facilitates the participation of citizens in social life and assists in the expression of diverse and relevant opinions, while avoiding harmful propaganda (McQuail, 1997).

This task evolves into something much more complex when the public interest presents in the form of competing claims. For example, the story of a gunman on a college campus demonstrates the concept of competing interests. We can easily agree that the loss of dozens of lives on a college campus is a tragedy that affects many people and, thus, is newsworthy. When a person committing the crime also suffers from a mental illness, tremendous media attention focuses on the act and its tragic consequences, all the while emphasizing the person's mental illness. This intense media glare reinforces the mistaken idea that all mentally ill persons are potentially violent killers. When the 24-hour news cycle moves to the next exciting and visually dramatic story, a contributing cause of the tragedy—an overwhelmed and underfunded mental health system—remains unexamined. Left untold is the story of inadequate mental health services and the impact this has on the lives, well-being, and productivity of millions of Americans.

> Cho Seung-Hui was a student at the Virginia Technical College in Pelham, Alabama. From a young age, family, friends and teachers had identified Seung-Hui as "troubled." As a college student, a judge ordered him to attend outpatient mental health treatment. Seung-Hui attended an initial evaluation but never made a second appointment. On April 17, 2007, Seung-Hui took his gun, went out on the campus shooting and ultimately killed 32 people. He then killed himself.
>
> (The Virginia Tech Review Panel, 2007.)

News coverage focused on the deaths and the horror of the incident. Self-made video images of Seung-Hui played on network, cable, and internet sites. These frightening images literally communicated the severity of the young man's illness. News reports failed to distinguish between criminal insanity and mental illness. There was a failure of the media to emphasize the overall small contribution of mental disorders to violence in society (Satcher, 2000). The Governor of Alabama convened a panel of experts to examine the tragedy. In addition to identifying weaknesses in the state's mental health services, the report identified a misinterpretation of state and federal law that led to a lack of shared communication between schools, mental health care providers, and, ultimately, the court. Because of this, the judicial system lacked vital cumulative information and, thus, could not force an unwilling young man into treatment (The Virginia Tech Review Panel Report, 2007).

Intolerance to persons with mental illness correlates positively with the number of hours spent watching television each week (Granello & Pauley, 2000). Fictional and news programming often inaccurately depict people with

Table 5.1 Media standards

- Act in the public interest
- Respect the rights of individuals
- Publish full, fair, and reliable information
- Express diverse and relevant opinions
- Abstain from harmful propaganda
- Objectivity
- Fairness
- Balance

mental illness as "psychos, sociopaths, and killers." While the media is capable of producing educational and sensitive portrayals of both mental illness and the mentally ill, these stories are too infrequent.

Journalists work under a set of voluntary standards (Table 5.1) which include avoiding stereotyping by race, gender, age, religion, ethnicity, geography, sexual orientation, physical appearance or social status (Schwitzer, 2004; Society of Professional Journalists). In 1983, entertainment industry leaders established the Entertainment Industries Council, Inc. (EIC), to provide information of major health and social issues to the film and television producers.

Most journalists adhere to the standards, working to write accurate stories, free from bias and editorial comment unless they clearly label the work as "commentary" or "editorial." In reality, the ability of any journalist to write in a completely objective manner is questionable. The French philosopher Michael Foucault (1980) argued that truth is not a universal absolute that exists independently of historical conditions. The idea that truth is in the eye of the beholder and subject to the bias of the beholder's vision explains much of media-based stigmatization of the mentally ill.

This leads us to ask, "who is the beholder (Corrigan, 1998, 2000; Corrigan, Backs, Green, Diwan, & Penn, 2001; Corrigan et al., 2001(a); Corrigan, Markowitz, Watson, Rowan, & Kubiak, 2003)?" Are reporters able to understand the concerns of racial and ethnic minorities with mental illness? Compared to 30 years ago, today's average newsroom is much more likely to reflect racial, gender, and ethnic diversity. Minority journalists comprise 13.4% of all journalists while minorities comprise one-third of the U.S. population (Center for Integration and Improvement of Journalism, 1994; Grieco & Cassidy, 2001). Minority reporters come from the same middle-class background as the other 86.6% of journalists. Groups of colleagues tend to think and act similarly. Regardless of journalists' commitment to objectivity, they are subject to the psychological function of their own minds and by the minds of their editors, news directors, and "spinmeisters" (Myrick, 2002). Journalists may not recognize their own biases, including a lack of understanding of the issues faced by fellow ethnic and racial minorities with mental illness.

Regardless of who writes the stories, the mass media is an important source of public knowledge about health and mental illness (Brodie, Hamel, Altman,

Blendon, & Benson, 2003; Pribble et al., 2006; Wahl, 2001; Wallack & Dorf-man, 1992). Large majorities of whites, African Americans, and Latinos rely heavily on the media for information about health and health care and take personal action because of media health coverage (Brodie, Kjellsoon, Hoff, & Parker, 1999). NBC Today host Katie Couric discussed colon cancer screening on NBC's *Today Show in 2000*. Following this broadcast colonoscopies increased by 27% (Cram et al., 2003).

Simultaneously, trust of media as a health information source is moderate-to-low (Brodie et al., 1999). We know little about the media as a source of information about mental illness for Asian, American Indian, Alaskan Native, Eastern Indian, and other minority populations. The media occasionally addresses the unique concerns of minority populations. While specialized elec-tronic and print media abound in racial and ethnic communities, few studies examine the images of mental illness in these specialized communications.

The Surgeon General summarized our current understanding of African American, Asian American, Native American, and Asian Indian American cultural beliefs about mental illness (Satcher, 2001). Each group reflects the cultural beliefs of their native culture and the diversity of values and beliefs in that culture. There may not even be a word for mental illness in the indigenous languages of some of these groups. As a result, a minority person with mental illness must confront both the stigma of minority status, as well as the stigma of mental illness in ethnic communities that may consider mental illness, "bad" or "evil." The Asian Indian American will not view mental illness in the same way as someone of Pakistani descent. The black community includes the descen-dents of slaves, as well as recent immigrants from Jamaica, Haiti, and Kenya. Perceptions of mental illness vary in each of these communities.

The absence of content analysis studies of images of the mentally ill person in the ethnic media leads us to examine existing studies of black and Latino attitudes toward the media. African Americans and Latinos believe that the general media speaks primarily to a white audience while ignoring health problems affecting minorities. A majority of African Americans and Latinos use ethnic media for health information (Brodie et al., 1999). African Amer-icans think the black media is more sensitive to their concerns and do a better job covering the health problems of African Americans (Sylvester, 1993; Krish-nan, Durrah & Winkler, 1997). In spite of this, African Americans and Latinos use general market media outlets more frequently than minority-oriented media sources. Thus, minority media are an important but less frequently used source of health information.

Nicholson, Grason, and Powe (2003) studied the impact of race on women's use of health information resources via health organizations, print, broadcast, and internet media. They found black women less likely to seek health information through health organizations, print news, or internet compared to white women.

Both print and broadcast media are less attentive to diseases that burden blacks more than whites. A 2006 study concluded that who dies, as well as how many die, are critical factors in determining what diseases receive mass media attention. This study did not address mental illness in the black population. However, the authors noted that diseases disproportionately affecting blacks, such as stroke and diabetes, received less media attention, and thus study participants perceived these diseases as less serious (Armstrong, Carpenter, & Hojnacki, 2006).

The black media differ from mainstream media in that there is limited coverage of health behaviors posing risk to the African American population such as diabetes, cardiovascular disease, or cancer. Mainstream media reporting on the black community tended to focus less on these widespread public health issues and more on AIDS and infant mortality (Amzel & Ghosh, 2007; Hoffman-Goetz, Gerlack, Marino, & Mills, 1997).

Making Change

There is limited research focusing on strategies for changing mental illness stigma. Corrigan and Penn (1999) identified three approaches to changing stigma: **protest, education,** and **contact.** The media potentially plays a role in each strategy.

Protest strategies publicly confront stigma and draw attention to injustice while providing education about the reality of mental illness. The National Stigma Clearinghouse identifies and protests negative media images of mental illness while promoting accurate portrayals of mental illness. The National Alliance for the Mentally Ill (NAMI) engages its members in monitoring television, film, and other media for degrading images of mental illness that they actively challenge. NAMI "Stigmabusters" played a significant role in the 2000 cancellation of the ABC program "Wonderland." In the program's first episode, a person with mental illness shot several police officers and stabbed a pregnant psychiatrist in the abdomen with a hypodermic needle. NAMI joined with a coalition of mental health organizations appealing to the producers, network management, and commercial sponsors. The network canceled the program.

Even if the result of protest is the removal of just one stigmatizing program, protest efforts empower organizations and members while, if only briefly, raising the consciousness of media, advertisers, and consumers. These active efforts that rectify inaccurate portrayals of mental illness are vital to destigmatization efforts.

Even as mental health advocates criticize the media for fostering stigma and discrimination, the media can be an ally in educating the public by challenging prejudice, initiating public discussion, and projecting positive stories about people living with mental illness (Stuart, 2003) *(Sidebar B)*.

Educational campaigns use the media to provide public education to targeted groups with the goal of dispelling stigma (Watson & Corrigan, 2005). The Substance Abuse and Mental Health Services Administration (SAMHSA) launched the Campaign for Mental Health Recovery in 2008 to encourage, educate, and inspire people between the ages of 18 and 25 to support their friends experiencing mental health problems. The campaign utilizes the internet, radio, and television. The American Psychiatric Association (APA) in 2006 launched a public awareness campaign, "Healthy Minds, Healthy Lives" which reaches out to members of racial and ethnic minorities. This campaign includes nationally broadcast interviews with psychiatrists, public service advertisements on radio and television, and a web site (American Psychiatric Association, 2008). The World Psychiatric Association acts as a global watchdog for persons with mental illness, alerting the media when global attention may contribute to improvement.

The National Mental Health Awareness Campaign is a nationwide nonpartisan public education campaign, launched as part of the 1999 White House Conference on Mental Health. It encourages people to identify, discuss, and seek help for mental health problems and create a more accepting environment for them to do so. The campaign sponsors a bureau of individuals with mental illness who publicly speak about their illness.

Contact with a person with mental illness may be more successful in changing stigma than other approaches (Corrigan et al., 2001(b)). Before speaking openly, the mentally ill person must first overcome self-stigma and concerns that others will consider them weak, dangerous, unemployable, or unworthy for promotion if their illness is known. Celebrities openly discussing mental illness increase public awareness and make it easier for others to talk about their own mental illness. When Yankees third baseman Alex Rodriquez acknowledged that he was in psychotherapy, he admitted that he was initially reluctant to enter therapy because, "in many ways therapy is synonymous with a bad thing." He also called therapy "an incredible thing" that helped him discover a different life (Associated Press, 2005).

Author and motivational speaker, Terrie Williams, admits that it was difficult for her to talk about her depression. She describes her journey in her book, *Black Pain*. Reflecting on hip-hop music, she proposes a direct connection between depression and the pain reflected in hip-hop. She states,

> *It is especially troublesome that the only examples of how Black people rise above hardship come from highly paid performers—athletes, singers, and rappers. And it pains me that so many of these images rest on violence, the putting down of women and the promotion of expensive things as sexy*

(Williams, 2008, p. 166).

Recommendations

Encouraging realistic depictions of minorities with mental illness in the media is a complicated task. It requires research, improved training for journalists, and those involved in program development, coalition building between advocacy groups, active protest of unfair images, and education for media consumers starting at the preschool age. Perhaps most important is support and encouragement for those individuals who courageously choose to speak about their mental illness to their families, friends, and the media.

Researchers cataloguing media representations of mental illness establish clear evidence of the perpetuation of negative stereotypes of persons with mental illness. We know little about the depiction of mental illness in the media specifically produced for the minority viewer or the impact of these images on the ethnic or racial minority person with mental illness. Much more is known about the attitudes of racial and ethnic minorities toward mental illness.

There is continued need for targeted media communication and education reflecting different cultural ideas about mental illness and health in a manner that respects cultural diversity, while encouraging acceptance and support of persons with mental illness. Preliminary evidence suggests that these programs can diminish stigmatizing attitudes (Corrigan & Gelb, 2006). Studies measuring message effectiveness must accompany these efforts for the purpose of message refinement. Public relations and marketing professionals are experts at message placement across multiple forms of media. Their involvement in the development and implementation of communication campaigns would add much to the success of these efforts (Sullivan, Hamilton, & Allen, 2005).

Informed journalists influence our understanding of mental health issues. Their work stimulates discussion amongst the public that can reduce stigma and discrimination. Aside from college-level psychology courses and courses on science writing, reporters generally have little training in the complexities of the mental health system, the people it affects, or the unique set of laws that make up the mental health code in each state. They are ill-equipped to cover the complex story of mental illness. This is likely why so much of the news coverage is relegated to the sensational and dramatic aspects of mental illness. Improved training would help reporters broaden their understanding of mental illness. They would learn that the story of mental illness is not just one person, but rather many people, families, friends, communities, advocates, and treatment providers confronting mental illness and stigma, while promoting the dignity and self-respect of the mentally ill person. The Rosalynn Carter Fellowships for Mental Health Journalism gives journalists this specialized training. It is a rare opportunity few practicing journalists access.

Summary

Stigma hurts. It leads to discrimination, exclusion, and injustice.

Members of a racial or ethnic minority with mental illness confront double stigma. The media contributes to this stigma by communicating negative portrayals of the person with mental illness. These portrayals reinforce existing cultural stereotypes of race, ethnicity, and mental illness and are contrary to the communication industry's own code of ethics. They persist because intensely dramatic and visual stories attract viewers, while it is difficult for a stigmatized minority to rise up and demand change. Through the efforts of courageous citizens and advocacy groups, the media is becoming more aware and willing to communicate a more positive image of the mentally ill person. There is much work to be done.

Acknowledgments The author wishes to gratefully acknowledge the invaluable comments and suggestions of Patrick W. Corrigan, Psy.D., Molly Mulligan, M.D., Deirdre Tannen, Psy.D., and Kenneth Stefancich. in the preparation of this chapter.

Side Bar A: Education on the Internet

Sam Harris's Story

"At the age of 14, I started having serious hallucinations and blackouts. I'm half African American and half Native American, and I didn't try to get help because, in both communities, they called that 'going to the white man.' But I became an outcast, because my symptoms got so bad that none of my friends wanted to have anything to do with me.

Instead, I lived with these symptoms for 4 years. My mental illness got so bad that I couldn't cope with school and they asked me to leave. I went to Miami to live with my father, but he threw me out, and from the age of 15 until I was 18 I lived on the streets of Miami, with constant hallucinations and delusions.

At 19, I joined the military. But I was still sick and, after basic training, they gave me an honorable discharge and directed me to get mental health treatment, so I did. After taking medication and seeing therapists, I went back to work two years later, as a cook. Four years after that, I got an associate's degree from the Restaurant School of Philadelphia and became a chef.

I worked as a chef for about 15 years. But there was a lot of stigma around mental illness in the restaurant business. Every restaurant I worked at, I saw other people disclose about themselves and they wound up being badly harassed and losing their jobs. So I hid my illness.

In 1995, I started working part time for the Chester City Consumer Center. After attending the Center for 6 months, I asked the director if there were openings, and she said she had wanted to hire me for the past 6 months. I'm still at the Center, now as its director, and it will be 10 years in November. Working with the Mental Health Association of Southeastern Pennsylvania, which is out there advocating for consumers, has helped me. Until I started working here, I felt like no one really cared."

(SAMHSA)

Side Bar B: Television Portrayal

During the CNN program House Call with Dr. Sanjay Gupta, correspondent Elizabeth Cohen presented a story demonstrating the potential of television as a tool for education.

Cohen spoke with Shawn Nguyen about her depression. "I fell in a very, very, deep black hole." Admitting or even talking about depression is taboo in many Asian cultures. Nguyen fled her home in Vietnam after the fall of Saigon. At age 19, she led a group of 20 refugees from Vietnam to the Philippines to Guam and finally to a camp in Arkansas. "It was very traumatizing," she recalls. Nguyen became a successful financial planner but left everything behind when she says she had to flee again, this time from her marriage. A diagnosis of colon cancer and then a heart attack further added to her stress. Her community expected her to be stoic. "In Asia, you know, any time we talk about depression, it's a sign of weakness. Weaknesses should be well hidden, you know, behind closed doors," Nguyen stated. In the Asian culture, asking for counseling is shameful for the person and their entire family.

"There were times when I came very close to taking my life one way or another. There is a tiny, little voice at the end that said, no, you remember, you've been taught that you can't do that. That's not the way out," (Holmes, Gupta, & Cohen, 2007).

References

American Psychiatric Association. (2008). Healthy minds. Healthy lives. Retrieved May 23, 2008; Available at http://www.healthyminds.org/.

Amzel, A., & Ghosh, C. (2007). National newspaper coverage of minority health disparities. *Journal of the National Medical Association, 10,* 1120–1125.

Anderson, M. (2003). One flew over the psychiatric unit: Mental illness and the media. *Journal of Psychiatric Mental Health Nursing, 10,* 297–306.

Armstrong, E. M., Carpenter, D. P., & Hojnacki, M. (2006). Whose deaths matter? Mortality, advocacy, and attention to disease in the mass media. *Journal of Health Politics, Policy and Law, 31,* 729–772.

Associated Press. (2005). *A-Rod: Therapy Helps Avoid 'Train Wreck.'* Last accessed May 23, 2008; Available at MSNBC, http://nbcsports.msnbc.com/id/7978062/.

Biagi, S., & Kern-Foxworth, M. (1997). *Facing difference: Race, gender and mass media.* Thousand Oaks, CA: Pine Forge Press.

Brodie, M., Flournoy, R. E., Altman, D. E., Blendon, R. J., Benson, J. M., & Rosenbaum, M. D. (2000). Health information, the internet, and the digital divide. *Health Affairs, 19,* 255–265.

Brodie, M., Hamel, E. C., Altman, D. E., Blendon, R. J., & Benson, J. M. (2003). Health news and the American public, 1996–2002. *Journal of Health, Politics, Policy and Law, 28,* 927–950.

Brodie, M., Kjellsoon, N., Hoff, T., & Parker, M. (1999). Perceptions of Latinos, African Americans, and Whites on media as a health information source. *Howard Journal of Communications, 10,* 147–167. http://www.informaworld.com/smpp/title~content= t713771688~db=all~tab=issueslist~branches=10 - v10.

Center for Integration and Improvement of Journalism. (1994). *News Watch: A critical look at coverage of people of color.* San Francisco, CA: San Francisco State University.

Chu, F. D., & Falkson, J. L. (1978). The President's Commission on Mental Health. *Journal of Health, Politics, Policy & Law, 3,* 141–144.

Corrigan, P. W. (1998). The impact of stigma on severe mental illness. *Cognitive and Behavioral Practice, 5,* 201–222.

Corrigan, P. W. (2000). Mental health stigma as social attribution: Implications for research methods and attitude change. *Clinical Psychology: Science and Practice, 7*, 48–67.

Corrigan, P. W. (Ed.). (2005). *On the stigma of mental illness: Practical strategies for research and social change* (pp. 239–256). Washington, DC: American Psychological Association.

Corrigan, P.W., Treen, A., Lundin, R., Kubiak, M.A. & Penn, D. (2001a). Familiarity with and social distance from people with serious mental illness. *Psychiatric Services, 52*, 953–958.

Corrigan, P., Backs, A., Green, A., Diwan, S., & Penn, D. (2001b). Prejudice, social distance and familiarity with mental illness. *Psychiatric Service, 27*, 219–226.

Corrigan, P., & Gelb, B. (2006). Three programs that use mass approaches to challenge the stigma of mental illness. *Psychiatric Services, 57*, 393–398.

Corrigan, P., Markowitz, F. E., Watson, A., Rowan, D., & Kubiak, M. A. (2003). An attribution model of public discrimination towards persons with mental illness. *Journal of Health and Social Behavior, 44*, 1–69.

Corrigan, P. W. & Penn, D. L. (1999). Lessons from social psychology on discrediting psychiatric stigma. *American Psychologist, 54*, 765–776.

Corrigan, P. W., River, L., Lundin, R. K., Penn, D. L., Upoff-Wasowski, K., Campion, J., et al. (2002). Three strategies for changing attributions about severe mental illness. *Schizophrenia Bulletin, 27*, 187–197.

Corrigan, P. W., Watson, A. C., Gracia, G., Slopen, N., Rasinski, K., & Hall, L. L. (2005). Newspaper stories as measures of Structural Stigma. *Psychiatric Services, 56*, 551–556.

Cotten, S. R., & Gupta, S. S. (2004). Characteristics of online and offline health information seekers and factors that discriminate between them. *Social Science & Medicine, 59*, 1795–1806.

Coverdale, J., Nairn, R., & Claasen, D. (2000). A legal opinion's consequences for the stigmatization of the mentally ill: Case analysis. *Psychiatry Psychology Law, 7*, 192–197.

Cram, P., Fendrick, A. M., Inadomi, J., Cowen, M. E., Carpenter, D., & Vijan, S. (2003). The impact of a celebrity promotional campaign on the use of colon cancer screening: The Katie Couric effect. *Archives of Internal Medicine, 163*, 1601–1605.

Entertainment Industries Council, Inc. Last accessed May 23, 2008; Available at http://www.eiconline.org.

Foucault, M. (1980). *Power/knowledge: Selected interviews and other writings, 1972–1977*. New York: Pantheon Books.

Freeman, H. (2001). Commentary. *Current Opinion in Psychiatry, 14*, 529–530.

Goffman, E. (1963). *Stigma: Notes on management of spoiled identity*. Harmondsworth: Penguin.

Granello, D. H., & Pauley, P. S. (2000). Television viewing habits and their relationship to tolerance toward people with mental illness. *Journal of Mental Health Counselling, 22*, 162–175.

Grieco, E. M., & Cassidy, R. C. (2001). *U.S. Census Bureau overview of race and Hispanic origin; Census 2000*. Washington, DC: United States Census Bureau.

Haghighat, R. (2001). A unitary theory of stigmatisation. *British Journal of Psychiatry, 177*, 207–215.

Hinshaw, S. P. (2005). The stigmatization of mental illness in children and parents: Developmental issues, family concerns, and research needs. *Journal of Child Psychology and Psychiatry, 46*, 714–734.

Hinshaw, S. P. (2006). Stigma and mental illness: Developmental issues. In D. Cichetti & D. Cohen (Eds.), *Developmental psychopatholgy: Vol. 3. Risk and adaptation* (2nd ed., pp. 841–881). New York: Wiley.

Hinshaw, S. P. (Ed.). (2007). *The mark of shame* (pp. 117–120). New York: Oxford University Press.

Hockenberry, J. (2003). Mental health and the media. In "The Infinite Mind," National Public Radio. Last accessed February 25, 2008; Available at http://www.lcmedia.com/mind279.htm.

Hoffman-Goetz, L., Gerlack, K., Marino, C., & Mills, S. (1997). Cancer coverage and tobacco advertising in African-American women's popular magazines. *Journal of Community Health, 22*, 261–270.

Hogan, M. F. (2003). New Freedom Commission Report: *The President's New Freedom Commission*: Recommendations to transform mental health care in America. *Psychiatric Services, 54*, 1467–1474.

Holmes, T. J., Gupta, S., & Cohen, E. (2007). Hiding the shame of mental illness. [Cable television series episode]. In, House Call with Dr. Sanjay Gupta. Atlanta: Cable News Network (CNN). Last accessed May 23, 2008; Available at http://transcripts.cnn.com/TRANSCRIPTS/0705/12/hcsg.01.html.

Krishnan, S. P., Durrah, T., & Winkler, K. (1997). Coverage of AIDS in popular African-American magazines. *Health Communication, 9*, 273–288.

Lawson, A., & Fouts, G. (2004). Mental illness in Disney animated films. *Canadian Journal of Psychiatry, 49*, 310–314.

McQuail, D. (1997). Accountability of media to society: Principles and means. *European Journal of Communication, 12*, 511–529.

McQuail, D. (2005). *McQuail's mass communication theory*. Thousand Oaks, CA: Sage.

Monahan, J. (1992). Mental disorder and violent behavior: Perceptions and evidence. *American Psychologist, 47*, 511–521.

Morris, G. (2006). *Mental health issues and the media*. New York: Routledge.

Myrick, H. (2002). The search for objectivity in journalism. USA Today. November, 2002. Last accessed May 23, 2008; Available at http://findarticles.com/p/articles/mi_m1272/is_2690_131/ai_94384327

National Alliance for the Mentally Ill. (March 30, 2000). Last accessed May 19, 2008; Available at http://www.nami.org/Content/ContentGroups/Press_Room1/20001/March_2000/Wonderland_Premiere_Brings_Call_On_White_House_To_Fight_Stigma_In_Entertainment_Industry.htm

Nicholson, W. K., Grason, H. A., & Powe, N. R. (2003). The relationship of race to women's use of health information resources. *American Journal of Obstetrics and Gynecology, 188*, 580–585.

Nunnally, J. (1957). The communication of mental health information: A comparison of the opinions of experts and the public with mass media presentations. *Behavioral Science, 2*, 222–230.

Olstead, R. (2002). Contesting the text: Canadian media depictions of the conflation of mental illness and criminality. *Sociology of Health and Illness, 24*, 621–643.

Otey, E., & Fenton, W. S. (2004). Editors' introduction: Building mental illness stigma research. *Schizophrenia Bulletin, 30*, 473–475.

President's New Freedom Commission. (2003). *Final report: Achieving the Promise: Transforming Mental Health Care in America*. Last accessed May 23, 2008; Available at http://www.mentalhealthcommission.gov/

Pribble, J. M., Goldstein, K. M., Fowler, E. F., Greenberg, M. J., Neol, S. K., & Howell, J. D. (2006). Medical news for the public to use? What's on local TV news. *American Journal of Managed Care, 12*, 170–176.

Ritterfeld, U., & Jin, S. A. (2006). Addressing media stigma for people experiencing mental illness using an entertainment-education strategy. *Journal of Health Psychology, 11*(2), 247–267.

Satcher, D. (2000). Executive summary: A report of the Surgeon General on mental health. *Public Health Reports, 115*, 89–101.

Satcher, D. (2001). *Mental health: Culture, race, and ethnicity: A supplement to mental health: A report of the Surgeon General*. Rockville, MD: U.S. Department of Health and Human Services, Substance Abuse and Mental Health Services Administration, Center for Mental Health Services, National Institute of Mental Health. Last accessed May 23, 2008; Available at http://mentalhealth.samhsa.gov/cre/toc.asp.

Schwitzer, G. (2004). A statement of principles for health care journalists. *American Journal of Bioethics, 4*, W9–W13.

Signorielli, N. (1989). The stigma of mental illness on television. *Journal of Broadcasting & Electronic Media, 33*, 325–331.

Society of Professional Journalists. *Code of Ethics*. Last accessed May 22, 2008; Available at http://www.spj.org/ethicscode.asp.

Stout, P., Villegas, J., & Jennings, N. A. (2004). Images of mental illness in the media: Identifying gaps in the research. *Schizophrenia Bulletin, 30*, 543–561.

Stuart, H. (2003). Stigma and the daily news: Evaluation of a newspaper intervention. *Canadian Journal of Psychiatry, 48*, 651–656.

Substance Abuse and Mental Health Services Administration. *What a difference a friend makes. Mental Health Campaign for Mental Health Recovery*. Last accessed May 23, 2008; Available at http://www.whatadifference.samhsa.gov.

Sullivan, M., Hamilton, T., & Allen, A. (2005). Changing stigma through the media. In P. W. Corrigan (Ed.), *On the stigma of mental illness: Practical strategies for research and social change* (pp. 297–312). Washington DC: American Psychological Association.

Sylvester, J. (1993). Media research bureau Black newspaper readership report. In F. Black (Ed.), *Milestones in black newspaper research* (pp. 11–13, 56–81). Washington, DC: National Newspaper Publishers Association.

Thornton, J. A., & Wahl, O. F. (1996). Impact of a newspaper article on attitudes toward mental illness. *Journal of Community Psychology, 24*, 17–25.

Tu, H.T., Cohen, G.R. Striking jump in consumers seeking health care information. Center for Studying Health System Change. August, 2008. Last accessed September 28, 2008. Available at www.rwjf.org/files/research/3431.3374.pdf.

U.S. Department of Health and Human Services. (1999). *Mental health: A report of the Surgeon General*. Rockville, MD: Author.

U.S. Department of Health and Human Services. (2001). *Mental health: Culture, race, and ethnicity, a supplement to mental health: A report of the Surgeon General*. Rockville, MD: Author.

Virginia Tech Review Panel. (2007). *The Virginia Tech review panel report*. Last accessed May 22, 2008; Available at http://www.vtreviewpanel.org/report/index.html accessed 5/19/2008.

Wahl, O. F. (1992). Mass media images of mental illness: A review of the literature. *Journal of Community Psychology, 20*, 343–352.

Wahl, O. F. 1995. *Media madness*. New Brunswick, NJ: Rutgers University Press.

Wahl, O. F. (2001). Mass media and psychiatry. *Current Opinion in Psychiatry, 14*, 530–531.

Wahl, O. F. (2003). Depictions of mental illnesses in children's media. *Journal of Mental Health, 12*, 249–258.

Wahl, O. F., Wood, A., & Richards, R. (2002). Newspaper coverage of mental illness: Is it changing? *American Journal of Psychiatric Rehabilitation, 6*, 9–31.

Wallack, L., & Dorfman, L. 1992. Television news, hegemony, and health. *American Journal of Public Health, 82*, 125–126.

Watson, A. C., & Corrigan, P. W. (2005). In P. W. Corrigan (Ed.), *On the stigma of mental illness: Practical strategies for research and social change* (pp. 289–290). Washington, DC: American Psychological Association.

Williams, M., & Taylor, J. (1995). Mental illness: Media perpetuation of stigma. *Contemporary Nurse, 4*, 41–46.

Williams, T. (2008). *Black pain*. New York: Scribner.

Wilson, C., Nairn, R., Coverdale, J., & Panapa, A. (2000). How mental illness is portrayed in children's television: A prospective study. *British Journal of Psychiatry, 176*, 440–443.

Chapter 6
Minority Mental Health and Wellness: A Perspective from Health Care Systems

Siran M. Koroukian

Disparities in the use of mental health services and outcomes by ethnic and/or minority status have been well documented. Recent efforts by health care systems in developed countries have aimed at enhancing cultural and linguistic competence to better address the mental health needs of growing ethnic and minority populations. This chapter presents a brief overview of the disparities in mental health service use; describes a framework discussing barriers to access and utilize mental health services in this population; and presents the recommendations offered by the Office of Minority Health with respect to the provision of culturally and linguistically sensitive health services, as it discusses their relevance in addressing each of the barriers.

Introduction

In the past several decades, developed countries witnessed a great influx of immigrants, creating a significant level of diversity in the population and an increasing representation of ethnic and minority individuals. According to Passel and Cohn of the Pew Research Center (2008), the total population in the United States is projected to grow from 296 million in year 2005 to 438 million in 2050, and the representation of non-Hispanic Whites is expected to decrease from 67% to 47%. Conversely, the representation of Hispanic/Latino and that of Asians and Pacific Islanders is expected to grow during that time period from nearly 14% to 29%, and from 5% to 9%, respectively. During that time period, the proportion of African Americans is expected to remain relatively stable at 13%. Data from the above-referenced source indicate that the 117 million people added during the 45-year period are represented by immigrants themselves and their U.S.-born children or grandchildren (67 million and

S.M. Koroukian (✉)
Case Western Reserve University, School of Medicine, Cleveland, OH
e-mail: skoroukian@case.edu

S. Loue, M. Sajatovic (eds.), *Determinants of Minority Mental Health and Wellness*, DOI 10.1007/978-0-387-75659-2_6,
© Springer Science+Business Media, LLC 2009

50 million individuals, respectively). In 2050, 19% of the U.S. population will be immigrants. This compares to 12% in 2005.

In this chapter, we use the term "minority" to refer not only to racial and ethnic minorities but also to gender and religious minorities. In gender minorities, including lesbian, gay, bisexual, and transgender (LGBT) individuals, the risk of mental illness is considerably higher than in the heterosexual population, due to the psychosocial stressors in their everyday life that are associated with anti-LGBT sentiments. Religious minorities include – among others – Muslims, who have been facing increased discrimination since the events of September 11, 2001, and individuals of the Older Order of the Amish, facing the difficulties of a sequestered lifestyle.

Addressing the mental health care needs of minority groups warrants changes at least at three levels. First, at the patient-provider level, the therapist needs to tailor the treatment in a culturally and linguistically competent manner. As noted by Hinton, Pich, and Pollack (2005, p. 59), "In designing the treatment for a particular cultural group, one must initially identify the main patterns of distress. One should then ascertain how that stress is generated in order to be able to design effective and culturally sensitive treatments." Therefore, a provider who is not aware of the sources generating distress in a patient will not be able to treat him/her effectively. The key is for the provider to be able to recognize the fact that the sources of distress will vary considerably across patients. To name a few, sources of distress include mistrust grown from decades of slavery and being disenfranchised among African Americans; a heightened level of discrimination at the workplace and elsewhere encountered on a day-to-day basis by individuals belonging to sexual minorities; and economic hardship, fragmentation of family support and social networks, and feelings of isolation experienced by immigrants. It is also extremely important for the provider to be cognizant of the variations by which distress will manifest itself in subgroups of minorities and of their help-seeking behaviors. For example, somatization will be an important sign of distress in Asian Americans and war refugees; and to seek help for mental distress, members of religious subgroups, such as the Amish or Muslims may resort to counseling by their clergy or Imams.

Next, at the organizational level, striving to adapt to the paradigm to deliver culturally and linguistically sensitive services will warrant important changes at the management level. As discussed below through the recommendations made by the Department of Health and Human Services, Office of Minority Health, this requires that organizations assess and gain a thorough understanding of the mental health needs of the communities that they serve; that they establish the necessary dialogue with community representatives; that they ensure the availability of providers that are prepared to deliver culturally and linguistically competent services; that they inform the community of the availability of culturally and linguistically sensitive services; and they continuously evaluate the services they provide.

Last, but not least, structural factors, including insurance coverage and lack thereof and fragmentation of care, constitute a major impediment to access mental health services. Inadequate health insurance coverage is generally associated with lower socioeconomic status, further complicating issues of access to such services.

As the former U.S. Surgeon General David Satcher noted in his report on mental health (2001), "Just as disparities are a cause of public concern, so is our diversity a national asset." However, much remains to be addressed in how minority groups' mental health care needs are addressed. As detailed below, disparities by minority status in how mental illness is diagnosed and treated are widespread and call for prompt action on behalf of the provider community.

Disparities in the Use of Mental Health Services and Outcomes

The Institute of Medicine (IOM) Report on disparities (2003, pp. 3–4) defines disparities as "racial or ethnic differences in the quality of healthcare that are not due to access-related factors or clinical needs, preferences, and appropriateness of intervention." The IOM report (2003, p. 4) focuses on the operation of health systems and discrimination at the individual, patient-provider level. Discrimination in that report refers to "differences in care that result from biases, prejudices, stereotyping, and uncertainty in clinical communication and decision-making."

There is a rich body of literature documenting the presence of ethnic and racial disparities in a wide range of illnesses. Disparities are manifested through the *underuse* of certain treatments and procedures, as is the case, for example, with cancer screening (Cooper & Koroukian, 2004), curative services (Cooper, Yuan, Landefeld, & Rimm, 1996), and use of analgesics (Bernabei et al., 1998). It is also demonstrated through the *overuse* of certain treatments and procedures, as in the case of bilateral orchiectomy and amputation in African Americans (Gornick et al., 1996). Some studies have shown that disparities are attenuated or even disappear when controlling for socioeconomic and insurance status, while others have demonstrated that disparities persist after accounting for such factors.

With regard to disparities in the use of mental health services, the Surgeon General's supplemental report *Mental Health: A Report of the Surgeon General* (1999, p. 3), summarizes disparities as follows: "Racial and ethnic minorities have less access to mental health services than do Whites. They are less likely to receive needed care. When they receive care, it is more likely to be poor in quality."

Sources of Disparities

The IOM report (2003) describes sources of disparities at three levels. First, at the patient level, disparities may exist because of patient preferences, treatment refusal, and clinical appropriateness of care. For example, some studies have documented greater rates of treatment refusal in minority patients than in their nonminority counterparts, possibly because of long-standing mistrust vis-à-vis the provider community, or because of prior negative experience with the health care system. However, differences in refusal rates have failed to account for the observed disparities. With respect to variations in clinical appropriateness of care, recent studies in ethnopharmacology have attempted to address differences in response to therapeutic agents across racial and ethnic groups, likely due to differences in "the distribution of polymorphic traits between population groups... rather than a trait unique to a particular racial or ethnic group" (Wood, 2001, p. 1394; article cited in the IOM Report, 2003). However, given that most studies document disparities in health services and interventions that are equally effective across all population groups, biological differences across ethnic and racial groups are unlikely to explain the observed disparities in care (IOM Report, 2003).

The second source of disparities relates to health-care systems, and the way by which they are organized and financed. Lack of adequate insurance presents one of the most important barriers to access mental health services. Additionally, health-care organizations' lack of or limited ability to provide adequate translation services constitutes an important impediment to nearly 14 million Americans with limited English proficiency to access health services. Similarly, time pressures on health care providers may impose another layer of difficulty in patient-provider communications, especially when cultural and language barriers are already present (IOM Report, 2003).

The third source of disparities refers to the role of bias and stereotyping in the actual process of delivering care. Provider prejudice or bias, or "an unjustified negative attitude based on a person's group membership" (Dovidio, Brigham, Johnson, & Gaertner, 1996, cited by the IOM Report, 2003, p. 10), manifesting itself in providers in various ways, has been shown to be associated with diagnostic and treatment decisions. In one experimental study, conscious and nonconscious African American stereotype-laden words were found to have a negative influence on a therapist's first impressions of a hypothetical patient whose race was not identified (Abreu, 1999, cited by the IOM Report, 2003). In turn, minority patients' negative impressions contribute to a greater level of mistrust, poor adherence, and refusal of treatment. Such reactions create and perpetuate a vicious circle, whereby providers become less engaged in the treatment process, and minority patients are less likely to receive the care they need.

Evidence of disparities in mental health care is shown through differentials in a number of measures, including prevalence rates of mental illnesses; rates of utilization of certain types of services, such as inpatient versus outpatient services and pharmacotherapy; and through the way by which they are treated.

Differentials in Prevalence Rates

Assessment of needs for mental health services is generally equated with prevalence (Surgeon General's Report (Supplement), 2001; Vega & Lopez, 2001).

In other words, we estimate the level of need for mental health services based on the rate of prevalence of mental health problems in a given community. However, there are important measurement issues that affect our assessment of prevalence and need. As a result, the true magnitude of unmet needs and disparities across subgroups of the population will always be difficult to quantify.

Undertreatment and underutilization of mental health services are often used as a proxy for the *true* prevalence rate of mental disorders. However, equating rates of undertreatment/underutilization with true prevalence rates poses major limitations. Undertreatment/underutilization result from a complex set of factors, including – but not encompassing – recognition of behaviors as part of a mental disorder, help-seeking behavior, and overcoming various barriers to access and utilize mental health services; however, these factors are not considered in assessing utilization. As a result, a number of individuals from a given community may not be identified as users of mental health services, when they actually need these services. In this case, the prevalence rate, reflected through the rate of undertreatment/underutilization, may be lower than the *true* prevalence rate in that community. Alternatively, members of another community may seek mental health services for relatively minor mental symptoms and experience little or no barriers in accessing and utilizing mental health services. Here, the prevalence rate obtained from the treatment/utilization rate may be higher than the *true* prevalence rate.

Even well-conducted household surveys may present deficiencies. In African American communities, for example, estimates of *true* prevalence may be artificially low, because such surveys fail to account for the homeless, those who are incarcerated, and those who are institutionalized (Snowden, 2001). In Hispanic communities, the magnitude of mental health problems may be severely underestimated, as many of the federal surveys are likely to miss potential respondents because they are not conducted in Spanish (Vega & Lopez, 2001).

Examining the distribution of mental health problems in various subgroups of the population has been problematic, with certain studies indicating greater prevalence of mental disorders in a given ethnic population compared to other ethnic populations, and other studies suggesting the opposite. Inconsistencies across studies may be attributed to differences in the methods employed to gather prevalence data, as discussed above, as well as measurement errors, sample size differences between large- and small-scale studies, and enumeration of symptoms versus symptom clusters. In particular, measurement errors may result from psychological instruments as well. Some items of a psychological instrument may be misunderstood and/or distorted because of the subject's educational attainment, and some behaviors may be perceived as pathological in one culture but not in another. Another reason may be a possible bias in the extent to which respondents are overcompliant in their answers or provide answers with varying degrees of social desirability (Rogler, Malgady, & Rodriguez, 1989).

Disparities in the Use of Mental Health Services

Because most studies are conducted in reliance on the definition of racial categories by the U.S. Census groups, the brief review of the literature on disparities in the use of mental health services is, accordingly, presented below. Such overgeneralizations are likely to lead to stereotyping, and as such, it is important to emphasize that these groups are far from being homogeneous (Atdjian & Vega, 2005), as noted below. For example, important within-group differences by country of origin exist both among Hispanics and Asian Americans. These differences are not shaped only by language, but also by geopolitical forces that prompted immigration from their country of origin to the United States (Vega & Lopez, 2001).

African Americans

Underutilization of mental health services by African Americans has been discussed in the context of misunderstanding and mistrust of health care providers (Suite, La Bril, Primm, & Harrison-Ross, 2007). Disparities in mental health care are evidenced by the overrepresentation of African Americans in inpatient settings and among those seeking psychiatric emergency care, as well their lower likelihood to receive outpatient mental health services (Lasser, Himmelstein, Woolhandler, McCromick, & Bor, 2002), or specialty mental health care (Alegria et al., 2002). Receipt of services in outpatient settings is an important measure because failure to receive such services early in episodes of mental illness is associated with greater use of inpatient care and longer lengths of stay (Chow, Jaffee, & Snowden, 2003). However, as with other minority groups, the increased likelihood relative to Whites to utilize inpatient services was held true only for those residing in low-poverty areas. Also, once they initiate care, African Americans have been found to be more likely to terminate it prematurely (Sue, Zane, & Young, 1994).

African Americans – especially younger men – are more likely to be coercively placed into mental health facilities compared to members of other groups (Takeuchi & Cheung, 1998). Additionally, as evidenced in a study by Chow et al. (2003), African Americans are more likely than Whites to be referred to mental health services through social service agencies. This finding held true both in high- and low-poverty areas. For African Americans residing in low-poverty areas, the likelihood of referral to mental health services through the criminal justice system was 4 times greater than that of Whites.

In African Americans and Hispanics alike, low income has been shown to be associated with a lower likelihood to visit a mental health professional (Dobalian & Rivers, 2008). For example, results from the National Comorbidity Study indicated that only 16% of African Americans saw a mental health specialist, and less than one in three consulted any kind of provider (Kessler et al., 1994).

African Americans rely heavily on public safety net programs. The gap between African Americans and Whites in utilization of outpatient mental health services narrows in community-based and in public programs such as Medicaid and widens in privately financed programs, be it fee-for-service or managed care (Snowden & Thomas, 2000) – a finding that implies that socioeconomic status alone cannot explain African Americans' underrepresentation in outpatient settings.

Hispanics '

Hispanics, many of whom are foreign-born, have lower income and educational attainment than Whites. Important differences that may exist in the demographic and social/political factors across Latino subgroups likely affect their mental health care access.

Lower utilization of mental health services in the Hispanic community is likely associated with low rates of health insurance coverage, as it is the case for many immigrant communities. Persistent low socioeconomic status, low educational attainment, and stagnation in the income level from the second to the third generation, as evidenced by the unchanged median income (U.S. Census Bureau, 1998, cited by Vega & Lopez, 2001), further contributes to the problem of limited health care access (Vega & Lopez, 2001). Because of fear of detection, the status of undocumented immigrants is a particularly important impeding factor relative to seeking health services. For example, given the lower proportions of immigrants among Cubans, they are more likely to be eligible for Medicare and Medicaid than are Mexicans or other immigrants from Central America (Vega & Lopez, 2001) and, therefore, have greater access to mental health services.

Hispanics are also more likely to be uninsured or enrolled in the Medicaid program. If insured, they have less mental health coverage than Whites and are less likely to be enrolled in managed care programs (McGuire, Alegria, Cook, Wells, & Zaslavsky, 2006). Yet, even after adjusting for insurance status, some of the factors that were identified as important indicators to access mental health specialty care were perceived need and decisions to seek care (Kimerling & Baumrind, 2005). In a study of managed care enrollees with regular source of care, rates of depression care and quality of care were lower in Latinos than in their White counterparts (Lagomasino et al., 2005), suggesting that other patient and/or provider attributes may be responsible for disparities. As such, Latinos were less than half as likely to report receiving any depression care, or care that met guideline criteria, and rates of care did not vary with the ethnic composition of the clinic patient population.

Hispanics are more likely than their White counterparts to be diagnosed with major depression (Minsky, Vega, Miskimen, Gara, & Escobar, 2003) but less likely to be diagnosed with schizophrenia (Chow et al., 2003). Those residing in low-poverty areas are more likely than Whites to be referred to mental health services through the criminal justice system. Similarly, their likelihood relative to Whites to utilize inpatient and emergency services is greater among those residing in low-poverty areas but lower among those residing in high-poverty areas (Chow et al., 2003). Differences in access to specialty mental health care between Hispanics and non-Hispanics persist after adjusting for socioeconomic status. Alegria et al. (2002) have identified at least five factors contributing to the lower rates of use of specialty services by Hispanics, including language fluency, the culture of self-reliance and mechanisms of coping with mental disorders, access to Medicaid specialty services in Hispanic neighborhoods, differences in recognition of mental health problems, and previous experience with low-quality of mental health care.

Temporal trends in disparities are not reassuring. Findings from a recent study indicate that mental health care disparities between Hispanics and non-Hispanics increased during the period from 1993 through 2002, as measured through the rate of diagnosis, type of mental health visit, type of treatment received, rate of psychotropic medications prescription, and specialty of the treating physician (Blanco et al., 2007). Similarly, widening Hispanic-White disparities in total mental health expenditures between 2000 and 2001 and 2003 and 2004 have been documented (Cook, McGuire, & Miranda, 2007).

Asian Americans/Pacific Islanders (AA/PI)

Asian Americans/Pacific Islanders (AA/PIs), the fastest-growing minority group in the United States, comprise individuals originating from 43 different ethnic subgroups, speaking over 100 languages and dialects (Surgeon General's Report (Supplement), 2001). Asian Americans are three times as likely as Whites to be diagnosed with schizophrenia (Chow et al., 2003).

Although AA/PIs are not overrepresented among the homeless, the incarcerated, or those who experience problems of substance abuse, they are overrepresented in the refugee population. Most such refugees, especially survivors of Pol Pot's concentration camps, have experienced posttraumatic stress disorder (PTSD), and many continue to suffer from depression several years after leaving Cambodia (Surgeon General's Report (Supplement), 2001).

Relative to their representation in the population, use of inpatient services by AA/PIs has been documented to be low. Use of outpatient services has been shown to have great variability across the different subgroups, with Japanese and Chinese Americans utilizing less outpatient care than expected, and Filipino Americans using these services at expected rates (Surgeon General's Report (Supplement), 2001). Use of emergency services has been reported to be at higher rates than Whites (Chow et al., 2003).

A number of factors pose barriers to accessing mental health services. In addition to limited English proficiency, it has been asserted that AA/PIs share a belief that mental health can be achieved through willpower and, because emotional and behavioral problems are a source of shame and stigma, they should remain within the family (Herrick & Brown, 1998). Of note is that AA/PIs are likely to express their mental distress in somatic symptoms. As a result, mental health conditions may be undetected, if the provider relies solely on Western diagnostic categories (Surgeon General's Report (Supplement), 2001). These factors, combined with high rates of uninsurance in certain subgroups, lower than expected rates of enrollment in Medicaid even among those residing in high poverty areas possibly because of immigrant status, mistrust of the system, and limited availability of culturally sensitive mental health services, contribute to delay of treatment until they are very ill.

American Indians and Alaska Natives (AI/AN)

American Indians and Alaska Natives (AI/AN) represent less than 1.5% of the U.S. population, and many live in rural isolation and experience economic hardship. Nearly 4 in 10 reside in rural areas, and 14% of adults are unemployed. According to a report by the Indian Health System, the rate of suicide in the 15–24 age group is nearly three times that in their nonnative counterparts. In addition, AI/AN adolescents have higher rates of depression, drug and alcohol use, delinquency, and out-of-home placements than their nonnative counterparts (Indian Health Services, 2001; Yates, 1987; cited by Johnson & Cameron, 2001).

Studies of AI/ANs' use of mental health services are few and yield inconsistent results as to the rates of use of different types of services. For example, while some studies have found higher rates of admission to state and county hospitals compared to Whites, others have suggested that AI/ANs' use of inpatient care is comparable to that of the general population (Surgeon General's Report (Supplement), 2001). Same inconsistencies across studies were found relative to their use of outpatient services.

Findings from an analysis of the Behavioral Risk Factor Surveillance System (BRFSS) by the Centers for Disease Control and Prevention (2004) indicated that frequent mental distress was most commonly reported by AI/ANs (14.4% unadjusted and 11.4% multivariable-adjusted), followed by non-Hispanics of "Other" race (12.9% unadjusted, and 12.3% multivariable-adjusted). Individuals of "Other" race, possibly of multiple race/ethnicity, are those who did not identify as one of the predefined race/ethnicity categories of the U.S. Census. In the 2002 National Survey on Drug Use and Health, rates of mental health treatment were found to be the highest among AN/AIs and those reporting more than one race (Barker et al., 2004). Interestingly, however, persons of these two racial categories reported the highest rates of unmet need for mental health treatment (Barker et al., 2004).

An important factor in AI/ANs' help-seeking behavior is their belief that culturally traditional practices, including seeking advice from family members and elders or care from traditional healers, would be more effective than professional services rendered on- or off-reservation (Walls, Johnson, Whitbeck, & Hoyt, 2006). Walls et al. (2006) also demonstrated that the use of informal traditional services was associated with *enculturation*, a construct that reflects the extent to which an individual participates in traditional activities, identifies with the American Indian culture, and practices traditional spirituality. Additionally, they showed that higher rates of perceived discrimination would be associated with preferences for informal or traditional care. However, those who lived off-reservation were more likely to use formal services.

Reliance on and presence of traditional care reflects a system parallel to the one providing formal care by clinicians. The integration of these two systems remains a challenge, as clinicians develop the sensitivity to demonstrate their respect for traditional healers and offer to consult them if their patient gives permission, and as policy makers consider issues of whether and how to reimburse for services provided by traditional healers (Walls et al., 2006).

Disparities in Pharmacotherapy

Disparities have been noted in antipsychotic prescription patterns and medication use, even among publicly insured patients (Kuno & Rothbard, 2002; Opolka, Rascati, Brown, Barner, et al., 2003), as well as in medication adherence (Opolka, Rascati, Brown, & Gibson, 2003). Other studies have suggested, however, that treatment disparities lie mainly in the rates of initiation of treatment, as is the case in the treatment of depression, and that rates of adequate treatment do not differ across sociodemographic groups once treatment was initiated (Harman, Edlund, & Fortney, 2004). It has also been shown that a greater representation of African Americans and Hispanic patients in substance abuse treatment centers is negatively associated with the availability of serotonin reuptake inhibitors (Knudsen, Ducharme, & Roman, 2007).

Disparities have also been noted in the receipt of newer antipsychotics that have fewer side effects (Opolka et al., 2004; Herbeck et al., 2004). Side effects may contribute to lower rates of adherence and to more frequent use of emergency department visits and psychiatric hospitalizations (Herbeck et al., 2004). In addition to side effects, a number of patient-related factors may contribute to low levels of adherence to medications. In a group of patients with bipolar disorders, for example, African American patients reported non-adherence to medications because of fear of addiction or because the medications were symbols of mental illness (Fleck, Keck, Corey, & Strakowski, 2005).

Findings from a temporal study have shown positive trends relative to narrowing, or even closing gaps in receipt of prescriptions for atypical antipsychotics that offer the advantage of fewer adverse effects compared with traditional antipsychotics. In examining data from the National Ambulatory Medical Care Survey and National Hospital Ambulatory Medical Care Survey, Daumit et al. (2003) showed that while African American and Hispanic patients had significantly lower odds than Whites of receiving a prescription for an atypical antipsychotic in the early 1990s, that disparity became smaller and the adjusted odds approached that of Whites by the late 1990s. However, disparities relative to Whites persisted for African Americans with the diagnosis of psychotic disorders, although it was smaller than that observed in earlier years. This trend was observed in parallel with a more widespread use of such therapies during the decade.

Additional Factors Hindering Access to Mental Health Services

Lack of Insurance and Unavailability of Providers

Adequate insurance coverage is considered one of the most important factors associated with seeking and utilizing mental health services. Unfortunately, most insurance programs providing coverage for medical conditions do not provide comparable coverage for behavioral problems, and the Bill on Mental Health Parity passed recently by the House of Representatives requires that coverage for treatment of mental and physical illnesses be comparable (Pear, 2008). Even with universal health care coverage in Canada, however, those with higher socioeconomic status are more likely than those with lower socioeconomic status to receive psychiatric care (Steele, Glazier, & Lin, 2006).

Community factors, including the availability of mental health services and specialists in a geographic area (Ronzio, Guagliardo, & Persaud, 2006), as well as HMO penetration have been found to be associated with use of alcohol, drug, and mental health services. However, while residence in areas with higher HMO penetration is associated with a greater likelihood to use such services in individuals with Medicare, Medicaid, or private managed care, it is associated with lower likelihood to use such services in individuals with other or no insurance plan (Stockdale et al., 2007).

Geographic location and residence in low-poverty neighborhoods have been found to be associated with the use of emergency and inpatient mental health services and coercive referrals as well (Chow et al., 2003). Compared with their urban counterparts, residents of rural areas experience greater psychiatric disease burden (Wallace, Weeks, Wang, Lee, & Kazis, 2006), a lower likelihood to receive any specialized mental health treatment (Hauenstein et al., 2007), and considerable unmet needs for mental health services (Hauenstein et al., 2006).

Limited English Proficiency (LEP)

LEP has been implicated in ethnic disparities, although results from various studies have been mixed. While a few studies have shown favorable access outcomes among patients with LEP, compared with their non-LEP counterparts (Gilmer et al., 2007; Marshall et al., 2006), the presumed association between LEP and compromised access to mental health services has been evidenced elsewhere by the lower use of mental health care among Hispanic and Asian/Pacific Islander LEP patients than among their English-speaking counterparts (Sentell, Shumway, & Snowden, 2007).

Mechanisms by which language use contributes to disparities are not well elucidated. Further, it is unclear whether LEP is the critical measure for access barriers, or a proxy for a number of variables that may not have been measured

– or measured well – in the numerous studies on LEP and access to care. For example, the effects of language proficiency have not been completely disentangled from that of acculturation, which plays a particularly important role relative to definitions of mental illness, stigma, and perceptions of mental health care (Sentell et al., 2007). Also, compared to the use of general health care services, which is also associated with LEP (Cheng, Chen, & Cunningham, 2007), use of mental health services is likely to be particularly affected by LEP, because mental health diagnosis and treatment rely heavily on communication. Thus, linguistic barriers diminish a patient's likelihood to participate in psychotherapy or to use specialist mental health services (Stuart, Minas, Klimidis, & O'Connell, 1996).

Social Support

Family involvement and social support play an important role in helping individuals develop mechanisms to cope with adversity (Surgeon General's Report (Supplement), 2001). A number of family- and social/community-level factors have been identified as risk factors for mental health problems. At the family level, these factors include severe marital discord, socio-economic disadvantage, history of criminality in the father, and mental disorders in the mother (Surgeon General's Report (Supplement) 2001). In the case of a child, many of these factors are also associated with foster care, which may impact his/her mental wellness. At the social/community level, the Surgeon's General report (2001) lists among risk factors violence, poverty, lack of adequate schools, and racism/discrimination.

There are a number of individual-level traits that are protective against mental illness. Resilience has been identified as one of the most important factors to cope with adversity, whether in minority groups, or among immigrants. Spirituality and religion have been implicated in improved self-perception and life satisfaction, although the findings from relevant research have not been consistent across studies (Surgeon General's Report (Supplement), 2001). Even as the mechanisms by which spirituality and religion may affect health are not well elucidated, the support gained from the community of individuals who share similar religious and spiritual traditions such as church groups likely contributes to mental wellness. In addition, as noted elsewhere in this chapter, when facing mental health problems, guidance and counseling are sometimes sought from spiritual leaders such as the Priest, Minister, or Bishop in the case of Christians, the Imam in the case of Muslims, or the traditional healer in the case of Native Americans. Depending on the individual's preferences, the role of such leaders should be acknowledged and accorded its proper place in therapy.

The extent to which faith-based social groups and spiritual leaders are relied upon likely varies not only across individuals but also across minority and ethnic groups. In the case of African Americans, for example, it is believed that social support and coping assistance obtained from their church and "voluntary support networks" consisting of family and friends counterbalance the effects of high levels of stress that African Americans experience on a daily basis (Snowden, 1998). However, contrary to the general belief, when troubled by mental health problems, African Americans are less likely than Whites to seek help from family and friends and from religious figures (Snowden, 1998). Additionally, when they do seek help from their voluntary support networks, they do so in conjunction with – but not as a substitute for – professional mental health programs. Families, friends, and religious figures may act as facilitators for help-seeking, by directing the person to seek professional help or are turned to after having an emotional problem clarified through professional intervention (Snowden, 1998).

Barriers to Providing Effective Mental Health Services for Racial and Ethnic Minority Groups in the Context of Research Framework

To better understand the barriers faced by minority patients, we refer to the framework proposed by Rogler et al. (1989). Although these barriers were described in the context of Hispanic patients, they are likely generalizable to most minority groups, given the many parameters that are in common across these groups. Most notable of these parameters are the mistrust vis-à-vis the health care system; the bias, prejudice, and stereotyping that providers exhibit when caring for these patients; and the type of mental stressors, such as discrimination, that they encounter on a day-to-day basis. Additional variables, including limited English proficiency, come into play for ethnic minority groups as well. These barriers are presented in a temporal sequence, as follows.

Emergence of Mental Health Problems in the Community (Cultural Variations in the Conceptions of Normality and Mental Illness)

How a person reacts to the mental stressors depends not only on one's personality and family/social support but also on cultural factors and teachings of what the norms are in that particular minority group relative to various behaviors and the individual's ability to cope with stress. In other words, whether a certain behavior is indeed considered as a mental disorder will depend on community-specific norms.

Well known in cross-cultural psychiatry is the inconsistent relationship between professional and lay conceptualizations of mental illness (Heurtin-Roberts, Snowden, & Miller, 1997), which vary widely across minority groups. Consequently, certain behaviors that may be considered as outside the norm by some communities, may be viewed as well within the norms by others. For example, African Americans tend to express their anxiety in somatic terms (Heurtin-Robers et al., 1997), rather than as symptoms that may be recognized by others as that of mental illness; the Amish demonstrate a greater level of tolerance than others for certain sexual behaviors during the adolescent period (Cates, 2005); homosexuality may be perceived as pathological by members of some communities but not by others. Since many of the epidemiological studies aimed at measuring the prevalence of mental disorders rely on self-reported data, the lay conceptualization of mental illness will undoubtedly contribute to the assessment of mental illness-related community burden.

Help-Seeking Behavior or Mental Health Service Utilization, Which Is Dependent on Individual's Conception of Normality

Lay conceptualization of mental illness will, in great part, dictate whether and when an individual might seek mental health care. Considerations include cultural factors and strategies to cope with stress; the family and social support structure and the individual's reliance on it; the degree of assimilation by minorities or acculturation by immigrants to the dominant culture; knowledge of mental health resources; and ability to access those services through insurance coverage

Wide variations in lay conceptualization of mental illness and help-seeking behaviors exist across subgroups of broadly defined categories of minority populations, and overgeneralization of some of the observations may lead to stereotyping. Bearing these variations in mind, following are a few examples of help-seeking behaviors: Studies suggest that in subgroups of Asian Americans, behaviors may be perceived as signs of mental illness only if they are psychotic, disruptive, or dangerous. Therefore, the tendency is not to seek care for personal problems or distress (Leong & Lau, 2001), since the culture views persons as hardy if they are in control of their lives and if they have the ability to welcome change as an exciting challenge (Kuo & Tsai, 1986, cited in Rogler et al., 1989). Help-seeking behavior in some communities is further hindered by feelings of shame and stigmatization. It is believed that such ailments can and should be remedied by willpower. Further, because symptoms are somaticized and because of the belief that mental disorders are linked to organic factors, help is sought from general medical professionals or alternative healers, rather than mental health providers (Leong & Lau, 2001). African Americans, on the other hand, tend to turn to informal help from family and friends and prefer indirect assistance, general encouragement, and prayers (Snowden, 2001). Similarly, LGBT individuals may choose to seek help through informal networks within their community due to fear of encountering anti-LGBT bias (Willging, Salvador, & Kano, 2006). Muslims often resort to their Imams for their counseling needs, although the extent to which Imams are equipped to offer adequate help to address mental disorders is unknown (Ali, Milstein, & Marzuk, 2005).

Previous negative experiences with the health care system are likely to greatly influence future help-seeking behaviors. Institutional barriers to utilize mental health services have also been identified. The lack of mental health professionals who are Spanish-speaking or who have an understanding of "folk beliefs" have been noted by Hispanics as one such barrier (Rogler et al., 1989). Differences in socioeconomic status between lower-class patients and higher-class mental health professionals may also pose a major barrier, even if the patient and mental health professional belong to the same minority or ethnic group.

Trust is an additional important element that needs to be taken into account when considering help-seeking behaviors. For example, because of injustices committed toward their ancestors and sometimes persisting discrimination, African Americans and Indian Americans tend to deny mental health problems and/or mistrust the good that may be offered by the dominant culture (Johnson & Cameron, 2001; Snowden, 2001).

Additional barriers that have been identified among immigrants in Canada include a perceived overwillingness of physicians to rely on prescription drugs as interventions; perceived dismissive attitude and lack of time from physicians in previous encounters; and a belief in the curative ability of nonmedical factors, including God and folk medicine (Whitley, Kirmayer, & Groleau, 2006).

Diagnosis and Evaluation of Mental Health – Cultural Biases and Misdiagnoses

Leong and Lau (2001) have identified five factors that can pose a threat to the cultural validity of psychological instruments used in assessing mental health: therapist bias in cultural judgment, inappropriate use of diagnostic and personality tests, cultural factors influencing symptom expression, language capability of the client, and pathoplasticity of psychological disorders. Most psychological tests have been standardized to nonminority, English-speaking individuals. Confounding this problem is that of the *category fallacy*, or the "unwarranted assumption that psychiatric categories and disorders have the same meaning when carried over to a new cultural context" (Kleinman, 1977, 1987, cited in Kirmayer, 2006, p. 129).

Two issues can arise when administering standardized tests to minority individuals and immigrants. The first originates from language proficiency, issues of translation, and equivalence in semantics (Leong & Lau, 2001). The other arises from differences in cultural backgrounds, since these tests typically involve a comparison of the behavior of the examinee with that of others from the normative group.

From a clinician's perspective, the greater the divergence of these behaviors from what she/he considers normal, the more pathologically the examinee is judged. *Over*diagnosis can happen when a clinician incorrectly judges normal variations in beliefs, behaviors, and experience that may be specific to the examinee's culture (Leong & Lau, 2001). Examples include hearing or seeing a deceased person during the bereavement period among subgroups of Asian

Americans that are interpreted as hallucinations, or symptoms of psychotic disorder; or the practice of spiritualism by Puerto Ricans, which believes in the existence of an invisible world of spirits that may influence human lives (Rogler & Hollingshead, 1985, cited in Rogler et al., 1989). Conversely, *under*diagnosis occurs when the clinician mistakenly attributes psychiatric symptoms to cultural differences (Leong & Lau, 2001).

Even outside the context of standardized tests, interviewing patients in their nonnative language may present the danger of misdiagnosis. This phenomenon was documented nearly 40 years ago in an article describing cases in which Hispanic patients showed psychotic symptoms when they were interviewed in their native language, but not when they were interviewed in their second language (Del Castillo, 1970, cited in Rogler et al., 1989).

Receipt of Psychotherapeutic Services

There is ongoing debate about whether and how culturally sensitive psychotherapeutic services bridge differences between the patient's native culture and that of the majority (Rogler et al., 1989). This debate has been motivated by minority patients' early attrition from therapy and the ineffectiveness of traditional treatment modalities. The relevant research attempts to identify the combination of several elements yielding the best outcome possible in a given patient, including the type of therapy, provider, and set of circumstances in which therapy is delivered (Paul, 1967, cited in Rogler et al., 1989).

Early attrition has been associated with a number of factors, including low acculturation, low socioeconomic status, and negative attitudes toward therapists, and the benefits of therapy. With respect to racial and ethnic matching of client and therapist, research has yielded inconsistent results concerning therapeutic outcomes. For example, a study by Sue, Fujino, Hu, Takeuchi, and Zane (1991) demonstrated that racial and ethnic therapy-client matching in Asian American patients was associated with increased mental health services utilization, as well as length and outcome of treatment, while another study by Ying and Hu (1994) failed to show the presence of association between such matching and increased mental health services utilization. From mental health clinicians' perspective, ethnic matching between clinician and patient was perceived to be difficult to implement in a highly integrated patient population (Ton, Koike, Hales, Johnson, & Hilty, 2005).

At a practical level, culturally sensitive care may be viewed as individualized care. The patient's level of acculturation should be assessed along a continuum, and cultural sensitivity in counseling should be pegged to the degree of the individual's commitment to and identification with his/her own culture versus that of the majority (Ruis & Casas, 1981, cited in Rogler et al., 1989). Kreisman (1975, cited in Rogler et al., 1989) has advocated the approach of incorporating the patient's cultural conception of his/her illness into the treatment. In doing so, the therapist should not abandon or compromise his/her own purpose of therapy (Rogler et al., 1989). Some have even supported the notion that the therapist should change culturally prescribed behavior. For example, by training Mexican American women to be more assertive, Boulette targeted the culturally prevalent behavior of submissiveness to overcome the related symptoms of somatic complaints, depression, and anxiety (Boulette, 1976, cited in Rogler et al., 1989).

Posttreatment Adjustment of the Individual and Return to the Community

There are two major points to consider in posttreatment adjustment, which is particularly difficult in individuals with severe mental illness: (a) reintegration into the family and community and (b) use of posttreatment services. The movement of deinstitutionalization has brought a series of challenges relative to posttreatment adjustment, in that patients are discharged from the hospital to a "non-system community aftercare" (Bessuk and Gerson, 1978, cited in Rogler et al., 1989, p. 120) The inadequacy of this community aftercare implies that the families would assume the responsibility of providing custodial care to these patients (Rogler et al., 1989).

Outcome studies, which are almost nonexistent in some groups like the Native Americans (Johnson & Cameron, 2001), are based on the criteria of employment and rehospitalization (Rogler et al., 1989). Employment status has been used as a proxy measure for "wellness" and reflective of at least a minimal level of functioning. Hospital readmissions, occurring frequently in patients with severe mental illness, have been interpreted as indicators of the individual's difficulties to adjust to the family and community lives. However, this may not always hold true, as difficulties in adjustment could also result from dysfunction in the family as well. Of note is that posttreatment care is often maintenance-oriented, rather than rehabilitation-oriented, as it fails to provide the kind of social and/or vocational training needed by patients with severe mental illness to reduce dependence and increase functioning (Rogler et al., 1989).

Previous studies have indicated that the percentage of patients returning to live with their families is rather small. Many become homeless or find different kinds of living arrangement, including boarding houses and nursing homes (Pepper & Ryglewicz, 1982, cited in Rogler et al., 1989). An important predictor of outcomes is the patient's socioeconomic status. High educational and occupational attainment, as well as good employment and marital status in the period preceding hospitalization, are also associated with favorable post-discharge outcomes. These findings, documented as early as five decades ago (Zigler & Phillips, 1960, cited in Rogler et al., 1989), are likely to be observed at varying degrees among various minority groups. In particular, isolation from family and friends and other supportive networks, which is also associated with unfavorable posttreatment outcomes, is likely to occur in individuals experiencing migrations and stresses of acculturation (Hammer, 1981, cited in Rogler et al., 1989).

Rogler et al. (1989) correctly point out that factors predicting posttreatment care utilization are often the same as the determinants of help-seeking behavior by psychologically distressed individuals. These factors include various barriers, including mistrust and sometimes lack of mental health providers, who can provide culturally and linguistically appropriate services.

Cultural Competence in the Delivery of Mental Health Services

The level of cultural diversity in our societies today calls for the need to develop culturally and linguistically appropriate services (CLAS). Although there is a dearth of empirical studies documenting the evidence that such services are indeed beneficial, CLAS are believed to have the potential to greatly improve health outcomes, patient satisfaction, as well as the efficiency and the cost-effectiveness of health services (Puebla Fortier, Convissor, & Pacheco, 1999).

Cultural and linguistic competence is defined as the "ability by health care providers and health care organizations to understand and respond effectively to the cultural and linguistic needs brought by patients to the health care encounter" (Puebla Fortier et al., 1999, p. 6).

As noted above, rather than relying on assumptions relative to the cultural and linguistic needs of the individual that are generally based on somewhat artificial categories of race and ethnicity defined by the U.S. Census, the approach discussed here emphasizes the extent to which an individual identifies himself/herself with his/her own culture versus that of the majority. The individual- versus racial/ethnic category-based approach in mental illness diagnosis and treatment constitutes a crucial step away from stereotyping.

Despite all the attention given to the notion of CLAS, there is a lack of comprehensive standards of cultural and linguistic competence in the delivery of health care services at the national level (Puebla Fortier et al., 1999). As a result, there is wide variation in the way in which various organizations have incorporated cultural and linguistic competence in their services. Some have limited their scope of cultural competence to linguistic competence. Others have focused on collecting data on the patient's race, ethnicity, and language (Puebla Fortier et al., 1999). These data, which were nearly nonexistent in the past, are currently gathered by health care systems that serve highly diverse patient populations. Despite the idiosyncrasies and variations in data-collection efforts, these data will help identify the cultural and linguistic needs of patients and, thus, likely shape the delivery of health services in future years.

Of note is the greater emphasis in these efforts on linguistic, rather than cultural competence (Puebla Fortier et al., 1999). This emphasis is driven by two factors. First, as noted above, there is no universal definition of cultural competence. Rather, it is broadly referred to in such terms as cultural awareness and cultural sensitivity. Additionally, much of the language in the existing literature is definitional and details on implementation are sorely lacking.

Second, the emphasis on linguistic competence is driven by the Federal requirement to provide interpreter services and translated written materials, as discussed below. The assessment of linguistically competent services usually involves easily attainable data, such as the number of translators, the existence of translated materials, and the number of patients with limited English proficiency.

In this section, the recommendations by Puebla Fortier et al. (1999) to the Office of Minority Health (OMH), U.S. Department of Health and Human Services, with regard to the provision of CLAS are reviewed in the context of the framework by Rogler, Malgady, and Rodriguez presented above. The discussion below focuses on how a given recommendation may help address one or more barriers described by Rogler, Malgady, and Rodriguez. These recommendations, which are presented below in broad thematic areas, were made to the OMH based on the review of a number of pertinent documents, including the Consumer Bill of Rights, the standards of the Joint Commission of Accreditation of Health Organizations, and the Health and Human Services Office for Civil Rights 1998 guidance.

Education of Mental Health Providers

Education on cultural competence should ideally be integrated in the earliest phases of health professionals' training to demonstrate that cultural competency is "foundational for practice" (Gabard, 2007, p. 166). Such education is best delivered in the presence of a diverse student body and exposure to a "critical mass of minorities" (Gabard, 2007, p. 166).

A number of relevant programs in various institutions, such as the cross-cultural nursing track at the University of Washington-Seattle, have been in existence for several decades (Puebla Fortier et al., 1999). However, not every health professional or administrator has received training in cultural competence. In fact, as reported in one study from England, "no attention was given in their initial education to the health care needs of minority ethnic groups" (Chevannes, 2002, p. 290), and many of the study participants reported engaging in self-initiated learning to improve their knowledge and understanding of minority health care needs.

Such foundation being absent in earlier phases of professional training, health care organizations should ensure that mental health providers are educated on normative and help-seeking behaviors of ethnic and other minorities, especially of the population residing in their service area. Such education should be provided on an ongoing basis, and the information gained incorporated into the providers' day-to-day interactions with the patient population.

A number of issues concerning education on cultural competence have yet to be addressed. Because of the lack of a universal definition of, and a standard curriculum to teach, cultural competence, educational materials on cultural competence are likely to vary widely across trainers (Puebla Fortier et al., 1999). Trainers themselves vary in the training they have received to educate others on cultural competence. Some may have experience in diversity training or even formal, doctoral-level training, while others may have no formal training in the subject matter at all. Often, such training is likely to provide a general overview of cultural competence in health services delivery and focus on the health beliefs, attitudes, and behaviors of specific ethnic subgroups (Puebla Fortier et al., 1999).

While it is important for health care providers to gain relevant knowledge about specific ethnic groups at a general level, this approach is likely to create stereotypes in caregivers' minds. A more important goal that should be achieved in staff training is to help caregivers understand the equivalence between individualized and culturally competent care. As noted above, cultural sensitivity in mental health care should be pegged to the patient's level of acculturation and to his/her level of cultural and linguistic needs.

Such education will help mental health providers to be cognizant of variations in mental illness presentation across minority subgroups, such as somatization, as well as variations in patients' and their families' beliefs about mental illness and therapeutic approach. In Asian American communities, for example, a discussion on biological etiology of mental illness could trigger shame and anxiety relative to the "marriageability" of the patient's offspring, and learning that mental illness would require lifelong pharmacotherapy could surprise or disappoint them (Ito & Maramba, 2002). In one study, therapists addressed the patients' and families' resistance to the mental illness label by changing "their professional diagnosis into that of a more social or practical problem that clients and families can accept and work toward some alleviation of the distress with the potential to return to school, work, or better social relationships" (Ito & Maramba, 2002, p. 46).

Knowledge about such perceptions and the therapist's willingness to accommodate patients' and families' beliefs about mental illness and the therapeutic process by making adjustments in their therapeutic approaches are essential components of culturally sensitive mental health care. This would help to address the barriers related to the diagnosis of mental illness, psychotherapeutic services, and return of the patient to the community. As for the emergence of mental health symptoms and help-seeking behavior, these barriers are addressed over longer periods of time, when the staff, along with the organization of which they are a part, are able to establish trust and dialogue with the community.

Comprehensive Management Strategy

Because linguistically and culturally sensitive services are most successful when they are not delivered on an ad hoc basis, the recommendations to the OMH call for a structured approach to diversity management, including the development of written policies and procedures and the designation of an administrative body responsible for cultural competence (Puebla Fortier et al., 1999).

Organizations can implement a number of effective strategies to address various barriers and to provide an environment that is inviting to minority subgroups. In addition to staff education, such strategies include language education, recruitment and retention of staff from the minority community, and establishing a dialogue with the members of the community that they serve. An example is how a clinic in Los Angeles providing mental health services to a predominantly Asian American community has addressed stigma by giving itself the ambiguous name of *Asian Pacific Family Clinic (APFC)* (Ito & Maramba, 2002). Since the clinic's name does not include any reference to mental health care, members of the community feel less inhibited to seek services there. Similarly, APFC, which served members of an Asian American community, employed staff who shared the same countries of origin and spoke the same language as that of the patients. In addition, to inspire an ambiance of cultural familiarity, APFC was decorated with pictures from various Asian countries (Ito & Maramba, 2002), and receptionists often knew the clients by their name and greeted them in their own home language. This contributed to the more informal, personal environment in which care is provided. More interestingly, some clients were hired to do clerical work on a part-time basis, so they were both clients and staff.

The culturally congruent match between client and therapist is likely to address the problem of overdiagnosis or underdiagnosis of mental disorders, at least partially. Furthermore, steps such as the ones described above have the potential to break barriers hindering help-seeking behaviors, receipt of psychotherapeutic services, and return to the community. In particular, the informal and personalized approach to communicate with patients is likely to increase patient retention and decrease discontinuation of care.

As the organization becomes better connected with and more attuned to the linguistic and cultural needs of the community, it will also become increasingly aware of how the community perceives and deals with psychiatric symptoms. In turn, this will help to develop and/or improve relevant educational and outreach programs.

Establishing connection with the community requires that issues of mistrust and imbalance of power and authority in the patient-provider relationship be addressed. Shared decision making involves trust and mutual respect, and engagement in a dialogue on values and preferences (Briss et al., 2004, cited by Allen, Kennedy, Wilson-Grover, & Gilligan, 2007). It can be achieved through provider education on communication and cultural competence, as well as the recruitment, training, and retention of providers from the same minority group as the patient population being served, discussed below in greater detail. These suggestions, which were made by African American men in the context of informed decision making for prostate cancer screening and treatment (Allen et al., 2007), are also relevant to mental health care, as is the emphasis on patient empowerment.

Consumer Representation and Empowerment

Consumer involvement is key to opening and maintaining a dialogue between health care organizations and the communities that they serve. Although such a dialogue may invite criticism and sometimes unachievable demands from the community, it is the only means by which the organization can gain in-depth understanding of the culture and make the necessary adjustments to the services that it provides.

At the individual level, collaborative relationship with the provider is important for effective treatment (Alegria et al., 2008), and consumer empowerment is an essential component of psychiatric rehabilitation and for the development of a positive sense of self and control over one's life and destiny. It encourages individuals to actively participate in the management of psychiatric symptoms and therapeutic decisions (Stromwall & Hurdle, 2003). An additional factor that enhances collaboration with health care providers is patient activation, consisting of developing the ability to formulate questions and to build information-seeking skills (Alegria et al., 2008). It is believed that increased activation and empowerment may prevent minority patients from prematurely terminating mental health treatment when such treatment does not fulfill expectations (Alegria et al., 2008).

Participation in peer support programs is another program believed to be associated with better community adjustment (Yanos, Primavera, & Knight, 2001), as well as with enhanced empowerment, albeit in small measures (Corrigan, 2006). Peer support, rendered in the form of consumer-operated services, fosters the "helper principle" that enhances self-esteem and reduces self-stigma by giving assistance to others (Corrigan and Watson, 2002, cited in Corrigan, 2006).

From the perspective of the community, empowerment is achieved through the development of social support systems and advocacy for patient rights and improved programs (Stromwall & Hurdle, 2003). Dialogue is an essential component of empowerment, and participants of the prostate cancer study referenced above have suggested that the dialogue take place in community settings such as school, fraternal and civic organizations, and even prisons, to reach individuals who are in greatest need of the information being exchanged in the dialogue (Allen et al., 2007). Because of past mistrust between minority communities and providers, and because of the institutional, social, and cultural barriers, dialogue is likely to be more fruitful when taking place in a community setting than in the provider's premises.

Consumer empowerment will be instrumental in addressing all five barriers identified by Rogler et al. (1989), from the emergence of mental health problems to the patient's posttreatment adjustment and return to the community. In particular, the dialogue between the organization and consumer representatives will play a crucial role in the development of a mutual understanding of normative behavior and will likely result in a greater participation of the patient and the family in care decisions. This dialogue will also be important to bridge the community and ethnic providers, as well as various resources and linguistic services.

Recruitment and Retention of Minority Health Care Professionals

The availability of bilingual-bicultural administrators, clinicians, and staff is generally considered a very important condition for the delivery of culturally sensitive care. Language is very important to establish trust between the patient and therapist at the onset – *the number one thing* (Ito & Maramba, 2002, p. 53). It is not a sufficient condition, however, because despite being from the same country of origin or from the same minority group, the patient and therapist may differ on many parameters, including social class, religious practices, languages, as well as personal and cultural beliefs (Bhui, Warfa, Edonya, McKenzie, & Bhurga, 2007). Findings from one study indicated that the provision of ethnic-specific services requires more than a linguistic/cultural match between therapist and patient. It entails negotiations aimed at aligning the therapeutic approach to the patient's beliefs about mental illness that are invariably shaped by one's own cultural background (Ito & Maramba, 2002).

In order to make the organization's services well aligned with the cultural and linguistic needs of the community, the management must take a proactive role in ensuring the continued availability of staff members who are able to deliver services with a high level of cultural and linguistic competence. This will involve active engagement in recruiting individuals from the community as early as junior high school and training them to fill in the role of bicultural-bilingual mental health professionals in years to come. In addition, given the fierce competition that organizations are likely to face when serving highly diverse communities, the management needs to have sound strategies of staff retention as well (Puebla Fortier et al., 1999). The role of such professionals can be expanded over time to serve additionally as liaisons between the organization and the community.

Four proactive measures have been identified for the recruitment and retention of minority health care professionals: (1) outreach to K-12 and undergraduate programs with the aim of informing students about the merits of health care professions; (2) parallel outreach to high school and college career counselors, in addition to internship and/or other opportunities for students to see how health care professionals operate; (3) advertisements in student newspapers and community activities such as street fairs; and (4) the creation of partnerships between university schools of health professions and local school boards to establish curricula that help prepare students for study that leads to graduate work and possible careers in health professions (Gabard, 2007). While this strategy was initially designed to recruit physical therapists, it can also be applied to the development of future providers of mental health services. Over time, such efforts are also likely to lead to a greater representation of minority

individuals in institutional leadership which, in the longer term, will be instrumental to further reduce organizational barriers to access the health care system
(Betancourt, Green, Carrillo, & Ananeh-Firempong, 2003).

The recruitment, training, and retention of mental health professionals from
within the community will help overcome issues of mistrust, an element that
constitutes a key barrier in help seeking, diagnosis, treatment, and posttreatment care.

Language Services

Language services to individuals with limited English proficiency have been
associated not only with improved health care access and outcomes but also
with increased patient satisfaction and reduced injury and death. The provision
of services to bridge language gaps between patients and health care providers is
a federal requirement. Such services should be provided through the availability
of bilingual staff, face-to-face interpretation, or interpretation via the telephone
in order to reach individuals with limited English proficiency, those with low
literacy, and those with visual, developmental, and/or cognitive difficulties
(Puebla Fortier et al., 1999). The translation of educational materials to other
languages should be of professionally accepted quality, and involve trained
translators, back translation, and review by individuals from the target population, such as consumer representatives (Puebla Fortier et al., 1999).

Despite this requirement, many providers are still unaware of their obligation to provide such services. Determining the language(s) for which an organization should provide interpretation services has been problematic. Although
the federal requirement specifies that all individuals with limited English proficiency should receive language services, most organizations use a certain
threshold or an arbitrarily set percentage cutpoint based on the density of a
particular ethnic subgroup in the population that they serve (Puebla Fortier et
al., 1999). As a result, a large number of patients experience unavailability of
services in their own language. At the receiving end, many patients may also be
unaware of their right to receive language services and/or reluctant to request
the presence of an interpreter. Additionally, patients may not even be aware of
the availability of language services at an organization.

The lack of training for individuals serving in the role of interpreter (including family and friends), or their incompetence, has been found to be associated
with high rates of medical errors. Being able to converse in English does not
qualify someone to serve as a medical interpreter; even when an interpreter is
"trained," his/her training may be in court or conference interpretation, rather
than medical interpretation (Puebla Fortier et al., 1999). In addition, the
patient-provider dynamic is likely to be altered in the presence of an interpreter,
and the dynamic may differ depending on whether the interpreter is a member
of the family, a professional interpreter, a clinician, or an administrative

assistant. While the interpreter is expected to be impartial, she/he might introduce new meanings in the process of translation and intrude on the communication between the provider and the patient (Bolton, 2002).

Of note is that translation by bilingual health care professionals should not necessarily be considered of adequate quality either. When serving as interpreters, health care professionals may be condensing, omitting, or even distorting the communication between the patient and the provider (Puebla Fortier et al., 1999). While interpreter incompetence is easily recognized, it is difficult to determine what actually constitutes competence, because there is a lack of consensus on what exactly competence in medical interpretation means. The recommendations to the OMH call for the development and adoption of national standards and standardized competency assessments for medical interpretation (Puebla Fortier et al., 1999). Until then, health care organizations should ensure that bilingual staff and interpreters have received the appropriate level of skills based on the current practice standards.

Patient education with regard to the right to receive language services may address various barriers in important ways. From help-seeking behavior to diagnosis of mental disorders, therapy, and posttreatment care, these barriers will be reduced if the patient and his/her family are empowered with this information and demand to receive the language services that they have the right to receive. In turn, serving a patient population that is well-informed of its rights will prompt health care organizations to make the necessary changes to meet the needs and demands of their customers.

The provision of language services affects all of the barriers listed above, and the lack of such services creates a wide gap between the health care organization and the population that it serves. Of note is that cultural competence and linguistic competence go hand in hand; deficiency in cultural competence deeply affects linguistic competence, and vice versa.

Outcomes Studies and Evaluation of CLAS

Cultural competence has been looked upon very favorably, and its effectiveness presumed, rather than proven through a body of empirical, evidence-based research. The very few outcomes studies in this area are discussed below. The presumption of its effectiveness, however, is well grounded, because at a theoretical level, cultural competence has the potential to address many of the factors constituting barriers to receipt of adequate care by minority individuals. These include cultural nuances leading to differences across racial/ethnic minorities in mental symptom recognition, language proficiency, cultural and linguistic congruence of the patient and the therapist, and category fallacy resulting from the application of strict diagnostic definitions based on norms of Western cultures to other cultures.

CLAS outcomes studies will require the incorporation of data on patient race/ethnicity, culture, and language. As noted above, efforts to collect relevant data are currently underway. Whether collecting data on race and ethnicity should be mandatory, voluntary, or permissible has long been subject to debate. The current consensus is that collection of such data is in fact permissible, as long as it is voluntary (Puebla Fortier et al., 1999). Collecting data on the patient's language preference is far less controversial, in that it provides practical information to decide whether the patient needs interpreter services.

The availability of these data will not only help to understand the cultural and linguistic needs of the community that an organization serves but also in planning relevant services. Additionally, to some extent, these data will be instrumental in utilization and outcomes studies. However, because most research relies on Western research instruments that have not yet been validated for specific cultures, and in order to gain in-depth understanding of the cultural issues involved in providing adequate mental health services, the quantitative analysis of these data should be conducted in parallel with qualitative and survey research, as described below.

In preparation for larger epidemiological surveys, de Jong and van Ommeren (2002) have called for the collection of qualitative data as summarized below:

Stage I: Identifying problems among subpopulations through focus groups: The focus group approach is most helpful when formulating research questions. It may be employed to identify risk, as well as protective factors; to learn about the concerns or needs of a community; and to be informed about the customs and coping strategies, as well as about possible links between life events, social support, and the onset or exacerbation of a problem. However, this approach does present limitations, especially when used in certain cultural contexts, for example, when free expression of thoughts may be impeded because of hierarchical relationships among study participants (deJong & Von Ommeren, 2002).

Stage II: Studying individuals through in-depth interviews: In-depth interviews are employed to gain knowledge about individuals' subjective experience and psychological processes and to overcome the challenges of adapting instruments to other cultures. They are most useful to identify issues that are considered important to local communities and to ensure that the relevant research questions are indeed studied (deJong & Von Ommeren, 2002).

Stage III: Preparing for the epidemiological study: Preparation for the epidemiological study involves meetings with different parties, including members of the research team, and that of the study population, with the goal to achieve member validity, or "the potential that respondents are able to recognize themselves in the basic research results" (de Jong & van Ommeren, 2002, p. 428; Mehan & Wood, 1975, cited by de Jong & van Ommeren, 2002).

Preparation for the meeting should ensure *content equivalence*, meaning that each item of the instrument that was originally developed has relevance within the context of the culture being studied; *semantic equivalence,* to ensure that the meaning of an item is unchanged when translated; *concept equivalence*, or that the theoretical construct being measured is the same in the two cultures; *criterion equivalence* to ensure that outcomes measured are in agreement with other criteria in the instrument; and *technical equivalence* to examine the potential of an instrument to produce systematic biases when used in another culture (deJong & Von Ommeren, 2002).

Stage IV: Epidemiological survey: The survey is conducted after the instruments have been prepared and validated. Surveys yield various measures, including prevalence, identification of risk and protective factors, comorbidity, and remission rates. However, individual-level variability will be difficult to measure at the population or subpopulation levels, even when qualitative techniques have been used (deJong & Von Ommeren, 2002).

To monitor changes and evaluate success in mental health services' adaptation to suit clients from different cultures, de Jong and van Ommeren (2005) have further proposed *both qualitative and quantitative* measures in four of the following contexts.

The clinical interface or the relations between the immigrant patient, the health care workers, and the treatment team: The areas to concentrate on include training the staff with regard to diagnostics and training, as assessed through participant observation, amount and content of training; integration/segregation, measured through the representativeness of various minority subgroups in the patient population being served; appointment of immigrant (minority) healthcare workers examined through the distribution of immigrant (minority) staff in the institution; ability to express preference regarding background of staff by evaluating the extent to which there is a cultural match between patient and staff; quality of relationship with interpreter reflected through the staff's ability and techniques to work with the interpreter; number of drop-out patients by minority status, by monitoring the number of and reason for drop-outs; patient satisfaction and clinical outcomes by conducting effectiveness research; and reliability of culture-specific diagnostics, by measuring diagnostic sensitivity and specificity with validated instrument and expert opinion in a random sample of patients (deJong & Von Ommeren, 2005).

Organizational adaptations required in the treatment context of the mental healthcare facility: The main areas of attention include the following: cultural ways of expression, by examining the linguistic and media diversity by which the staff communicate with the patient; the organization's orientation level of respect vis-à-vis cultural variations in various mores such as sexuality, conflict management, use of rituals and culture-specific healers; personnel policy toward immigrants (minority groups), as measured by the representation of minority staff in the organization; training curriculum; and the size and distribution of budget allocated to immigrant (minority) care (deJong & Von Ommeren, 2005).

The relation between the mental health facility and the ethnic communities: This context can be measured by looking at the level of satisfaction of the ethnic (minority) community with the services rendered by the organization, assessed through interviews with key informants; the level of acceptance of the institution by the ethnic (minority) community, as reflected by the increase (or decrease) of immigrant (minority) care seekers at the institution over time; and the extent to which the organization is in contact with the community, as reflected through the nature and frequency of contact between the organization and minority subgroups (deJong & Von Ommeren, 2005).

The relation between the mental healthcare system, other facilities, and the society at large: This context reflects health care consumption and patients' health-seeking behavior across the primary, secondary, and tertiary health care settings; network development, including referrals, coordination of care, and transfer of information between the organization and various other entities, such as the social welfare department, public housing authorities, and social workers (deJong & Von Ommeren, 2005).

As for any type of service, CLAS should undergo ongoing evaluation to monitor its progress in performance over time and to identify areas of improvement. Examples of trends that organizations might monitor include – among others – utilization of language services and that of mental health services; outcomes, including rehospitalization in the posttreatment period; and patient satisfaction. Results from such analyses would help organizations fine-tune mental health services, both in content and in the way in which they are delivered to special populations.

This recommendation pertains to all of the barriers identified by Rogler et al. (1989), from the emergence of mental disorders to posttreatment care. Careful, ongoing evaluations of measurements relative to each of the barriers would help minimize factors hindering access to culturally and linguistically sensitive mental heath services over time.

Evaluating the Effectiveness of Culturally Competent Services

As noted above, each of these recommendations provides a very sensible approach to providing culturally competent services and to reducing the barriers described by Rogler et al. (1989). However, none would be effective when applied without combining with the other approaches. From a theoretical standpoint, it appears that "packaging" these approaches and offering them in one setting would yield the best possible outcomes. Unfortunately, empirical research in this area is sorely lacking, and few of the studies conducting a systematic review of the literature either demonstrated the effectiveness of culturally competent services and the components thereof or identified the cultural consultation model as one that was proven effective and associated with great clinician satisfaction (Bhui et al., 2007).

A systematic review conducted by the Task Force on Community Preventive Services concluded that the effectiveness of five interventions to improve the cultural competence of health care systems could not be determined in their systematic review, because of a lack of both quantity and quality of relevant studies (Anderson et al., 2003). The five interventions that were reviewed included programs to recruit and retain staff members who reflect the cultural diversity in the community served; use of interpreter services by bilingual providers for clients with limited English proficiency; cultural competency training for health care providers; use of linguistically and culturally appropriate health education materials; and culturally specific health care settings.

On the other hand, two other studies independently documented the benefits of one intervention, that of cultural consultations. The first of these was developed in Montreal, Quebec (Canada), through an intervention "integrating anthropology perspectives with conventional psychiatry, cognitive-behavioral, and family systems perspectives" (Kirmayer, Groleau, Guzder, Blake, & Jarvis, 2003, p. 146). This intervention was designed to provide the following: specific cultural information; links to community resources or to formal cultural psychiatric or psychological assessment; and recommendations for treatment. Diagnostic assessment, treatment planning, and service delivery were guided by the social, cultural, and political context in which symptoms and behaviors were presented. Special attention was given to avoid making generalizations or cultural stereotypes, and focus was kept on detailed histories and local cultural issues. The most common recommendations emanating from the cultural consultations included reassessing or changing treatment; using additional treatment; and change in diagnosis. Clinician satisfaction with the cultural consultation services was high (over 80%). These services resulted in increased knowledge of the social, cultural, or religious aspects of their cases; increased knowledge of the psychiatric or psychological aspects of their cases; improved treatment; improved communication; and increased confidence in diagnosis or treatment. In less than 15% of the cases, clinicians reported difficulties or dissatisfaction relative to the lack of follow-up; unavailability or inappropriateness of community resources; concerns about the cultural broker; and the impression that greater focus was given to the social context than to psychiatric issues (Kirmayer, Groleau, Guzder, Blake, & Jarvis, 2003).

The second study, conducted in Sacramento, California (United States), consisted of a qualitative study based on interviews and focus groups with clinicians. The study sought to identify participants' perceptions of the availability and efficacy of services for ethnic minorities and the adequacy of cultural-competence training workshops (Ton et al., 2005). The investigators identified many barriers in implementing culturally sensitive services. They reported that while training workshops were helpful, there were difficulties translating principles of cultural competence into actual practice. Also, while the use of ethnic matching has been proven successful in areas with ethnic enclaves, such as Los Angeles and San Francisco, it proved to be less practical in an area like Sacramento, where the vastly diverse patient population precluded ethnic matching or the cultivation of a predominant enthnocultural setting. Cultural consultation services would make it possible to benefit from the knowledge of interpreters and cultural brokers, as these individuals collaborate closely with the referring physician throughout the course of the evaluation (Ton et al., 2005).

Concluding Remarks

This chapter presented disparities in mental health services utilization across various subgroups of the population, as well as barriers to access and use these services in the framework by Rogler et al. (1989). In its latter part, the chapter discussed the recommendations put forth to the Office of Minority Health by Puebla Fortier et al. (1999) for assuring cultural competence in health care.

Unfortunately, as important as each of these recommendations seems, we still lack empirical evidence to support their effectiveness relative to improving outcomes of health care in general, and mental health care in particular. Many in the field remain skeptical, referring to cultural competence as "an ideology or a set of guiding principles" (Vega & Lopez, 2001). Skepticism is also nurtured by the lack of standards in the operationalization of cultural competence and its many facets. Rather than "cultural competence," which focuses on the inter-personal skills of the provider, some prefer to speak of the "interculturization of mental health services," defined as the "adaptation of mental health services to suit clients from different cultures" (de Jong & van Ommeren, 2005, p. 438).

The chapter adhered to the framework by Rogler et al. (1989), focusing on the recognition of behaviors as part of a mental disorder, mental health help-seeking behaviors, the deficiency of diagnostic tools, initiation of psychiatric treatment, and posttreatment of care. Because of its strong focus on the barriers associated with cultural and linguistic competence in the delivery of mental health services, the chapter did not include any in-depth discussions pertaining to financial barriers to accessing and utilizing mental health services. Also absent from this chapter was a discussion of the deficiencies in the delivery of mental health services, including the fragmentation of care.

These structural problems affect minority patients in important ways. Immigrant patients, for instance, may lack the know-how to navigate across the various systems and find a way to have mental health care coverage or to find a provider within their geographical and financial reach that would best meet their cultural and linguistic needs. As a result, these patients may be likely to seek care from a number of mental health providers before they can designate one as their "usual source of mental health care." The optimal goal is the identification of a provider as a "usual source of mental health care." Unfortunately, many patients are unlikely to find such a "home" and end up seeking care from multiple providers.

Another aspect of fragmented care is the lack of coordination of care between the systems providing *mental* health services and the ones providing medical care for *physical* conditions. Medical comorbidities in patients with mental health conditions are often undiagnosed or diagnosed late (Koranyi, 1979) – a factor that leads to increased morbidity and mortality in this population, compared with those who do not present psychiatric conditions.

Last, but not least, a major challenge lies in the development and provision of wellness programs. The responsibility to provide such services rests not only with health care systems but with the society as a whole. Among other places, such services must be integrated with diversity management programs in schools and in the workplace to prevent harassment, bullying, and overt/covert discrimination, which may lead to stress and insidious deterioration of mental health.

References

Alegria, M., Canino, G., Rios, R., Vera, M., Calderon, J., Rusch, D.,et al. (2002). Inequalities in use of specialty mental health services among Latinos, African Americans, and Non-Latino Whites. *Psychiatric Services, 53*(12), 1547–1555.

Alegria, M., Polo, A., Gao, S., Santana, L., Rothstein, D., Jimenez, A.,et al. (2008). Evaluation of a patient activation and empowerment intervention in mental health care. *Medical Care, 46*(3), 247–256.

Ali, O. M., Milstein, G., & Marzuk, P. M. (2005). The Imam's role in meeting the counseling needs of Muslim communities in the United States. *Psychiatric Services, 56*(2), 202–205.

Allen, J. D., Kennedy, M., Wilson-Grover, A., & Gilligan, T. D. (2007). African-American men's perceptions about prostate cancer: Implications for designing educational intervention. *Social Science & Medicine, 64*, 2189–2200.

Anderson, L. M., Scrimshaw, S. C., Fullilove, M. T., Fielding, J. E., Normand, J., & the Task Force on Community Preventive Services. (2003). Culturally competent healthcare systems. A systematic review. *American Journal of Preventive Medicine, 24*(3S), 68–79.

Atdjian, S., & Vega, W. A. (2005). Disparities in mental health treatment in U.S. racial and ethnic minority groups: Implications for psychiatrists. *Psychiatric Services, 56*(12), 1600–1602.

Barker, P. R., Epstein, J. F., Hourani, L. L., Gfroerer, J., Clinton-Sherrod, A. M., West, N., et al. (2004). *Patterns of mental health services utilization among adults, 2000 and 2001.* Department of Health and Human Services, Substance Abuse and Mental Health Services Administration, Office of Applied Studies. Last accessed March 9, 2008; Available at http://www.oas.samhsa.gov/mhtx/PDFW/2 k-2k1mentalhealthW.pdf

Bernabei, R., Gambassi, G., Lapane, K., Landi, F., Gatsonis, C., Dunlop, R.,et al. (1998). Management of pain in elderly patients with cancer. SAGE Study Group. Systematic assessment of geriatric drug use via epidemiology. *Journal of the American Medical Association, 279*(23), 1877–1882.

Betancourt, J. R., Green, A. R., Carrillo, J. E., & Ananeh-Firempong, O. (2003). Defining cultural competence: A practical framework for addressing racial/ethnic disparities in health and health care. *Public Health Reports, 118*, 293–302.

Bhui, K., Warfa, N., Edonya, P., McKenzie, K., & Bhurga, D. (2007). Cultural competence in mental health care: A review of model evaluations. *BMC Health Services Research, 7*(Jan. 31), 15.

Blanco, C., Patel, S. R., Jiang, H., Lewis-Fernandez, R., Schmidt, A. B., Liebowitz, M. R., et al. (2007). National trends in ethnic disparities in mental health care. *Medical Care, 45*(11), 1012–1019.

Bolton, J. (2002). The third presence: A psychiatrist's experience of working with non-English speaking patients and interpreters. *Transcultural Psychiatry, 39*(1), 97–114.

Cates, J. A. (2005). Facing away: Mental health treatment with the Old Order Amish. *American Journal of Psychotherapy, 59*(4), 371–383.

Centers for Disease Control and Prevention. (2004). Self-reported frequent mental distress among adults – United States, 1993–2001. *Morbidity and Mortality Weekly Report, 53*(41), 963–966.

Cheng, E. M., Chen, A., & Cunningham, W. (2007). Primary language and receipt of recommended health care among Hispanics in the United States. *Journal of General Internal Medicine, 22*(Suppl 2), 283–288.

Chevannes, M. (2002). Issues in educating health professionals to meet the diverse needs of patients and other service users from ethnic minority groups. *Journal of Advanced Nursing, 39*(3), 290–298.

Chow, J. C., Jaffee, K., & Snowden, L. (2003). Racial/ethnic disparities in the use of mental health services in poverty areas. *American Journal of Public Health, 93,* 792–797.

Cooper, G. S., Yuan, Z., Landefeld, C. S., & Rimm, A. A. (1996). Surgery for colorectal cancer: Race-related differences in rates and survival among Medicare beneficiaries. *American Journal of Public Health, 86*(4), 582–586.

Cooper, G. S., & Koroukian, S. M. (2004). Racial disparities in the use of and indications for colorectal procedures in Medicare beneficiaries. *Cancer, 100*(2), 418–424.

Cook, B. L., McGuire, T., & Miranda, J. (2007). Measuring trends in mental health care disparities. *Psychiatric Services, 58*(12), 1533–1540.

Corrigan, P. W. (2006). Impact of Consumer-Operated Services on empowerment and recovery of people with psychiatric disabilities. *Psychiatric Services, 57*(10), 1493–1496.

Daumit, G. L., Crum, R. M., Guallar, E., Powe, N. R., Primm, A. B., Steinwachs, D. M.,et al. (2003). Outpatient prescriptions for atypical antipsychotics for African Americans, Hispanics, and Whites in the United States. *Archives of General Psychiatry, 60,* 121–128.

Dobalian, A., & Rivers, P. A. (2008). Racial and ethnic disparities in the use of mental health services. *Journal of Behavioral Health Services Research,* 35(2): 128–141.

de Jong, J. T. V. M., & van Ommeren, M. (2002). Toward a culture-informed epidemiology: Combining qualitative and quantitative research in transcultural contexts. *Transcultural Psychiatry, 39*(4), 422–433.

de Jong, J. T. V. M., & van Ommeren, M.(2005). Mental health services in a multicultural society: Interculturization and its quality surveillance. *Transcultural Psychiatry, 42*(3), 437–456.

Dovidio, J. F., Brigham, J. C., Johnson, B. T., & Gaertner, S. L. (1996). Stereotyping, prejudice, and discrimination: Another look. In N. Macrae, C. Stangor, & M. Hewstone (Eds.), *Stereotypes and stereotyping.* New York: Guilford.

Fleck, D. E., Keck, P. E. Jr., Corey, K. B., Strakowski, S. M. (2005). Factors associated with medication adherence in African American and white patients with bipolar disorder. *Journal of Clinical Psychiatry, 66*(5), 646–652.

Gabard, D. L. (2007). Increasing minority representation in health care professions. *Journal of Allied Health, 36*(3), 165–175.

Gilmer, T. P., Ojeda, V. D., Folsom, D. P., Fuentes, D., Garcia, P., & Jeste, D. V. (2007). Initiation and use of public mental health services by persons with severe mental illness and limited English proficiency. *Psychiatric Services, 58*(12), 1555–1562.

Gornick, M. E., Eggers, P. W., Reilly, T. W., Mentnech, R. M., Fitterman, L. K., Kucken, L. E., et al. (1996). Effects of race and income on mortality and use of services among Medicare beneficiaries. *New England Journal of Medicine, 335*(11), 791–799.

Harman, J. S., Edlund, M. J., & Fortney, J. C. (2004). Disparities in the adequacy of depression treatment in the United States. *Psychiatric Services, 55*(12), 1379–1385.

Hauenstein, E. J., Petterson, S., Merwin, E., Rovnyak, V., Heise, B., & Wagner, D. (2006). Rurality, gender, and mental health treatment. *Family and Community Health, 29*(3), 169–185.

Hauenstein, E. J., Petterson, S., Rovnyak, V., Merwin, E., Heise, B., & Wagner, D. (2007). Rurality and mental health treatment. *Administration and Policy Mental Health, 34*(3), 255–267.

Herbeck, D. M., West, J. C., Ruditis, I., Duffy, F. F., Fitek, D. J., Bell, C. C.,et al. (2004). Variations in use of second-generation antipsychotic medication by race among adult psychiatric patients. *Psychiatric Services, 55*(6), 677–684.

Herrick, C. A., & Brown, H. N. (1998). Underutilization of mental health services by Asian Americans residing in the United States. *Issues in Mental Health Nursing, 19*, 225–240.

Heurtin-Roberts, S., Snowden, L., & Miller, L. (1997). Expressions of anxiety in African Americans: Ethnography and the epidemiological catchment area studies. *Culture, Medicine, and Psychiatry, 21*, 337–363.

Hinton, D. E., Pich, V., & Pollack, M. H. (2005). Panic attacks in traumatized Southeast Asian refugees. Mechanisms and treatment implications. In A. M. Georgiopoulos & J. F. Rosenbaum (Eds.), *Perspective in cross-cultural psychiatry* (pp. 37–62). Philadelphia, PA: Lippincott Williams & Wilkins.

Institute of Medicine (2003). Unequal treatment. Confronting racial and ethnic disparities in health care. Washington, D.C. The National Academies Press.

Ito, K. L., & Maramba, G. G. (2002). Therapeutic beliefs of Asian American therapists: View from an ethnic-specific clinic. *Transcultural Psychiatry, 39*(1), 33–73.

Johnson, J. L., & Cameron, M. C. (2001). Barriers to providing effective mental health services to American Indians. *Mental Health Services Research, 3*(4), 215–223.

Kessler, R. C., McGonagle, K. A., Zhao, S., Nelson, C. B., Hughes, M., Eshelman, S.,et al. (1994). Lifetime and 12-month prevalence of DSM-III-R disorders in the United States. *Archives of General Psychiatry, 51*(1), 8–19.

Kimerling, R., & Baumrind, N. (2005). Access to specialty mental health services among women in California. *Psychiatric Services, 56*(6), 729–734.

Kirmayer, L. J., Groleau, D., Guzder, J., Blake, C., & Jarvis, E. (2003). Cultural consultation: A model of mental health service for multicultural societies. *Canadian Journal of Psychiatry, 48*(3), 145–153.

Kirmayer, L. J. (2006). Beyond the "New Cross-cultural Psychiatry": Cultural biology, discursive psychology and the ironies of globalization. *Transcultural Psychiatry, 43*(1), 126–144.

Knudsen, H. K., Ducharme, L. J., & Roman, P. M. (2007). Racial and ethnic disparities in SSRI availability in substance abuse treatment. *Psychiatric Services, 58*(1), 55–62.

Koranyi, E.K. (1979). Morbidity and rate of undiagnosed physical illnesses in a psychiatric clinic population. *Archives of General Psychiatry*; 36: 414–419.

Kuno, E., & Rothbard, A. B. (2002). Racial disparities in antipsychotic prescription patterns for patients with schizophrenia. *American Journal of Psychiatry, 159*(4), 567–572.

Lagomasino, I. T., Dwight-Johnson, M., Miranda, J., Zhang, L., Liao, D., Duan, N.,et al. (2005). Disparities in depression treatment for Latinos and site of care. *Psychiatric Services, 56*(12), 1517–1523.

Lasser, K. E., Himmelstein, D. U., Woolhandler, S. J., McCromick, D., & Bor, D. H. (2002). Do minorities in the United States receive fewer mental health services than Whites? *International Journal of Health Services, 32*(3), 567–578.

Leong, F. T. L., & Lau, A. S. L. (2001). Barriers to providing effective mental health services to Asian Americans. *Mental Health Services Research, 3*(4), 201–214.

Marshall, G. N., Berthold, M., Schell, T. L., Elliott, M. N., Chun, C., & Hambarsoomians, K. (2006). Rates and correlates of seeking mental health services among Cambodian refugees. *American Journal of Public Health, 96*(10), 1829–1835.

McGuire, T. G., Alegria, M., Cook, B. L., Wells, K. B., & Zaslavsky, A. M. (2006). Implementing the Institute of Medicine definition of disparities: An application to mental health care. *Health Services Research, 41*(5), 1979–2005.

Minsky, S., Vega, W., Miskimen, T., Gara, M., & Escobar, J. (2003). Diagnostic patterns in Latino, African American, and European American psychiatric patients. *Archives of General Psychiatry, 60*(6), 637–644.

Opolka, J. L., Rascati, K. L., Brown, C. M., Barner, J. C., Johnsrud, M. T., & Gibson, P. J. (2003). Ethnic differences in use of antipsychotic medication among Texas Medicaid clients with schizophrenia. *Journal of Clinical Psychiatry, 64*(6), 635–639.

Opolka, J. L., Rascati, K. L., Brown, C. M., & Gibson, P. J. (2003). Role of ethnicity in predicting antipsychotic medication adherence. *Annals of Pharmacotherapy, 37*(5), 625–630.

Opolka, J. L., Rascati, K. L., Brown, C. M., & Gibson, P. J. (2004). Ethnicity and prescription patterns for Haloperidol, risperidone, and olanzapine. *Psychiatric Services, 55*(2), 151–156.

Passel, J. S., & Cohn, D. (2008). *U.S. population projections: 2005–2050.* Washington, DC: Pew Research Center, Social & Demographic Trends. Last accessed April 7, 2008; Available at http://pewhispanic.org/files/reports/85.pdf

Pear, R. (2008). House Approves Bill on Mental Health Parity. The New York Times. Last accessed April 9, 2008; Available at .http://www.nytimes.com/2008/03/06/washington/06health.html?_r=1&scp=1&sq=mental+health+parity&st=nyt&oref=slogin

Puebla Fortier, J., Convissor, R., & Pacheco, G. (1999). *Assuring cultural competence in health care: Recommendations for national standards and an outcomes-focused research agenda: Recommendations for national standards and a national public comment process.* Silver Spring, Maryland: Resources for Cross Cultural Health Care. Last accessed April 14, 2008; Available at http://www.omhrc.gov/Assets/pdf/checked/Assuring_Cultural_Competence_in_Health_Care-1999.pdf.

Rogler, L. H., Malgady, R. G., & Rodriguez, O. (1989). *Hispanics and mental health: A framework for research.* Malabar, FL: Robert E. Krieger Publishing Company.

Ronzio, C. R., Guagliardo, M. F., & Persaud, N. (2006). Disparity in location of urban mental service providers. *American Journal of Orthopsychiatry, 76*(1), 37–43.

Sentell, T., Shumway, M., & Snowden, L. (2007). Access to mental health treatment by English language proficiency and race/ethnicity. *Journal of General Internal Medicine, 22*(Suppl 2), 289–293.

Snowden, L. R. (1998). Racial differences in informal help seeking for mental health problems. *Journal of Community Psychology, 26*(5), 429–438.

Snowden, L. R., & Thomas, K. (2000). Medicaid and African American outpatient mental health treatment. *Mental Health Services Research, 2*(2), 115–120.

Snowden L. R. (2001). Barriers to effective mental health services for African Americans. *Mental Health Services Research, 3*(4), 181–187.

Steele, L. S., Glazier, R. H., & Lin, E. (2006). Inequity in mental health care under Canadian universal health coverage. *Psychiatric Services, 57*(3), 317–324.

Stockdale, S. E., Tang, L., Zhang, L., Belin, T. R., & Wells, K. B. (2007). The effects of health sector market factors and vulnerable group membership on access to alcohol, drug, and mental health care. *Health Services Research, 42*(3 Pt 1), 1020–1041.

Stromwall, L. K., & Hurdle, D. (2003). Psychiatric rehabilitation: An empowerment-based approach to mental health services. *Health & Social Work, 28*(3), 206–213.

Stuart, G. W., Minas, I. H., Klimidis, S., & O'Connell, S. (1996). English language ability and mental health service utilization. *Australian and New Zealand Journal of Psychiatry, 30*(2), 270–277.

Sue, S., Fujino, D. C., Hu, L., Takeuchi, D. T., & Zane, N. (1991). Community mental health services for ethnic minority groups: A test of cultural responsiveness hypothesis. *Journal of Consulting and Clinical Psychology, 59*(4), 533–540.

Sue, S., Zane, N., & Young, K. (1994). Research on psychotherapy on culturally diverse populations. In A. Bergin & S. Garfield (Eds.), *Handbook of psychotherapy and behavior change* (4th ed.). New York: Wiley.

Suite, D. H., La Bril, R., Primm, A., & Harrison-Ross, P. (2007). Beyond misdiagnosis, misunderstanding and mistrust: relevance of the historical perspective in the medical and mental health treatment of people of color. *Journal of the National Medical Association, 99*(8), 879–885.

Takeuchi, D. T., & Cheung, M. K. (1998). Coercive and voluntary referrals: How ethnic minority adults get into mental health treatment. *Ethnicity & Health, 3*(3), 149–158.

Ton, H., Koike, A., Hales, R. E., Johnson, J. A., & Hilty, D. M. (2005). A qualitative needs assessment for development of a cultural consultation service. *Transcultural Psychiatry, 42*(3), 491–504.

U.S. Department of Health and Human Services. (2001). *Mental health: Culture, race, and ethnicity – a supplement to mental health: A report of the Surgeon General.* Rockville, MD:

U.S. Department of Health and Human Services, Substance Abuse and Mental Health Services Administration, Center for Mental Health Services.

Vega, W. A., & Lopez, S. R. (2001). Priority issues in Latino mental health services research. *Mental Health Services Research, 3*(4), 189–200.

Wallace, A. E., Weeks, W. B., Wang, S., Lee, A. F., & Kazis, L. E. (2006). Rural and urban disparities in health-related quality of life among veterans with psychiatric disorders. *Psychiatric Services, 57*(6), 851–856.

Walls, M. L., Johnson, K. D., Whitbeck, L. B., & Hoyt, D. R. (2006). Mental health and substance abuse services preferences among American Indian people of the Northern Midwest. *Community Mental Health Journal, 42*(6), 521–535.

Whitley, R., Kirmayer, L. J., & Groleau, D. (2006). Understanding immigrants' reluctance to use mental health services: A qualitative study from Montreal. *Canadian Journal of Psychiatry, 51*(4), 205–209.

Willging, C. E., Salvador, M., & Kano, M. (2006). Pragmatic help seeking: How sexual and gender minority groups access mental health care in a rural state. *Psychiatric Services, 57*(6), 871–874.

Wood, A. J. J. (2001). Racial differences in the response to drugs – pointers to genetic differences. *New England Journal of Medicine, 344*(18), 1394–1396.

Yanos, P. T., Primavera, L. H., & Knight, E. L. (2001). Consumer-Run Service participation, recovery of social functioning, and the mediating role of psychological factors. *Psychiatric Services, 52*(4), 493–500.

Ying, Y. W., & Hu, L. T. (1994). Public outpatient mental health services: Use and outcome among Asian Americans. *American Journal of Orthopsychiatry, 64*(3), 448–455.

Chapter 7
Social Support, Mental Health, Minorities, and Acculturative Stress

Deborah Goebert

The United States is experiencing a dramatic ethnic transformation, largely due to immigration rates and minority birth rates. Recent census data indicate that, by the year 2050, there will be an approximate 71% population increase among African Americans, a 213% increase for Asian Americans and Pacific Islanders, and a 188% increase for Hispanic Americans (U.S. Census Bureau, 2004). These population increases underscore the importance of understanding the process of psychological adjustment within minority populations and the factors that contribute to this process.

The rate of psychological adjustment among minorities has been extensively studied with contradictory findings. Some researchers report higher rates of psychological distress, depression, and anxiety among minorities when compared to non-Hispanic whites, while others find similar rates. Researchers have generally agreed that minorities face multiple stressors, particularly acculturative stress, which can have deleterious effects on their well-being. One possible explanation for the contradictory nature of at least some of these findings is that the relationship between acculturative stress and well-being may be mediated by contextual factors. One important potential mediator is social support. In this chapter, we explore the concepts of social support, stress and acculturative stress, and their relations on mental health and well-being among minorities.

Definition of the Social Support Construct

Social support is multidimensional (Thoits, 1982; Turner, 1981; Vaux, 1988). There is no single, adequate and simple definition of social support. Social support can be viewed as a complex process unfolding in an ecological context (Vaux, 1990). This process involves transactions between people and their social networks and is shaped by features of both the person and the social ecology.

D. Goebert (✉)
University of Hawaii, John A. Burns School of Medicine, Honolulu, Hawaii
e-mail: goebertd@dop.hawaii.edu

S. Loue, M. Sajatovic (eds.), *Determinants of Minority Mental Health and Wellness*, DOI 10.1007/978-0-387-75659-2_7,
© Springer Science+Business Media, LLC 2009

This ecological model of support allows a more complete understanding of support processes, including their relationship to stress and well-being. The model also serves as a framework for intervention, highlighting targets, and strategies for programs designed to facilitate social support.

Social support has been broadly defined as an individual's perception that she or he is connected to others and obtains emotional and instrumental assistance when needed. However, scholars have yet to reach consensus on the most appropriate way to conceptualize and define social support. In 2004, Williams, Barclay and Schmied reported on 30 definitions of social support from the literature used across disciplines and identified the commonalities amongst these definitions of social support. They grouped these definitions into several categories, including notions of time and timing, social ties and relationships, supportive resources, intentionality of support, impact of support, recognition of support need, and characteristics of providers and recipients. It was noted that definitions range from nonspecific to specific definitions. At the simplest level, the social support literature reveals two fundamental ways to conceptualize social support: (1) the *structure* of relationships and (2) the *functions* that they provide. Consequently, social support may refer to either the structural or functional aspects of social relationships or both (Cohen & Syme, 1985).

Social Support Structure

With respect to structure, social support can come from a variety of informal and formal sources. *Informal social support* can be obtained from members of an individual's informal network, such as family, friends, coworkers, and neighbors. *Formal social support* may come from institutions such as schools, religious institutions, social services, and mental health services (Hill, 1993).

Social integration and social networks are terms that have often been used in the literature to describe structural elements of social relationships. Social integration, for example, usually refers to the existence and quantity of social relationships. The term social network is used to refer to the structural properties of social relationships.

Social integration includes formal and informal social ties such as family, friends, and social and religious groups (Berkman, 1995). Social integration can also connote ties to the community and culture and can, therefore, include the process of combining a group of persons like minority groups, ethnic minorities, refugees, and underprivileged sections of the society, to integrate into the mainstream of society. Measurement of social integration can be used to determine whether a respondent is socially isolated or has social ties and summarizes the number of available social contacts. Social integration measures the number of social ties and not the quality of the potential interactions represented by those ties.

Social networks represent the ways in which social support is exchanged. Networks consist of a set of points (people) and the ties of support that connect them (Antonucci, 1985). Social networks include structure, composition, and component relationships (Vaux, 1988). The structure of a social network is determined by both its size (the number of individuals who make up the networks) and its density (the level of interconnectedness among members) (Antonucci, 1985; Vaux, 1988). Network composition examines who is involved in the network, such as family members, friends, and neighbors. The relationships within a social network can be assessed according to many factors such as the frequency with which contact occurs, the geographic proximity of its members, and the intensity and resiliency of the relationships. In addition, researchers often examine the context in which social support exchanges take place, the degree of reciprocity involved, as well as whether the relationship consists of one or more different types of exchange (Vaux, 1988).

Social Support Function

In examining the functions of social support, researchers have studied individuals' perceptions regarding the level of different types of social support they receive. Some definitions emphasize functions related to needs. For example, Cobb (1976) defined social support as information that leads to the belief that an individual is cared for and loved, is valued and esteemed, and belongs to a network of communication and mutual obligation. Thoits (1982) viewed social support as the degree to which a person's basic social needs for affection, esteem, belonging, identity, and security are gratified through interaction with others through socio-emotional aid and instrumental aid. House (1981) suggested that social support is an interpersonal transaction involving (1) emotional concern such as liking, love, and empathy; (2) instrumental aid such as goods and services; (3) information; and (4) appraisal necessary for self-evaluation.

Research focuses on categories of supportive behaviors and/or actions (Antonucci, 1985). Functional social support includes the provision of emotional or affective support, affirmative support, and tangible aid (Antonucci, Fuhrer, & Dartigues, 1997; Cohen & Syme, 1985; House, 1987; House & Kahn, 1985; Kahn & Antonucci, 1980; Koblinsky & Anderson, 1993). Emotional or affirmative support refers to expressions of liking, admiration, respect, love, or acknowledgment of the appropriateness of some act or statements of another person. It can include feelings of being cared for and esteemed, as well as offering care or sympathy, listening to someone, and/or being available to another person. In addition, it is used to refer to the more qualitative aspects of social relationships, such as the level of satisfaction that people feel regarding the support that they receive. It can be further conceptualized as validation through providing praise or positive affirmations to another. Instrumental or tangible support include transactions in which direct aid or assistance is given, including things, money, information, time, and entitlements is described as the provision of financial resources, transportation, and/or assistance with cooking, cleaning, and shopping, as well as providing information about resources or giving advice.

Social support has been extensively studied and has conceptualized in ways that include different aspects of social support. Two domains of social support are often investigated: structure and function.

Social Support Measures

The first social support measures began appearing in the literature during the 1970s. Since that time, a multitude of scales have been developed, adapted, and/or translated. A few of the more common scales with documented psychometric properties and the perceived usefulness of the measures in empirical research are mentioned herein.

Some measures assess both structural and functional aspects of social support. For example, the Norbeck Social Support Questionnaire (NSSQ) measures the structural and functional dimensions of social support, with affect, affirmation, and aid proposed as three types of supportive transactions. The measure asks respondents to list significant people in their lives who provide social support and to rate those people regarding affect, affirmation, and aid provided. Additional items assess the aggregate social support network and losses of social support. The Social Support Questionnaire (SSQ) (Sarason, Levine, Bashman, & Sarason, 1983) evaluates satisfaction with support across twenty-seven situations, each of which requires a two-part answer: a list of the people who provide support in the specified circumstances and a rating of satisfaction with that support. Two scores are provided – an N score (for the number of supports) and an S score (for the satisfaction with the supports). The Social Support Resources (SS-R) (Vaux, 1982, *Measures of three levels of social support: Resources, behaviors and feelings,* unpublished) assesses an individual's satisfaction on five modes of social support (emotional, socializing, practical assistance, financial assistance, and advice or guidance), and the Arizona Social Support Interview Schedule (ASSIS) (Barrera, 1981) examines the satisfaction with six modes of support including material aid, physical assistance, intimate interaction, guidance, feedback, and social participation. The Social Relationship Scale (SRS) (McFarlane, Neale, Norman, Roy, & Streiner, 1981) focuses on rating helpfulness or unhelpfulness with support across a range of potentially stressful situations. The Inventory of Socially Supportive Behaviors (ISSB) was developed out of a need to expand understanding of social support in terms of discrete behaviors (Barrera, 1986). Respondents report the frequency with which they were recipients of 40 supportive actions. The Child and Adolescent Social Support Scale (CASSS) (Malecki, Demaray, & Elliott, 2000) assesses the four types of support (emotional, informational, appraisal, and instrumental) from different sources of support (parents, teachers, classmates, and friends).

Other measures of social support focus specifically on structure. Different aspects of the network have been measured by a number of existing instruments. Network size measures the number of members (e.g., family, friends, and neighbors) involved in the network, whereas network density measures the interrelationship of members involved in the network. The Social Network Questionnaire (SNQ) (Hirsch, 1979) focuses on assessing both the size and density. The Social Support Resources (SS-R) (Vaux, 1982, *Measures of three levels of social support: Resources, behaviors and feelings,* unpublished) and the Social Support Network Interview (SSNI) (Fischer, 1982) measure network composition.

Given the numerous typologies in the modes and function of social support, multiple measures are available. For example, the Perceived Social Support instrument from Friends and Family (PSS-Fr) (PSS-Fa) (Procidano & Heller, 1983) examines the extent to which an individual perceives his/her needs for support, information, and feedback are fulfilled and is available in multiple languages. The Multidimensional Scale of Perceived Social Support (MSPSS) (Zimet et al., 1988) measures the perceived adequacy of social Support from family, friends, and significant others. The Inventory of Socially Supportive Behaviour (ISSB) (Barrera, Sandler, & Ramsay, 1981) measures activities directed at assisting in mastering emotional distress, sharing tasks, giving advice, teaching skills, and providing material aid. The Social Support Behaviour (SS-B) (Vaux, 1982, *Measures of three levels of social support: Resources, behaviors and feelings,* unpublished) measures supportive behavior including emotional, socializing, practical assistance, financial assistance, and advice or guidance. The Social Support Appraisals (SS-A) (Vaux, 1982, *Measures of three levels of social support: Resources, behaviors and feelings,* unpublished) measures the degree to which an individual feels cared for, respected, and involved. Three scores are computed, one each for appraisal of family, friends, and others.

Social Support and Mental Health and Well-Being

The link between well-being and social support dates back to Durkheim (1897, 1951). Over the past several decades, the relation between social support, mental health, and well-being has been investigated. There is now an extensive literature on the relationship between social support and mental health showing mostly beneficial effects (see reviews by Berkman, 1995; Berkman, Glass, Brissette, & Seeman, 2000; Seeman, 2000, 2001). Research has demonstrated that social support can reduce the risk of mental illness and improve well-being (e.g., Cohen & Wills, 1985; Hogan, Linden, & Najarian, 2002). Several researchers have reported a negative relation between social support and internalizing problems such as anxiety and depression (Bienenfeld, Koenig, Larson, & Sherill, 1997; Compas, Slavin, Wagner, & Vannatta, 1986; George, 1996; Kahn & Antonucci, 1980; Martire, Stephens, & Townsen, 1998; Russell & Cutrona,

1991). In addition, Demaray and Malecki (2002) found that perceived social support was positively associated with a wide range of positive adjustment indicators such as social skills, self-concept, and adaptive skills; and was negatively associated with problematic behavioral indicators such as externalizing and internalizing behaviors. These results demonstrate that social support can reduce problematic behavior and negative affect as well as promote adjustment. The beneficial impact of social relations on psychosocial functioning has been shown in both cross-sectional and longitudinal designs (see Jakobsson & Hallberg, 2002; Revenson, 1993 for reviews).

Social support has been found to be an important factor in child and adolescent well-being. Overall, research findings have shown that social support is negatively related to depression and anxiety in adolescents (Barrera & Garrison-Jones, 1992; Caldwell, Antonucci, Jackson, Wolford, & Osofsky, 1997; Cheng, 1997, 1998; Compas et al., 1986; Licitra-Kleckler & Waas, 1993; Ostrander, Weinfurt, & Nay, 1998; Patten et al., 1997; White, Bruce, Farrell, & Kliewer, 1998). Furthermore, poor social support has been correlated with high levels of delinquency and poor school performance in high risk students (Rosenfeld, Richman, & Bowen, 1998). Hamburg (1991) suggested that poor social supports are major factors in violence and illegal behavior among adolescents. Conversely, Markstrom, Marshall, and Tryon (2000) found that social support was a significant predictor of resiliency in a sample of low-income Caucasian and African American adolescents. Social support has also been found to be an important variable in predicting hopefulness and self-esteem in adolescents (Yarcheski, Mahon, & Yarcheski, 2001). For families with disabled children, early intervention and development of strong social support networks are strong predictors of well-being and health within the family unit (Dunst, Leet, & Trivelle, 1988; Dunst, Travelle, Hamby, & Pollock, 1990). Finally, Letourneau and colleagues (2001) conducted randomized control trials of providing structured parental social support in 34 families of children at high-risk for mental health problems due to poverty or parents' lack of education and their youth and inexperience. Fewer mental health problems arose when social supports were developed.

Social support may also be especially beneficial for the elderly. Continuous changes, the aging process, chronic illnesses, and multiple losses increase the need for social support in elders (Johnson, 1998). Studies demonstrate that elders with high levels of social support perform more health promotion activities and have higher perceived health status (Adams, Bowden, Humphrey, & McAdams, 2000; Martin & Panicucci, 1996). Much of the research on social support has been done on an individual level, or looking at individuals within the family unit. Fink (1995) found that individuals sought support from within the family unit when caring for elderly parents. Social support, in addition to hardiness and socioeconomic factors, explained 65% of the variance for well-being in family caregivers. However, current research indicates that social support networks may not solely result in benefits for the elderly. For some older individuals, social support may exert a detrimental impact on mental health (Silverstein, Chen, & Heller, 1996).

Social Support, Mental Health, and Minorities

There is an increasing amount of research examining the role of social networks and the effects of social support in blacks, Hispanics, and white families (Hashima & Amato, 1994; Letiecq & Koblinsky, 2003; McLoyd, 1990; Raikes & Thompson, 2005). Kim and McKenry (1998) compared social support and social network patterns in European, American, and three large U.S. ethnic minority groups – Asian Americans, African Americans, and Hispanics. Using a large national data set, the researchers found differences in the salient social activities and social networks of the four groups. Asian Americans were more likely than other groups to spend a social evening with friends and relatives; Asian American and European Americans were most likely to engage in group recreation; African Americans and European Americans were more likely to visit a bar or tavern; and African Americans were most likely to attend a church-related social event. When questioned about borrowing money for an emergency, African American, Hispanic, and Asian Americans were more likely than European Americans to ask children or their own parents for money and were less likely than European Americans to ask for a loan from friends, neighbors, coworkers, siblings, or other relatives. Jayakody, Chatters and Taylor (1993) investigated kin as providers of emotional support, finding that 80% received support from their extended families. Kim and McKenry (1998) also demonstrated that African Americans have larger family networks and receive more support from extended family than European Americans. While Hispanic families also tend to have large, close-knit social networks (MacPhee, Fritz, & Miller-Heyl, 1996; Zambrana, Silva-Palacios, & Powell, 1992), Hispanics may receive less emotional support from their extended families compared to white families (MacPhee et al., 1996).

Higher rates of symptomatology and depressive symptoms among blacks have consistently been found in early research. These higher rates of distress in blacks compared to whites have been attributed to characteristics of their social situation, such as a greater number of life stressors (Kessler, 1979),and higher levels of alienation (Mirowsky & Ross, 1989). Kessler and Neighbors (1986) meta-analyzed data from eight epidemiologic surveys and demonstrated that while controlling for socioeconomic status (SES) reduced the association between race and psychological distress, blacks with lower SES had higher rates of distress than whites with lower SES. More recent, large studies like the Epidemiologic Catchment Area study (ECA) (Robins & Regier, 1991) and the National Comorbidity Study (NCS) (Kessler et al. 1994) have demonstrated that blacks did not have higher rates than whites. In fact, lower rates for blacks than whites were particularly pronounced for the affective disorders (depression) and the substance use disorders (alcohol and drug abuse). However, African Americans are overrepresented in vulnerable, high-need populations because of homelessness, incarceration, and, for children, placement in foster care. The rates of mental illness in high-need populations are much higher. Additionally, African American women report more depressive symptoms than African American men or European American women or men, and these women have a depression rate twice that of European American women (Brown, 1990; Kessler et al., 1994). African American women have a triple jeopardy status which places them at risk for developing depression – their ethnicity, culture, and gender are devalued by the dominant culture (Carrington, 1980; Taylor, 1992). This can intensify the amount of stress in their lives and erode their social support systems and health (Warren, 1994).

According to several studies, such as Hispanic Health and Nutrition Examination Survey (HHANES), the Epidemiologic Catchment Area Study (ECA), and the National Co-morbidity Survey (NCS), Hispanics are at high risk for depressive episodes within their lifetimes, with the NCS reporting that 17.7% of Latinos will suffer from major depression in their lifetimes (Hough, Landsverk, & Karno, 1987). A national study comparing the incidence of mental illness among recent immigrant Mexicans and whites in comparison to their native-born counterparts demonstrated that the immigrants, regardless of ethnicity, experienced fewer mental health disorders (Grant et al., 2004). Using data from the National Latino and Asian American Study, Mulvaney-Day, Alegria & Sribney (2007) explore the relationships of family support, friend support, family cultural conflict, and neighborhood social cohesion with mental health. They found that family support and family cultural conflict were strongly associated with self-rated mental health, but neighborhood social cohesion was not, after controlling for language, education, income, and other demographic measures.

Research findings have suggested that the mental health levels among Asians do not differ significantly from those of the general population. For example, the Chinese American Psychiatric Epidemiological Study (CAPES), a comprehensive epidemiological survey involving the largest number of respondents ever found in a mental health survey of any Asian group in the United States, showed that Chinese in the United States had moderate levels of depressive disorders (7% lifetime and 3% during the past year (U.S. Department of Health and Human Services, 2001). These rates were lower than those found in the general population. However, Pernice, and Brook (1994), in their study of mental health levels among community samples of Indo-Chinese refugees, Pacific Island immigrants, and British immigrants, reported finding higher rates of emotional distress among Indo-Chinese refugees (25%) and Pacific Island immigrants (18%) when compared to British immigrants (4%). The strongest predictors of symptomatology were having experienced discrimination, not having close friends, being unemployed and spending most of one's time with one's own ethnic group (Pernice & Brook, 1996a, 1996b). Abbott, Wong, Williams, Au, and Young (2000) identified risk factors for depression and found that lower emotional support and low dominant cultural orientation increase the risk of being depressed.

Southeast Asian refugees are also at risk for posttraumatic stress disorder associated with the trauma they experienced prior to resettlement (Chung & Kagawa-Singer, 1993). Many Indo-Chinese refugees experienced family separation and its adverse effects at various stages of flight and during resettlement (Beiser, Dion, Gotowiec, Hyman, & Vu., 1995). After resettlement, many Indo-Chinese refugees may be socially and culturally isolated if the local ethnic community is not well established. Social support is a major protective factor, helps newcomers cope with the stress of migration, and reduces the risk of emotional disorders.

Less research has been conducted with Pacific Islanders. Nahulu and colleagues (1996) found that Native Hawaiian adolescents had higher levels of perceived family and friends' support than their non-Hawaiian counterparts (primarily Caucasians, Filipinos, Japanese, and those of mixed ancestry). Gender, ethnicity (Hawaiian vs. non-Hawaiian), family support, friends' support, and discussing problems adequately predicted symptoms of depression and anxiety, accounting for 17% and 16% of the variance, respectively. Utilizing the same database of Hawaiian adolescents, Yuen, Nahulu, Hishinuma, & Miyamoto (1996) found that family support was one of the best predictors of 6-month suicide attempts. Goebert et al. (2000) reported from their examination of a larger data set from this study that for both the Hawaiian and non-Hawaiian groups, family support was the best unique predictor of dichotomized levels of psychiatric symptoms (i.e. depression, anxiety, aggression-conduct problems, substance use) compared to low SES, family discord, family criminality, and poor family health. Using this same data set, Hishinuma et al. (2004) found that the quality of the social supports, including family relations, is related to adolescents' psychiatric adjustment while demographic variables, with particular emphases on ethnicity and culture, must be considered when considering school-related outcomes.

Social Support and Culture

While there is substantial evidence demonstrating the influence of social support on mental health and well-being, there is less research on the cultural context of social support (Taylor et al., 2004). Cultural differences have been shown in the ways in which groups view their relationships and use social support when stressed (Lin, 1999). In more individualistic cultures, such as in the United States, the dominant model of the self is an independent self that regards a person as possessing a set of self-defining attributes, which are used to take action in the expression of personal beliefs and the achievement of personal goals (Markus & Kitayama, 1991; Markus, Mullally, & Kitayama, 1997; Morris & Peng, 1994). Individuals are expected to make their own decisions based on their own volition (Markus & Kitayama, 1991). Relationships also take an independent form and are thought to be freely chosen and with relatively few obligations (Adams & Plaut, 2003). Given that relationships are construed to be voluntary, people from individualistic cultures are encouraged to directly and verbally express their own thoughts and needs (Holtgraves, 1997; Kim & Ko, 2007; Kim & Sherman, 2007). There is also an expectation that others also will reciprocate with responses based on their own volitions and needs. Thus, in the individualistic cultural context, one can ask for social support with relatively little caution; support seeking generally leads to positive outcomes for both receiver and provider, as the voluminous research on social support attests.

By contrast, in more collectivistic cultures, the self-view is one of interdependence. As such, a person is fundamentally connected to others, conforming to relational norms, and viewing group goals as primary and personal beliefs, needs, and goals as secondary (Kim & Markus, 1999; Kitayama & Uchida, 2005; Markus & Kitayama, 1991; Morling, Kitayama, & Miyamoto, 2003; Triandis, 1989). In these cultures, relationships also take an interdependent form in which relationships with others are less voluntary and more prearranged. These interdependent relationships come with a greater sense of obligation (Adams & Plaut, 2003). In this context, bringing personal problems to others for their help is done cautiously (Iyengar, Lepper, & Ross, 1999). Thus, individuals may be extremely cautious about the negative relational implications of asking for social support because they are more concerned about upsetting relationships, disrupting group harmony, and making the problem worse.

Research shows that European Americans are more likely to report needing and receiving social support than are Asians and Asian Americans (Hsieh, 2000; Shin, 2002; Wellisch et al., 1999). Moreover, one study (Liang & Bogat, 1994) found that received social support had negative buffering effects for Asians (i.e., it made Asians feel more stressed). To examine cultural differences in social coping, Taylor et al. (2004) conducted three studies that found that Asians and Asian Americans were significantly less likely to report drawing on social support for coping with stress than were European Americans, a pattern that was especially true for Asian nationals and Asian immigrants. When asked why they might not seek social support or help from others when dealing with a stressor, Asians and Asian Americans indicated that the primary reason was concern with their relationships. Specifically, they indicated that they were concerned about worrying others, disrupting the harmony of the group, losing face, and making the problem worse.

Latino culture emphasizes *familismo*, which involves strong feelings of attachment, shared identity, and loyalty among family members (Marín & Marín, 1991). Latino families are thought to provide emotional support, which protects members against external stressors (Fuligni, Tseng, & Lam, 1999; Vega, Kolody, Valle, & Weir, 1991). Consistent with this notion, better family functioning and emotional support from family members have been linked to lower levels of depressive symptoms among Latino adolescents and adults (Hovey & King, 1996; Vega et al., 1991) and to better emotional adjustment among Latino college students (Schneider & Ward, 2003). Additionally, peer support may be important for Latino college students. Like parents, friends can provide emotional, informational, and instrumental support; however, they are more likely to be immediately available (on campus) and more likely to have information relevant to negotiating the college environment (Rodriguez, Mira, Myers, Monis, & Cardoza, 2003). In line with this hypothesis, studies of Latino college students found that emotional support from peers was associated with better social adjustment (Schneider & Ward, 2003) and that support from friends, but not family, predicted lower psychological distress (Rodriguez et al., 2003).

Social Support and Stress

The benefit of social support in relation to health and well-being may stem from a reduction in the psychological impact of stress, although investigators have also reported direct benefits of support, regardless of stress levels (see Cohen & Wills, 1985, for a review of direct and interactive effects). For example, people with high levels of social support experience less stress when in stressful situations and are able to cope with stress more successfully (Taylor, 1995). Studies have shown that social support provides individuals with security, worthiness, and a sense of identity during times of crisis (Reinhardt, 1996) and decreases feelings of hopelessness (Van Servellen, Sarna, Padilla, & Brecht, 1996). While immigration does not necessarily compromise psychological well-being among immigrants, it can involve factors that are highly stressful such as language barriers, financial difficulties, racial/ethnic discrimination, homesickness, alienation, and loneliness (Dao, Lee, & Chang, 2007; Leong & Chou, 1994; Mori, 2000). The stress process model is frequently used to explain higher rates of psychological distress, anxiety, and depression among immigrant and minority populations.

Scholars have proposed the stress process model as a theoretical approach that highlights the social factors that mediate and moderate the impact of stress on health and well-being. This approach defines stress as a demanding level of environmental strain placed on a person (Wheaton, 1983). The stress process model focuses on stressors, the consequences or outcomes of stress, and mediators (Pearlin, 1989). Historically, researchers have concentrated on two types of stressors – major life events and chronic stressors. Major life events refer to discrete events that are undesired, unplanned, and uncontrolled, typically carrying harmful consequences. Chronic stressors, on the other hand, refer to continuous, ongoing sources of stress, such as conflicts and problems that individuals encounter in their day-to-day lives (Pearlin, Lieberman, Menaghan, & Mullin, 1981). Research suggests that such persistent stress results in more deleterious outcomes than acute events (Aneshensel, 1992). Outcomes refer to the consequences of stress on the individual. Typically, past research has focused on the manifestation of stress on physical and mental health (Pearlin et al., 1981). Stress has been found to impact, the immunological and endocrine systems, anxiety, depression, and mental health and well-being. Mediators are resources that influence how individuals react to stressors. Social support can limit the severity of outcomes that follow a stressor by lessening the detrimental outcomes resulting from individuals' responses to stress, particularly in terms of mortality, as well as physical and mental health (Turner, Frankel, & Levin, 1983; Pearlin, 1989). Social support, which involves the provision of psychological and material resources, may serve as a buffer against stress by preventing a situation from being appraised as stressful in the first place or by providing a solution to a stressful problem, minimizing its perceived importance, or facilitating healthy behavioral responses (Cohen & Wills, 1985; Kessler & McLeod, 1985; Turner & Turner, 1999).

Past research examining the main versus buffering debate has produced mixed results. Some studies have found that social support impacts health regardless of stress level. Other research, however, indicates that social support is only significant during periods of high stress (Turner, 1983, Turner & Noh, 1983). For the most part, research findings suggest that, while social support has a clear impact on mental health status regardless of stress levels, it has a greater impact in times of high stress (Turner & Turner, 1999). There is also evidence of a relationship between an individual's social location (i.e., SES, gender, age, marital status, ethnicity, etc.), social support, and stress. For example, stress is more likely to result in psychological distress among individuals with low SES (Turner & Marino, 1994; Turner & Turner, 1999). Social support partially accounts for the increased susceptibility to stress found among lower-class individuals (Turner & Noh, 1983). However, among the middle-class, social support is a significant predictor of psychological distress, regardless of stress level. Overall, research using the stress process model suggests that the social context in which an individual is located carries important implications for the stress process, including the role that social support plays in this process.

Acculturative Stress

Acculturation is the process by which individuals and their families learn and adopt the language, values, beliefs, attitudes, and behaviors of the dominant sociocultural environment (Berry, 1980; Berry & Sam, 1996; Lee, 1988; Phinney, Horenczyk, Liebkind, & Vedder, 2001; Redfield, Linton, & Herskovitz, 1936). Typically, it refers to immigrants but can also include indigenous peoples. The process of acculturation takes place over time, and it involves changes that result from sustained contact between two distinct cultures (Redfield et al., 1936). Acculturation occurs on both the cultural and psychological levels (Berry, Trimble, & Olmedo, 1986). At the cultural level, acculturation refers to collective changes in social structure, social climate, economic base, and political organization (Berry, Poortinga, Segall, & Dasen, 1992). Psychological acculturation refers to changes in the behaviors, attitudes, values, and identities of individuals (Berry, 1980; Graves, 1967). Making the distinction between the cultural and psychological levels is required for the identification of individual differences in acculturation (Berry, 2003).When examining the relationship between psychological acculturation and specific health issues, researchers often regard acculturation at the cultural level as a confounding factor (Borrayo & Jenkins, 2003).

Psychological acculturation is a core construct in health research among minority ethnic groups (Tomomi, 2006). Substantial evidence has linked psychological acculturation to mental health (Dyal & Dyal, 1981; Murphy, 1977; Shin & Shin, 1999), psychiatric symptoms (Hsu, 1999; Kim, Li, & Kim, 1999; Kirmayer, 2001; Yeh, 2003), and conceptualization of illness (Kim-Goh, 1993; Murguia, Zea, Reisen, & Peterson, 2000; Pang, 1998; Ying, Lee, Tsai, Yeh, & Huang, 2000). Furthermore, research has shown that individuals with a same-ethnicity social network have less distress than those with a weak support system (Beiser, 1999; Fawzy, Fawzy, Arndt, & Pasnau, 1995; Kessler et al., 1994; Terry, Rawle, & Callan-Victor, 1995). It should be noted, however, that several studies have not found evidence that acculturation is distressful (e.g., Inkeles, 1969; Rudmin, 2003). In fact, in a study of 55 samples in 13 nations, Sam, Vedder, Ward, and Horenczyk (2006) found that immigrant adolescents had better mental health than their nonimmigrant classmates. Other researchers have also found that those with close ties to their cultural group tend to suffer more distress compared to those with supports for the dominant culture (Boehnlein et al., 1995; Brugha, 1995).

One of the key processes of acculturation is acculturative stress (Berry, 1980; Born, 1970). Acculturative stress refers to the psychological, somatic, and social difficulties that may accompany acculturation processes. This "psychic conflict" between cultural norms was first noted by Redfield et al. (1936, p. 152). According to Ying, Lee, and Tsai (2000), reframing perspectives from a collective-oriented culture to an individualistic culture presents considerable challenges for individuals. This then may affect an individual's health (Dressler, 1996). Berry, Kim and Williams identified psychological and social factors that may account for levels of acculturative stress such as social support found within the new community – immediate and extended family support networks, SES, pre-migration variables such as adaptive functioning and knowledge of the new language and culture, cognitive attributes, and the degree of tolerance for and acceptance of cultural diversity (Berry & Kim, 1988; Williams & Berry, 1991). Thus, acculturative stress can stem from incongruent cultural values and practices, language difficulties, and discrimination (Gil, Vega, & Dimas, 1994).

Families immigrating to a new country with different cultural values are at risk of facing weaker social support networks than those built in their country of origin (Liu & Li, 2006). Some families may continue to experience strong emotional and instrumental support, whereas others may struggle with a sense of isolation stemming from poverty, language barriers, neighbors from different cultures, and the challenges of adjusting to a new community. Thus, acculturative stress is a significant problem for many minority people (e.g., Berry, Kim, Minde, & Mok, 1983; Burnam, Hough, Karno, Escobar, & Telles, 1987; Hovey, 2000). Although immigrants are most likely to experience this form of stress, it may also be seen in later generations (Mena, Padilla, & Maldonado, 1987; Padilla, Alvarez, & Lindholm, 1986). Because the children of immigrants acculturate more quickly than their parents, second-generation youth may feel caught between the opposing values of their parents and peers or experience conflict between their own values and those of their less acculturated parents (Miranda, Bilot, Peluso, Berman, & Van Meek, 2006; Padilla et al., 1986). Such discrepant expectations can create family tension (Szapocznik, Scopetta, Kurtines, & Arnalde, 1978).

Pressures to assimilate, lack of intercultural competence, or discrimination also can lead to a perception of stress and to negative emotions (Williams & Berry, 1991). Several studies have supported an association between acculturative stress and negative affect such as anxiety or depression. For example, acculturative stress has been linked to more depressive symptoms and anxiety symptoms, as well as higher levels of general psychological distress even after controlling for other forms of stress in adult Latino samples (Hovey & King, 1996; Hovey & Magaña, 2002; Rodriguez, Myers, Morris, & Cardoza, 2000; Salgado de Snyder, 1987). Other research indicates that Latino adolescents and adults experience high levels of depressive and anxiety symptoms, often exceeding levels reported by non-Hispanic whites (e.g., Roberts & Sobhan, 1992; Torres Stone, Rivera, & Berdahl, 2004; Varela et al., 2004).

Research has demonstrated that a well-functioning and supportive family environment serves as a buffer from acculturative stress, particularly in the initial periods of acculturation (Miranda & Matheny, 2000; Cortes, 1995; Miranda, Estrada, & Firpo-Jimenez, 2000). Vega, Hough, and Miranda (1985) proposed a model of Latino mental health in which factors such as social support moderate the relations between stress and adjustment. In their model, persistent strain (e.g., acculturative stress) is more likely to be associated with elevated symptomatology if social support is low. Solberg and Villarreal (1997) found that social support moderated the association between stress and psychological distress among college students reporting low levels of social support but not among those reporting high social support. Finch and Vega (2003) explored the effect of social support mechanisms as potential moderators and mediators between stressful acculturation experiences and health among Mexican immigrants. They found that health was negatively associated with acculturation stressors and positively associated with social support.

Oppedal, Røysamb, and Sam (2004) examined the mediating and moderating roles of social support in the acculturation – mental health link among junior high school students. Acculturation was described in positive terms as a developmental process toward gaining competence within more than one sociocultural setting. Perceived discrimination and ethnic identity crisis were included as risk factors in this process. A model of structural relations was tested, with results supporting an indirect path for the effect of acculturation on mental health change. Based on the integrative concept of social support, Lee, Crittenden, and Yu (1996) investigated the effects of quantitative, structural, and functional aspects of social support on the level of depressive symptoms among elderly Korean immigrants, taking into account their level of acculturation and life stress. They found that Korean elders having more close persons and more frequent contacts with them exhibited fewer depressive symptoms. Furthermore, emotional support was found to moderate the harmful effect of life stress and, thus, to be more relevant than instrumental support to mental health.

Summary

As minority and immigrant populations continue to grow, mental health status becomes not only an integral part of the development of healthy communities but also fundamental to the overall health of our nation. Mental health and well-being must be adequately addressed. Initial signs and symptoms of acculturative stress may include negative psychological consequences, such as emotional distress, depression, and anxiety. Social support appears to be a robust buffer of acculturative stress, making it one of many dimensions that should be examined.

References

Abbott, M. W., Wong, S., Williams, M., Au, M. K., & Young, W. (2000). Recent Chinese migrants' health, adjustment to life in New Zealand and primary health care utilization. *Disability and Rehabilitation, 22*, 43–56.

Adams, M. H., Bowden, A. G., Humphrey, D. S., & McAdams, L. B. (2000). Social support and health-promotion lifestyle of rural women. *Online Journal of Rural Nursing and Health Care, 1*, 1.

Adams, G., & Plaut, V. C. (2003). The cultural grounding of personal relationship: Friendship in North American and West African worlds. *Personal Relationships, 10*, 333–348.

Aneshensel, C. S. (1992). Social stress: Theory and research. *Annual Review of Sociology, 18*, 15–38.

Antonucci, T. C. (1985). Personal characteristics, social support and social behavior. In R. H. Binstock & E. Shanas (Eds.), *Handbook of aging and the social sciences*, (2nd ed., pp. 94–128). New York: Van Nostrand Reinhold.

Antonucci, T. C., Fuhrer, R., & Dartigues, J. F. (1997). Social relations and depressive symptomatology in a sample of community-dwelling French older adults. *Psychology and Aging, 12*, 189–195.

Barrera, M. Jr. (1981). Social support in the adjustment of pregnant adolescents: Assessment issues. In B. H. Gottlieb (Ed.), *Social networks and social support* (pp. 69–96). Beverly Hills: Sage Publications.

Barrera, M. Jr. (1986). Distinctions between social support concepts, measures, and models. *American Journal of Community Psychology, 14*, 413–445.

Barrera, M., Jr., & Garrison-Jones, C. (1992). Family and peer social support as specific correlates of adolescent depressive symptoms. *Journal of Abnormal Child Psychology, 20*, 1–16.

Barrera, M. Jr., Sandler, I. N., & Ramsay, T. B. (1981). Preliminary development of a scale of social support: Studies on college students. *American Journal of Community Psychology, 9*, 435–447.

Beiser, M., Dion, R., Gotowiec, A., Hyman, I., & Vu, N. (1995). Immigrant and refugee children in Canada. *Canadian Journal of Psychiatry, 40*, 67–72.

Berkman, L. F. (1995). The role of social relations in health promotion. *Psychosomatic Medicine, 57*, 245–254.

Berkman, L. F., Glass, T., Brissette, I., & Seeman, T. E. (2000). From social integration to health: Durkheim in the new millennium. *Social Science and Medicine, 51*, 843–857.

Berry, J. W. (1980). Acculturation as varieties of adaptation. In A. Padilla (Ed.), *Acculturation: Theory, models and findings* (pp. 9–25). Boulder: Westview.

Berry, J. W. (2003). Conceptual approaches to acculturation. In K. M. Chun, P. B. Organista, & G. Marin (Eds.), *Acculturation: Advances in theory, measurement and applied research* (pp. 17–36). Washington, DC: American Psychological Association.

Berry, J. W., & Kim, U. (1988). Acculturation and mental health. In P. Dasen, J. W. Berry, & N. Sartorius (Eds.), *Health and cross-cultural psychology: Towards applications* (pp. 207–236). London: Sage.

Berry, J. W., Kim, U., Minde, T., & Mok, D. (1987). Comparative studies of acculturative stress. *International Migration Review, 21*, 491–511.

Berry, J. W., Poortinga, Y. H., Segall, M. H., & Dasen, P. R. (1992). *Cross-cultural psychology: Research and applications*. Cambridge: Cambridge University Press.

Berry, J. W., & Sam, D. (1996). Acculturation and adaptation. In J. W. Berry, M. H. Segall, & C. Kagitcibask (Eds.), *Handbook of cross-cultural psychology: Vol. 3. Social behaviour and applications*. Boston: Allyn & Bacon.

Berry, J. W., Trimble, J. E., & Olmedo, E. L. (1986). Assessment of acculturation. In W. Lonner & J. W. Berry (Eds.), *Field methods in cross-cultural psychology* (pp. 291–324). Beverly Hills, CA: Sage

Bienenfeld, D., Koenig, H. G., Larson, D. B., & Sherrill, K. A. (1997). Psychosocial predictors of mental health in a population of elderly women. Test of an explanatory model. *American Journal of Geriatric Psychiatry 5*, 43–53.

Beiser, M. (1999) Strangers at the Gate: The Boat Peoples' First Ten Years in Canada (Toronto, University of Toronto Press).

Boehnlein, J. K., Tran, H.D., Riley, C., Vu, K.C., Tan, S., & Leung, P.K. (1995). A comparative study of family functioning among Vietnamese and Cambodian Refugees. *Journal of Nervous and Mental Diseases, 183*, 768–773.

Born, D. (1970). Psychological adaptation and development under acculturative stress: Toward a general model. *Social Science & Medicine, 3*, 529–547.

Borrayo, E. A., & Jenkins, S. R. (2003). Feeling frugal: Socioeconomic status, acculturation, and cultural health beliefs among women of Mexican descent. *Cultural Diversity and Ethnic Minority Psychology, 9*, 197–206.

Brown, D. R. (1990). Depression among Blacks: An epidemiological perspective. In D. S. Ruiz & J. P. Comer (Eds.), *Handbook of mental health and mental disorder among Black Americans* (pp. 71–93). New York: Greenwood Press.

Brugha, T. (1995). *Social support and psychiatric disorder: Research findings and guidelines for clinical practice*. London: Cambridge University Press.

Burnam, A., Hough, R. L., Karno, M., Escobar, J. I., & Telles, C. (1987). Acculturation and lifetime prevalence of psychiatric disorders among Mexican Americans in Los Angeles. *Journal of Health & Social Behavior, 28*, 89–102.

Caldwell, C. H., Antonucci, T. C., Jackson, J. S., Wolford, M. L., & Osofsky, J. D. (1997). Perceptions of parental support and depressive symptomatology among black and white adolescent mothers. *Journal of Emotional & Behavioral Disorders, 5*, 173–183.

Carrington, C. H. (1980). Depression in Black women: A theoretical perspective. In L. Rodgers-Rose (Ed.), *The Black woman* (pp. 265–271). Beverly Hills, CA: Sage Publications.

Cheng, C. (1997). Role of perceived social support on depression in Chinese adolescents: A prospective study examining the buffering model. *Journal of Applied Social Psychology, 27*, 800–820.

Cheng, C. (1998). Getting the right kind of support: Functional differences in the types of social support on depression for Chinese adolescents. *Journal of Clinical Psychology, 54*, 845–849.

Chung, R. C., & Kagawa-Singer, M. (1993). Predictors of psychological distress among Southeast Asian refugees. *Social Science and Medicine, 36*, 631–639.

Cobb, S. (1976). Social support as a moderator of life stress. *Psychosomatic Medicine, 38*, 300–314.

Cohen, S., & Syme, S. L. (1985). Issues in the study and application of social support. In S. Cohen & S. L. Syme (Eds.), *Social support and health* (pp. 3–22). San Diego, CA: Academic Press.

Cohen, S., & Wills, T. A. (1985). Stress, social support, and the buffering hypothesis. *Psychological Bulletin 98*(2), 310–357.

Compas, B., Slavin, L., Wagner, B., & Vannatta, K. (1986). Relationship of life events and social support with psychological dysfunction among adolescents. *Journal of Youth & Adolescence, 15*(3), 205–221.

Cortes, D. E. (1995). Variations in familism in two generations of Puerto Ricans. *Hispanic Journal of Behavioral Sciences, 17*, 249–255.

Dao, T. K., Lee, D., & Chang, H. L. (2007). Acculturation level, perceived English fluency, perceived social support level and depression among Taiwanese international students. *College Student Journal, 41*, 287–295.

Demaray, M. K., & Malecki, C. K. (2002). The relationship between perceived social support and maladjustment for student at risk. *Psychology in the School, 39*(3), 305–316.

Dressler, W. W. (1996). Culture, stress, and disease. In S. F. Sargent & T. M. Johnson (Eds.), *Medical anthropology* (pp. 252–271). Westport, CT: Praeger.

Dunst, C. J., Leet, H. E. & Trivelle, C. M. (1988). Family resources, personal well being, and early intervention. *The Journal of Special Education, 22*, 108–116.

Dunst, C. J., Trivelle, C. M., Hamby, D. M., & Pollock, B. (1990). Family systems correlates of the behavior of young children with handicaps. *Journal of Early Intervention, 14*, 204–218.

Durkheim, E. (1897). Le Suicide: Étude de Sociologie. Paris: Alcan. 8vo, pp. 462.

Durkheim, E. (1951). *Suicide.* New York: Free Press. (Originally published 1897).

Dyal, J. A., & Dyal, R. Y. (1981). Acculturation, stress and coping. *International Journal of Intercultural Relations, 5*, 301–328.

Fawzy, F., Fawzy, N., Arndt, L., & Pasnau, R. (1995). Critical review of psychosocial interventions in cancer care. *Archives of General Psychiatry, 52*, 100–113.

Finch, B. K., & Vega, W. A. (2003). Acculturation stress, social support, and self-rated health among Latinos in California. *Journal of Immigrant Health, 5*, 109–117.

Fink, S. V. (1995). The influence of family resources and family demands on the strains and well being of caregiving families. *Nursing Research, 44*, 139–146.

Fischer, C. S. 1982. *To dwell among friends.* Chicago: University of Chicago Press.

Fuligni, A. J., Tseng, V., & Lam, M. (1999). Attitudes toward family obligations among American adolescents with Asian, Latin American, and European backgrounds. *Child Development, 70*, 1030–1044.

George, L. K., (1996). Social and economic factors related to psychiatric disorders in late life. In E. W. Busse & D. G. Blazer (Eds.), *Handbook of geriatric psychiatry* (pp. 129–153). Washington, DC: American Psychiatric Press.

Gil, A. G., Vega, W. A., & Dimas, J. M. (1994). Acculturative stress and personal adjustment among Hispanic adolescent boys. *Journal of Community Psychology, 22*, 43–54.

Goebert, D., Nahulu, L., Hishinuma, E., Bell, C., Yuen, N., Carlton, B., et al. (2000). Cumulative effect of family environment on psychiatric symptomatology among multi-ethnic adolescents. *Journal of Adolescent Health, 27*(1), 34–42.

Grant, B. F., Stinson, F. S., Hasin, D. S., Dawson, D. A., Chou, S. P., & Anderson, K. (2004). Immigration and lifetime prevalence of DSM-IV psychiatric disorders among Mexican

Americans and Non-Hispanic Whites in the United States. *Archives of General Psychiatry*, *61*, 1226–1233.

Graves, T. (1967). Psychological acculturation in a tri-ethnic community. *South-Western Journal of Anthropology*, *23*, 337–350.

Hamburg, D. A. (1991). Health and behavior: An evolutionary perspective on contemporary problems. In R. Jessor (Ed.), *Perspectives on behavioral science – the Colorado lecture* (pp. 177–200). New York: Westview.

Hashima, P. Y., & Amato, P. R. (1994). Poverty, social support, and parental behavior. *Child Development*, *65*, 394–403.

Hill, R. B. (1993). Dispelling myths and building strengths: Supporting African American families. *Family Resource Coalition Report 1*, 3–5.

Hirsch, B. J. (1979). Psychological dimensions of social networks: A multimethod analysis. *American Journal of Community Psychology*, *7*, 263–277.

Hishinuma, E. S., Johnson, R. C., Carlton, B. S., Andrade, N. N., Nishimura, S. T., Goebert, D. A., et al. (2004). Demographic and social variables associated with psychiatric and school–related indicators for Asian/Pacific–Islander adolescents. *International Journal of Social Psychiatry*, *50*, 301–318.

Hogan, B. E., Linden, W., & Najarian, B. (2002). Social support interventions. Do they work? *Clinical Psychology Review*, *22*, 381–440.

Holtgraves, T. (1997). Styles of language use: Individual and cultural variability in conversational indirectness. *Journal of Personality and Social Psychology*, *73*, 624–637.

Hough, R. L., Landsverk, J. A., & Karno, M. (1987). Utilization of health and mental health services by Los Angeles Mexican-American and non-Latino whites. *Archives of General Psychiatry*, *44*, 702–709.

House, J. S. (1981). *Work stress and social support*. Reading, MA: Addison-Wesley.

House, J. S. (1987). Social support and social structure. *Sociological Forum*, *2*, 135–146.

House, J. S., & Kahn, R. L. (1985). Measures and concepts of social support. In S. Cohen & S. L. Syme (Eds.), *Social support and health* (pp. 83–108). New York: Academic Press.

Hovey, J. (2000). Acculturative stress, depression, and suicidal ideation in Mexican Immigrants. *Cultural Diversity and Ethnic Minority Psychology*, *6*, 134–151.

Hovey, J. D., & King, C. A. (1996). Acculturative stress, depression, and suicidal ideation among immigrant and second-generation Latino adolescents. *Journal of the American Academy of Child & Adolescent Psychiatry*, *35*, 1183–1192.

Hovey, J. D., & Magaña, C. G. (2002). Exploring the mental health of Mexican migrant farm workers in the Midwest: Psychological predictors of psychological distress and suggestions for prevention and treatment. *Journal of Psychology 136*, 493–513.

Hsieh, C. (2000). Self-construals, coping, and the culture fit hypothesis: A cross-cultural study. *Dissertation Abstracts International*, *6*(1-B), 588 (UMI No. 95014-309).

Hsu, S. I. (1999). Somatisation among Asian refugees and immigrants as a culturally shaped illness behaviour. *Annals of the Academy of Medicine, Singapore*, *6*, 841–845.

Inkeles, A. (1969). Making men modern: On the causes and consequences of individual change in six developing countries. *American Journal of Sociology*, *75*(2), 208–225.

Iyengar, S. S., Lepper, M. R., & Ross, L. (1999). Independence from whom? Interdependence with whom? Cultural perspectives on ingroups versus outgroups. In D. Prentice & D. Miller (Eds.), *Cultural divides* (pp. 273–301). New York: Sage.

Jakobsson, U., & Hallberg, I. R. (2002). Pain and quality of life among older people with rheumatoid arthritis and/or osteoarthritis: A literature review. *Journal of Clinical Nursing*, *11*, 430–443.

Jayakody, R., Chatters, L. M., & Taylor, R. J. (1993). Family support to single and married African American mothers: The provision of financial, emotional, and child care assistance. *Journal of Marriage and the Family*, *55*, 261–276.

Johnson, J. E. (1998). Stress, social support and health in frontier elders. *Journal of Gerontological Nursing*, *24*(5), 29–35.

Kahn, R. L., & Antonucci, T. C. (1980). Convoys over the life course: Attachment, roles, and social support. *Life-span Development and Behavior, 3*, 253–286.

Kessler, R. C. (1979). Stress, Social Status, and Psychological Distress. *Journal of Health & Social Behaviour, 20*, 259–73.

Kessler, R. C., McGonagle, K. A., Zhao, S., Nelson, C. B., Hughes, M., Eshleman, S., et al. (1994). Lifetime and 12-month prevalence of DSM-III-R Psychiatric Disorders in the United States. *Archives of General Psychiatry, 51*, 8–19.

Kessler, R. C., & McLeod, J. D. (1985). Social support and mental health in community samples. In S. Cohen & S. L. Syme (Eds.), *Social support and health* (pp. 219–240). New York: Academic Press.

Kessler, R. C., & Neighbors, H. W. (1986). A new perspective on the relationships among race, social class and psychological distress. *Journal of Health and Social Behavior, 27*, 107–115.

Kim, H. S., & Ko, D. (2007). Culture and self-expression. In C. Sedikides & S. Spencer (Eds.), *Frontiers of social psychology: The self* (pp. 325–342). New York: Psychology Press.

Kim, K., Li, D., & Kim, D. (1999). Depressive symptoms in Koreans, Korean-Chinese and Chinese: A transcultural study. *Transcultural Psychiatry, 36*(3), 303–316.

Kim, H., & Markus, H. R. (1999). Deviance or uniqueness, harmony or conformity? A cultural analysis. *Journal of Personality and Social Psychology, 77*, 785–800.

Kim, H. K., & McKenry, P. C. (1998). Social networks and support: A comparison of African Americans, Asian Americans, Caucasians, and Hispanics. *Journal of Comparative Family Studies, 29*, 313–334.

Kim, H. S., & Sherman, D. K. (2007). "Express yourself": Culture and the effect of self-expression on choice. *Journal of Personality and Social Psychology, 92*, 1–11.

Kim-Goh, M. (1993). Conceptualization of mental illness among Korean-American clergymen and implications for mental health service delivery. *Community Mental Health Journal, 29*, 405–412.

Kirmayer, L. D. (2001). Cultural variations in the clinical presentation of depression and anxiety: Implications for diagnosis and treatment. *Journal of Clinical Psychiatry, 62*, 22–30.

Kitayama, S., & Uchida, Y. (2005). Interdependent agency: An alternative system for action. In R. M. Sorrentino & D. Cohen (Eds.), *The Ontario symposium: Vol 10. Cultural and social behavior* (pp. 137–164). Mahwah, NJ: Erlbaum.

Koblinsky, S. A., & Anderson, E. A. (1993). Serving homeless children and families in Head Start. *Children Today, 2*, 19–23, 36.

Lee, E. (1988). Cultural factors in working with Southeast Asian refugee adolescents. *Journal of Adolescence, 11*, 167–179.

Lee, M. S., Crittenden, K. S., & Yu, E. (1996). Social support and depression among elderly Korean immigrants in the United States. *International Journal of Aging & Human Development, 42*(4), 313–327.

Leong, F. L., & Chou, E. L. (1994). The role of ethnic identity and acculturation in the vocational behavior of Asian Americans: An integrative review. *Journal of Vocational Behavior, 44*, 155–172.

Letiecq, B. L., & Koblinsky, S. A. (2003). African American fathering of young children in violent neighborhoods: Paternal protective strategies and their predictors. *Fathering, 1*(3), 215–238.

Letourneau, N., Drummond, J., Fleming, D., Kysela, G. M., McDonald, L., & Stewart, M. (2001). Supporting parents: Can intervention improve parent-child relationships. *Journal of Family Nursing, 7*(2), 159–187.

Liang, B., & Bogat, G. A. (1994). Culture, control, and coping: New perspectives on social support. *American Journal of Community Psychology, 22*, 123–147.

Licitra-Kleckler, D. M., & Waas, G. A. (1993). Perceived social support among high-stress adolescents: The role of peers and family. *Journal of Adolescent Research, 8*, 381–402.

Lin, N. (1999). Social networks and status attainment. *Annual Review of Sociology, 23*, 467–487.

Liu, T. C., & Li, C. (2006). *Psychoeducation interventions with Southeast Asian students: An ecological approach.* Retrieved March 1, 2008, from www.ncela.gwu.edu/pathways/asian/Southeast.htm

MacPhee, D., Fritz, J., & Miller-Heyl, J. (1996). Ethnic variations in personal social networks and parenting. *Child Development, 67,* 3278–3295.

Malecki, C. K., Demaray, M. K., & Elliott, S. N. (2000). A working manual on the Development of the Child and Adolescent Social Support Scale – CASS 2000. DeKalb, IL: Northern Illinois University.

Marín, G., & Marín, B. V. (1991). *Research with Hispanic populations.* Newbury Park, CA: Sage.

Markstrom, C. A., Marshall, S. K., & Tryon, R. J. (2000). Resiliency, social support, and coping in rural low-income Appalachian adolescents from two racial groups. *Journal of Adolescence, 23,* 693–709.

Markus, H. R., & Kitayama, S. (1991). Culture and the self: Implications for cognition, emotion, and motivation. *Psychological Review, 98,* 224–253.

Markus, H. R., Mullally, P., & Kitayama, S. (1997). Selfways: Diversity in modes of cultural participation. In U. Neisser & D. A. Jopling (Eds.), *The conceptual self in context: Culture, experience, self-understanding* (pp. 13–61). Cambridge, UK: Cambridge University Press.

Martin, J. C., & Panicucci, C. L. (1996). Health-related practices and priorities: The health behaviors and beliefs of community-living Black older women. *Journal of Gerontological Nursing, 22,* 411–448.

Martire, L. M., Stephens, M. A., & Townsend, A. L. (1998). Emotional support and well being of mid-life women: Role specific mastery as a mediational mechanism. *Psychology & Aging, 13*(3), 396–404.

McFarlane, A. H., Neale, K. A., Norman, G. R., Roy, R. G., & Streiner, D. L. (1981). Methodological issues in developing a scale to measure social support. *Schizophrenia Bulletin, 7,* 90–100.

McLoyd, V. C. (1990). The impact of economic hardship on Black families and children: Psychological distress, parenting, and socio-emotional development. *Child Development, 61,* 311–346.

Mena, F. J., Padilla, A. M., & Maldonado, M. (1987). Acculturative stress and specific coping strategies among immigrant and later generation college students [Special issue]. *Hispanic Journal of Behavioral Sciences, 9,* 207–225.

Miranda, A. O., Bilot, J. M., Peluso, P. R., Berman, K., & Van Meek, L. G. (2006). Latino families: The relevance of the connection among acculturation, family dynamics, and health for family counseling research and practice. *The Family Journal: Counseling and Therapy for Couples and Families, 14,* 268–273.

Miranda, A. O., Estrada, E., & Firpo-Jimenez, M. (2000). Differences in family cohesion, adaptability, and environment among Latino families in dissimilar stages of acculturation. *Family Journal: Counseling & Therapy for Couples & Families, 8,* 341–350.

Miranda, A. O., & Matheny, K. B. (2000). Socio-psychological predictors of acculturative stress among Latino adults. *Journal of Mental Health Counseling, 22,* 306–317.

Mirowsky, J., & Ross, C. E. (1989). *Social causes of psychological distress.* New York: Aldine de Gruyter.

Mori, S. (2000). Addressing the mental health concerns of international students. *Journal of Counseling and Development, 78,* 137–144.

Morling, B., Kitayama, S., & Miyamoto, Y. (2003). American and Japanese women use different coping strategies during normal pregnancy. *Personality and Social Psychology Bulletin, 29,* 1533–1546.

Morris, M. W., & Peng, K. (1994). Culture and cause: American and Chinese attributions for social and physical events. *Journal of Personality and Social Psychology, 67,* 949–971.

Mulvaney-Day, N. E., Alegria, M., & Sribney, W. (2007). Social cohesion, social support, and health among Latinos in the United States. *Social Science & Medicine, 64,* 477–495.

Murguia, A., Zea, M. C., Reisen, C. A., & Peterson, R. A. (2000). The development of the Cultural Health Attributions Questionnaire (CHAQ). *Cultural Diversity and Ethnic Minority Psychology, 6*, 268–283.

Murphy, H. B. M. (1977). Migration, culture and mental health. *Psychological Medicine, 7*, 677–684.

Nahulu, L. B., McDermott, J. F., Jr., Andrade, N. N., Danko, G. P., Makini, G. K. Jr., Johnson, R. C., et al. (1996). Psychosocial risk and protective influences in Hawaiian adolescent psychopathology. *Cultural Diversity and Mental Health, 2*, 107–114.

Oppedal, B., Røysamb, E., & Sam, D. L. (2004). The effect of acculturation and social support on change in mental health among young immigrants *International Journal of Behavioral Development, 28*, 481–494.

Ostrander, R., Weinfurt, K. P., & Nay, W. R. (1998). The role of age, family support, and negative cognitions in the prediction of depressive symptoms. *School Psychology Review, 27*, 121–137.

Padilla, A. M., Alvarez, M., & Lindholm, K. J. (1986). Generational status and personality factors as predictors of stress in students. *Hispanic Journal of Behavioral Sciences, 8*, 275–288.

Pang, K. Y. C. (1998). Symptoms of depression in elderly Korean immigrants: Narration and the healing process. *Culture, Medicine and Psychiatry, 22*, 93–122.

Patten, C. A., Gillin, C., Farkas, A. J., Gilpin, E., Berry, C. C., & Pierce, J. P. (1997). Depressive symptoms in California adolescents: Family structure and parental support. *Journal of Adolescent Health, 20*, 271–278.

Pearlin, L. I. (1989). The sociological study of stress. *Journal of Health & Social Behavior, 30*, 241–256.

Pearlin, L. I., Lieberman, M. A., Menaghan, E. G., & Mullin, J. T. (1981). The stress process. *Journal of Health & Social Behavior, 22*, 337–356.

Pernice, R., & Brook, J. (1994). Relationship of migrant status (refugee or immigrant) to mental health. *International Journal of Social Psychiatry, 40*, 177–188.

Pernice, R., & Brook, J. (1996a). Refugees' and immigrants' mental health: Association of demographic and post-migration factors. *Journal of Social Psychology, 136*(4), 511–519.

Pernice, R., & Brook, J. (1996b). The mental health pattern of migrants: Is there a euphoric period followed by a mental health crisis? *International Journal of Social Psychiatry, 42*(1), 18–27.

Phinney, J., Horenczyk, G., Liebkind, K., & Vedder, P. (2001). Ethnic identity, immigration, and well-being: An interaction perspective. *Journal of Social Issues, 57*, 493–510.

Procidano, M. E., & Heller, K. (1983). Measures of perceived social support from friends and from family: Three validation studies. *American Journal of Community Psychology, 11*, 1–24.

Raikes, H. A., & Thompson, R. A. (2005). Efficacy and social support as predictors of parenting stress among families in poverty. *Infant Mental Health Journal, 26*, 177–190.

Redfield, R., Linton, R., & Herskovitz, M. (1936). Memorandum on the study of acculturation. *American Anthropologist, 38*, 149–152.

Reinhardt, J. P. (1996). The importance of friendship and family support in adaptation to chronic vision impairment. *Journal of Gerontology: Psychological Sciences, 5*, 268–278.

Revenson, T. A. (1993). The role of social support with rheumatic disease. *Baillieres Clinical Rheumatology, 7*, 377–396.

Roberts, R. E., & Sobhan, M. (1992). Symptoms of depression in adolescence: A comparison of Anglo, African, and Hispanic Americans. *Journal of Community Psychology, 25*, 639–651.

Robins, L. N., & Regier, D. A., (Eds.). (1991). *Psychiatric disorders in America: The Epidemiologic Catchment Area Study*. New York: Free Press.

Rodriguez, N., Mira, C. B., Myers, H. E., Monis, J. K., & Cardoza, D. (2003). Family or friends: Who plays a greater supportive role for Latino college students? *Cultural Diversity & Ethnic Minority Psychology, 9*, 236–250.

Rodriguez, N., Myers, H. F., Morris, J. K., & Cardoza, D. (2000). Latino college student adjustment: Does an increased presence offset minority-status and acculturative stresses? *Journal of Applied Social Psychology, 30*, 1523–1550.

Rosenfeld, L. B., Richman, J. M., & Bowen, G. L. (1998). Low social support among at-risk adolescents. *Social Work in Education, 20*, 245–260.

Rudmin, F. W. (2003). Critical history of the acculturation psychology of assimilation, separation, integration, and marginalization. *Review of General Psychology, 7*(1), 3–37.

Rudmin, F. W. (2006). Debate in science: The case of acculturation. *AnthroGlobe Journal.* Retrieved March 1, 2008 from http://www.anthroglobe.ca/docs/rudminf-acculturation-061204.pdf

Russell, D. W., & Cutrona, C. E. (1991). Social support, stress, and depressive symptoms among the elderly: Test of a process model. *Psychology and Aging, 6*, 190–201.

Salgado de Snyder, V. N. (1987). Factors associated with acculturative stress and depressive symptomatology among married Mexican immigrant women [Special issue]. *Psychology of Women Quarterly, 11*, 475–488.

Sam, D. L., Vedder, P., Ward, C., Horenczyk, G., Berry, J. W., & Phinney, J. S. (2006). Immigrant youth in cultural transition: Acculturation, identity, and adaptation across national contexts. In D. L. Sam & P. Vedder (Eds.), *Psychological and sociocultural adaptation of immigrant youth* (pp. 117–141). Mahwah, NJ: Lawrence Erlbaum.

Sarason, I. G., Levine, H. M., Bashman, R. B., & Sarason, B. R. (1983). Assessing social support: The Social Support Questionnaire. *Journal of Personality and Social Psychology, 44*(1), 127–139.

Schneider, M. E., & Ward, D. J. (2003). The role of ethnic identification and perceived social support in Latinos' adjustment to college. *Hispanic Journal of Behavioral Sciences, 25*, 539–554.

Seeman, T. E. (2000). Health promoting effects of friends and family on health outcomes in older adults. *American Journal of Health Promotion, 14*, 362–370.

Seeman, T. E. (2001). How do others get under our skin? Social relationships and health. In C. D. Ruff & B. H. Singer (Eds.), *Emotion, social relationships, and health* (pp. 189–210). New York: Oxford University Press.

Shin, J. Y. (2002). Social support for families of children with mental retardation: Comparison between Korea and the United States. *Mental Retardation, 40*, 103–118.

Shin, K. R., & Shin, C. (1999). The lived experience of Korean immigrant women acculturating into the United States. *Health Care for Women International, 20*, 603–617.

Silverstein, M., Chen, X., & Heller, K. (1996). Too much of a good thing? Intergenerational social support and the psychological well-being of aging parents. *Journal of Marriage and the Family, 58*, 970–982.

Solberg, V. S., & Villarreal, P. (1997). Examination of self-efficacy, social support, and stress as predictors of psychological and physical distress among Hispanic college students. *Hispanic Journal of Behavioral Sciences, 19*, 182–201.

Szapocznik, J., Scopetta, M. A., Kurtines, W. M., & Arnalde, M. A. (1978). Theory and measurement of acculturation. *Inter-American Journal of Psychology, 12*, 113–130.

Taylor, S. E. (1992). The mental health status of Black Americans: An overview. In R. L. Braithwate & S. E. Taylor (Eds.), *Health issues in the Black community* (pp. 20–34). San Francisco, CA: Jossey-Bass Publishers.

Taylor, S. E. (1995). *Health psychology* (3rd ed.). New York: McGraw Hill.

Taylor, S. E., Sherman, D. K., Kim, H. S., Jarcho, J., Takagi, K., & Dunagan, M. S. (2004). Culture and social support: Who seeks it and why. *Journal of Personality and Social Psychology, 87*, 354–362.

Terry, D. J., Rawle, R., & Callan-Victor, J. (1995). The effects of social support on adjustment to stress: The mediating role of coping. *Personal Relationships, 2*, 97–124.

Thoits, P. A. (1982). Conceptual, methodological, and theoretical problems in studying social support as a buffer against life stress. *Journal of Health and Social Behavior, 23*, 145–159.

Tomomi, M. (2006). Measures of psychological acculturation: A Review. *Transcultural Psychiatry, 43*(3), 462–483.

Torres Stone, R. A., Rivera, F., & Berdahl, T. (2004). Predictors of depression among non-Hispanic Whites, Mexicans and Puerto Ricans: A look at race/ethnicity as a reflection of social relations. *Race and Society, 7,* 79–94.

Triandis, H. C. (1989). The self and social behavior in differing cultural contexts. *Psychological Review, 96,* 506–520.

Turner, R. J. (1981). Social support as a contingency in psychological well-being. *Journal of Health and Social Behavior, 22,* 357–367.

Turner, R. (1983) Direct, indirect, and moderating effects of social support upon psychological distress and associated conditions. In B. Kaplan (Ed.). *Psychological stress* (pp. 105–155), New York: Academic Press.

Turner, R. J., Frankel, B. G., & Levin, D. M. (1983). Social support: Conceptualization, measurement, and implications for mental health. *Research in Community and Mental Health, 3,* 67–111.

Turner, R. J., & Marino, F. (1994). Social support and social structure: A descriptive epidemiology. *Journal of Health and Social Behavior, 35,* 193–212.

Turner, R. J., & Noh, S. (1983). Class and psychological vulnerability among women: The significance of social support and personal control. *Journal of Health & Social Behavior, 24,* 2–15.

Turner, R. J., & Turner, J. B. (1999). Social integration and support. In C. C. Aneshensel, S. Carol, & J. C. Phelan (Eds.), *Handbook of the sociology of mental health* (pp. 301–319). New York: Kluwer/Plenum.

U.S. Census Bureau. (2004). U.S. interim projections by age, sex, race, and Hispanic origin. Retrieved September 25, 2008, from http://www.census.gov/ipc/www/usinterimproj/

U.S. Department of Health and Human Services. Office of the Surgeon General. Substance Abuse and Mental Health Services Administration. (2001). *Mental health: Culture, race, and ethnicity. A supplement to mental health: A report of the Surgeon General* [(SMA)-013613].Rockville, MD: Authors.

Van Servellen, G., Sarna, L., Padilla, G., & Brecht, M. L. (1996). Emotional distress in men with life-threatening illnesses. *International Journal of Nursing Studies, 33,* 551–565.

Varela, R. E., Vernberg, E. M., Sanchez-Sosa, J. J., Riveros, A., Mitchell, M., & Mashunka-shey, J. (2004). Anxiety reporting and culturally associated interpretation biases and cognitive schemas: A comparison of Mexican, Mexican American, and European American families. *Journal of Clinical Child and Adolescent Psychology, 33,* 237–247.

Vaux, A. (1988). *Social support: Theory, Research and intervention.* New York: Praeger.

Vaux, A. (1990). An ecological approach to understanding and facilitating social support. *Journal of Social and Personal Relationships, 7,* 507–518.

Vega, W. A., Hough, R. L., & Miranda, M. R. (1985). Modeling crosscultural research in Hispanic mental health. In W. A. Vega & M. R. Miranda, (Eds.), *Stress & Hispanic mental health: Relating research to service delivery* (pp. 1–29). Rockville, MD: National Institute of Mental Health.

Vega, W. A., Kolody, B., Valle, R., & Weir, J. (1991). Social networks, social support, and their relationship to depression among immigrant Mexican women. *Human Organization, 50,* 154–162.

Warren, B. J. (1994). The experience of depression for African-American women. In B. J. McElmurry & R. S. Parker (Eds.), *Second annual review of women's health* (pp. 267–283). New York: National League for Nursing Press.

Wellisch, D., Kagawa-Singer, M., Reid, S. L., Lin, Y., Nishikawa-Lee, S., & Wellisch, M. (1999). An exploratory study of social support: A cross-cultural comparison of Chinese-, Japanese-, and Anglo-American breast cancer patients. *Psycho-Oncology, 8,* 207–219.

Wheaton, B. (1983). Stress, personal coping resources, and psychiatric symptoms: An investigation of interactive models. *Journal of Health and Social Behavior, 24,* 208–229.

White, K. S., Bruce, S. E., Farrell, A. D., & Kliewer, W. (1998). Impact of exposure to community violence on anxiety: A longitudinal study of family social support as a protective factor for urban children. *Journal of Child & Family Studies, 7*, 187–203.

Williams, P., Barclay, L., & Schmied, V. (2004). Defining social support in context: A necessary step in improving research, intervention, and practice. *Qualitative Health Research, 14*, 942–960.

Williams, C. L., & Berry, J. W. (1991). Primary prevention of acculturative stress among refugees: Application of psychological theory and practice. *American Psychologist, 46*, 632–641.

Yarcheski, A., Mahon, N. E., & Yarcheski, T. J. (2001). Social support and well-being in early adolescents: The role of mediating variables. *Clinical Nursing Research, 10*, 163–181.

Yeh, C. J. (2003). Age, acculturation, cultural adjustment, and mental health symptoms of Chinese, Korean, and Japanese immigrants youths. *Cultural Diversity and Ethnic Minority Psychology, 9*, 34–48.

Ying, Y., Lee, P. A. & Tsai, J. L. (2000). Cultural orientation and racial discrimination: Predictors of coherence in Chinese American young adults. *Journal of Community Psychology, 28*, 427–442.

Ying, Y. W., Lee, P. A., Tsai, J. L., Yeh, Y. Y., & Huang, J. S. (2000). The conception of depression in Chinese American college students. *Cultural Diversity and Ethnic Minority Psychology, 6*, 183–195.

Yuen, N. Y. C., Nahulu, L. B., Hishinuma, E. S., & Miyamoto, R. H. (1996). Cultural identification and attempted suicide in Native Hawaiian adolescents. *Journal of the American Academy of Child and Adolescent Psychiatry, 39*(3), 360–367.

Zambrana, R. E., Silva-Palacios, V., & Powell, D. R. (1992). Parenting concerns, family support systems and life problems in Mexican-origin women: A comparison by nativity. *Journal of Community Psychology, 20*, 276–288.

Zimet, G. D., Dahlem, N. W., Zimet, S. G., et al. (1988). The multidimensional scale of perceived social support. *Journal of Personality Assessment, 52*, 30–41.

Chapter 8
Religion and Mental Health Among Minorities and Immigrants in the U.S.

Anahí Viladrich and Ana F. Abraído-Lanza

Introduction

The impact of religion on mental health has long been debated, with religious organizations being the first that offered care to the mentally ill (Koening & Larson, 2001). And although until not so long ago religious beliefs and practices were considered to have pernicious effects on health, more recent research has pointed out the positive effects of religion and spirituality on both physical and mental health outcomes (see Holt & McClure, 2006; Seybold & Hill, 2001). National and international studies have shown the positive influence on psychological and physical health derived from church attendance and religious affiliation amidst diverse religious faiths (Campbell et al., 2007; Kark et al., 2006).[1] In the last decades, a prolific body of research on religion and mental health has been undertaken by various disciplines, ranging from the medical and health fields to the social sciences and humanities (e.g., religion studies). Innovative studies on diverse ethnic communities in the U.S. have assessed the role of local worship communities (including Catholic churches, Hindu temples, mosques, and Protestant congregations), in promoting civic engagement and in providing spiritual and social support to their members (see Foley & Hoge, 2007; Menjívar, 2006; Kim, 2002).

Despite this fertile literature, the pathways linking religiosity to both mental and physical health are not well understood, and additional research is needed on the potential mechanisms leading to both salubrious and detrimental health outcomes (Dull & Skokan, 1995; George, Ellison, & Larson, 2002; Holt & McClure, 2006; Shreve-Neiger & Edelstein, 2004). Caution is also recommended when assuming religious-health associations that may lead to erroneous conclusions regarding the role of faith in healing (Levin, Chatters, & Taylor, 2005). This is of particular importance when addressing the mental

A. Viladrich (✉)
The School of Health Sciences, The Schools of the Health Professions, Hunter College of the City of New York, School of Health Sciences, New York, NY
e-mail: aviladri@hunter.cuny.edu

S. Loue, M. Sajatovic (eds.), *Determinants of Minority Mental Health and Wellness*, DOI 10.1007/978-0-387-75659-2_8,
© Springer Science+Business Media, LLC 2009

health needs of minority groups, given their racial/ethnic, cultural and national differences (Loewenthal, 2007). Not only are religion and religiosity multi-dimensional constructs, but they also vary across cultures as shown in the anthropological and psychiatric literature (Kleinman, 1980).

Although religion and spirituality refer to different constructs, these concepts are often used interchangeably (Loue & Sajatovic, 2006; Fetzer Institute, 1999). Spirituality is mostly understood as the subjective side of the religious experience, defined as a search for an inward essential meaning toward a sense of transcendence and connection with others, including nature and/or a supreme being. This definition in itself may or may not involve adherence to religious structure or traditions (Chan, Ng, Ho, & Chow, 2006, Buck, 2006). Religion, on the other hand, is more often conceptualized as the operational dimension of faith (Loue & Sajatovic, 2006; Fowler, 1981) commonly used to represent the formal and institutional expression of the sacred outside the inner experience (Koenig, McCullough & Larson 2001). Even though religion and spirituality constitute two different theoretical concepts some argue that in practice, this separation becomes a misleading artifact. In fact, Hill and Pargament (2003) and Hill et al. (2000) point out that these are related rather that independent constructs and that their distinction ignores the organized forms that all spiritual experience takes places in a social context – meaning the religious domain.[2] Nevertheless, the notion of spirituality as a clearly separated sphere from religiosity may be relevant particularly when dealing with non-Western philosophies of thought, in which the notion of *spirit* has a unique and discrete meaning, as shown by research on minorities in the U.S., including native Americans, African Americans, and many immigrant populations including Latinos (see Holt & McClure, 2006; King, Burgess, Akinyela, Counts-Spriggs, Parker, 2005; Walters & Simoni, 2002).

Part of the discrepancies noted above reflect wide disparities in the measurement of religiosity and spirituality, with constructs that often overlap and lead to artificial simplifications, as in the case of single scales used to examine the effect of complex religious and spiritual beliefs (Fetzer Institute, 1999). As Loue and Sajatovic (2006) note, even when differences between religion and spirituality are provided, there is often an enormous variability regarding the definitions and operationalizations used. These distinctions become even more complex when addressing the religious and spiritual beliefs and practices of diverse ethnic communities, which hold their own indigenous conceptualizations of health and unique explanatory models of disease (Kleinman, 1980). For the purpose of analyzing the main trends in the literature on religion and religiosity, in this piece, we use the terms religion, religiosity, and spirituality interchangeably unless noted otherwise.

This chapter provides a brief overview of some of the most important research trends regarding the role of religion on the mental health of minorities in the U.S. To that end, we rely on two complementary perspectives: the analysis of community-level dimensions, specifically, the role of churches in service-delivery and religious counseling, and an individual-level examination of religiosity, including religious coping in the context of chronic illness. The bulk of our literature review particularly emphasizes mental health service delivery both from "traditional" institutions (i.e., churches) and "non-traditional" sources (i.e., folk healers). We begin by examining general theories on religion and health that are particularly relevant to ethnic minorities and immigrants in the U.S. We then discuss the literature on religiosity and religious coping to highlight research endeavors toward understanding patients' resilience in resisting and fighting illness and pain. Although there has been a great deal of work on formal mental health services for minorities in the U.S., we address the provision of alternative healing resources in the form of organized religion and folk healing practitioners. To that end, we first examine the importance of churches in meeting minorities' needs, with special attention to the role of the clergy as ad hoc mental health counselors. Second, we focus on the cultural variations of religious healing in mental health, for which we examine a specific case study: the role of Latino healers in providing informal mental health care services to the Latino population in New York City (NYC). We finally discuss some of our main findings and suggest implications for future research taking into account the vast, and complex, pathways that link religion with the mental health of minorities in the U.S.

Overview of Theories or Models on the Effect of Religiosity on Health

Recent reviews of the literature provide excellent summaries of theories and models proposed to explain the associations between religiosity and health (Chatters, 2000; George et al., 2002; Thoresen & Harris, 2002; see also a special issue of the *American Psychologist*, volume 58, number 1, 2003). Our intent here is to provide a brief overview of these theories particularly regarding minorities' mental health stressors and outcomes. We explicitly focus on behavioral, social, cognitive, psychological coping processes, and structural explanations for which there is some research relevant to ethnically diverse populations. Importantly, the models we describe below are not mutually exclusive, and a variety of factors may interact to produce salubrious outcomes. For example, social processes can interact with cognitive beliefs, as in cases where emotional support or tangible assistance from clergy leads to a greater sense of comfort and less psychological distress. We should also note that our focus on psychosocial and structural explanations excludes the discussion of other models, such as physiological (e.g., Seeman, Dubin, & Seeman, 2003; Dull & Skokan, 1995), and other more controversial mechanisms, for which there is limited research (e.g., divine intervention, as examined in studies of "intercessory prayers"; for a brief discussion see Thoresen & Harris, 2002, p. 8).

Behavioral Explanations

Behavioral theories suggest that religious individuals engage in healthier behaviors and lifestyles than do those who are less religious. According to these theories, proscriptions against risky behaviors, internalized moral codes, or adherence to other religious, philosophical doctrines (e.g., the belief that the body is the "temple of the Holy Spirit", see Hill, Ellison, Burdette, & Musick, 2007, p. 220) may lead to better health outcomes. For example, relative to other denominations, there are lower rates of cardiovascular disease and lung cancer among members of specific groups (e.g., the Church of Jesus Christ of Latter Day Saints) with strong proscriptions against smoking, a risk factor for these diseases (see Dull & Skokan, 1995; Levin, 1994). Behavioral theories do not focus exclusively on denominational characteristics, however. Instead, there is evidence that religiosity is associated with healthier behaviors in the general population. For example, Strawbridge, Shema, Cohen, and Kaplan (2001) analyzed data spanning 29 years from the Alameda County Study, a large, randomized household survey of residents living east of San Francisco Bay. Relative to those who attend less frequently, or not at all, individuals who seek weekly religious services are more likely to improve poor health behaviors, specifically, to quit smoking, become physically active, not become depressed, and increase social relationships. These relationships, however, are more evident in women than in men. Despite the longitudinal design and large sample size, ethnic minorities constituted only 15% of the sample in Strawbridge et al.'s (2001) study.

Although most studies on this issue focus on Whites, there is evidence that religiosity is associated with healthy behaviors among ethnic minorities. For example, in a large, multiethnic, statewide probability sample of Texas adults (N = 1,504), Hill et al. (2007) investigated, the hypothesis that involvement in religious activities is associated with healthier lifestyles. They assessed religious involvement with an index of six public (e.g., attendance of religious services) and private forms of religiosity (e.g., prayer, reading the Bible). A healthy lifestyle measure was assessed as an index of 12 items that included health promoting, risk, and screening behaviors (e.g., exercising, smoking, obtaining dental examinations). Adjusting for potential confounders, religious involvement was associated with healthier behaviors. Importantly, the effect did not vary by either gender or ethnic group (Blacks, Mexicans, other race/ethnicity, or non-Hispanic Whites), indicating that the association between religious involvements is similar for all groups. Therefore, despite the paucity of research on ethnic minorities, existing evidence supports the hypothesis that religious ethnic minority individuals engage in healthier behaviors than do those who are less religious.

Social Support and Social Capital

Another class of explanations focuses on social processes. A vast literature documents the beneficial effects of social support on physical and psychological well-being (Wills & Filer Fagen, 2001). Social support is conceptualized and measured in numerous ways, including the number of individuals in a social network, the resources that they provide, the adequacy of or satisfaction with those relationships or of their availability, a subjective perception by the recipient, or an observable behavior. A related concept is social capital, which is defined broadly as the aspects of social structures that provide resources to individuals (Kawachi & Berkman, 2000). Measures of social capital include membership and engagement in civic associations, levels of interpersonal trust, and perceptions of reciprocity. There is a growing body of evidence that social capital is an important resource for promoting health and well-being. Social capital may operate via several mechanisms, including the mobilization of social support, promotion of healthy behaviors, and other psychosocial processes (Kawachi & Berkman, 2000).

Because many religious denominations foster social networks through regular gatherings in places of worship (e.g., churches, synagogues, and mosques), the social support derived from being a member of a congregation could bestow a number of health benefits. Moreover, in at least two ways, religious support from congregation members, clergy, or other religious leaders might be qualitatively different from and provide added benefits over other sources of support (Hill & Pargament, 2003). First, although individual members of a congregation might change, the institutional and social structures remain, providing stable sources of support throughout the life course, through a "support convoy" process (Kahn & Antonucci, 1980; Hill & Pargament, 2003). Second, the religious content of the support (e.g., being surrounded by individuals who share a similar philosophy of life or world view, or who offer prayers) might provide additional comfort or other psychological benefits (Hill & Pargament, 2003). The social supportive functions of religious institutions might be particularly important for immigrants, for whom the need to reestablish social networks is a major source of psychological distress (Perez Foster, 2001). Nevertheless, the extent to and mechanisms by which religious organizations assist immigrants in rebuilding family and social networks deserves further investigation. We discuss some of these issues in the section on churches below.

Cognitive Processes

Various cognitive mechanisms are proposed to explain the relationship between religiosity and health (Dull & Skokan, 1995; George et al., 2002). Religious beliefs might offer a specific philosophy of life or worldview (Pargament, 1997). These belief systems could engender a sense of direction, purpose, and comfort. Spiritual frameworks could provide motivation and direction for living, especially during difficult times. Religious worldviews can also offer adaptive belief systems that can be useful particularly when confronting stressful circumstances. For example, religion is hypothesized to enhance a sense of control over stressful events (Dull & Skokan, 1995). For the faithful, for example,

prayer is a way of exerting some influence over the course of events (by achieving a sense of closeness with God or asking for divine intervention), or by
bestowing strength to tolerate hardship. In addition, religion provides a sense
of optimism and hope, and a purpose and meaning for disturbing events
or chronic adversity. Events are reinterpreted in terms of a greater purpose,
"grander plan," or simply as "meant to be" (Dull & Skokan, 1995, p. 55).

Despite an abundant number of hypotheses concerning cognitive mechanisms that may mediate the association between religiosity and mental health
outcomes, there is a paucity of research testing these effects particularly among
ethnic minorities. Moreover, the relatively few number of studies that specifically tested cognitive mediation processes yielded mixed results. For example, in
one study of bereaved non-Latino parents, religion contributed to finding
meaning in the child's death, which in turn, predicted psychological well-
being 18 months later (McIntosh, Silver, & Wortman, 1993). A study on
individuals undergoing kidney transplantation (Tix & Frazier, 1998) found
that religious coping predicted life satisfaction (but not psychological distress)
12 months after the surgery. Perceived control or cognitive restructuring of the
event, however, did not mediate this effect. Both studies examined mediation in
the context of an acute event rather than on ongoing health problems. Indeed,
this reflects the paucity of research testing these mechanisms in coping with
chronic, ongoing stressors. A study of Puerto Rican women living with HIV
found that self-esteem and a sense of mastery mediated the relationship between
religiosity and depressive symptoms (Simoni & Ortiz, 2003). In the context of
other chronic, ongoing stressful circumstances faced by ethnic minorities or
immigrant populations, religiosity may help individuals gain a sense of self-
efficacy over stressful life circumstances and perhaps accept events they cannot
change. These cognitive mechanisms may, in turn, lead to enhanced psychological well-being.

Religiosity as a Coping Strategy

Religiosity can also involve spiritual methods or strategies for coping with a
variety of life circumstances. These methods, referred to as *religious coping*,
involve cognitive (e.g., seeking comfort or strength from faith or God) or
behavioral strategies (e.g., praying) based on religious beliefs or practices.
Because religious coping relates to spiritual responses to or strategies used to
deal with or manage stressful situations, religious coping is distinct from global
religiosity (e.g., intrinsic or self-rated religiousness, church attendance). During
stressful periods, there is evidence of the positive effect of religious coping on
mental and physical health (see Pargament, 1997). This association remains
even after controlling for global religiosity (Pargament, 1997), although most of
this research has been based on ethnic majority populations.

The literature on religious coping is unique in its focus on both the positive and negative sides of coping. For example, individuals either may exhibit various religious reactions to stressful life circumstances, including either feeling anger or feel punished by God. There is evidence that such responses, in contrast to calling on God as a "partner" or benevolent being, are associated with worse psychological and physical well-being (Koenig, Pargament, & Nielsen, 1998; Pargament, Koenig, & Perez, 2000). It is also interesting to note theoretical discrepancies surrounding the concept of religious coping. Traditional coping theory, based predominantly on ethnic majority populations, frequently conceptualizes religion as a form of passive or palliative coping (e.g., Carver, Scheier, & Weintraub, 1989; Lazarus & Folkman, 1984), and these are considered less effective than active, behaviorally oriented strategies. The assumption that religious strategies are passive forms of coping is questionable, however. Pargament and Park's (1995) review concluded that there is little evidence to support the proposition that religious coping necessarily reflects passivity or avoidance. To the contrary, religious coping characterized by "a sense of partnership with God", in particular, engenders a sense of personal power and efficacy (Pargament & Park, 1995, p. 25).

To date, there is a limited but growing number of studies on religious coping among culturally diverse groups. For example, there is evidence that ethnic minorities frequently use religious forms of coping (e.g. prayer) in response to a variety of difficult circumstances (Abraído-Lanza, Guier, & Revenson, 1996; Connell & Gibson, 1997; Mellins & Ehrhardt, 1994). Furthermore, religiosity and spirituality are strong cultural values in studies of ethnic minorities, such as Latinos (Zuñiga Rojas, 1999; Guarnaccia et al., 1992). Because religious coping tends to be studied in the context of ongoing, stressful circumstances, we now turn to a specific case study of religious coping in the context of chronic illness. We focus much of our discussion on chronic pain conditions, where there is a substantial body of work on religious coping among ethnic minorities.

The Research Evidence: Religious Coping in the Context of Chronic Illness

Although religiosity may be an important resource in daily life experiences, various studies examined its association with psychological well-being in the context of a chronic illness. Chronic illness poses numerous difficulties that can adversely affect psychological well-being, including pain, discomfort, disability, other debilitating symptoms, and uncertainty about the future (Stanton, 2007). Given the potential role of religiosity to provide needed psychological, social, and other resources to promote wellness, various studies focus on religiosity among ethnic minorities with chronic illness. A general finding in the literature on chronic pain is that African Americans and Latinos use more praying/hoping than do Whites (Edwards, Moric, Husfeldt, Buvanendran, & Ivankovich, 2005; Jordan, Lumley, & Leisen, 1998; Novy, Nelson, Hetzel, Squitieri, & Kennington, 1998; Tan, Jensen, Thornby, & Anderson, 2005; Edwards et al., 2005). Results concerning pain and disability are somewhat mixed, in that religious coping/hope is associated with greater pain among African Americans in some studies (Edwards et al., 2005) but not others (Jordan et al., 1998; Tan et al., 2005), and with greater disability, especially among African Americans (Edwards et al., 2005; Jordan et al., 1998).

Finally, the findings on psychological well-being are also somewhat diverse. In one study, religious coping/hope was associated with greater distress among African Americans, not among Latinos or Whites (Edwards et al., 2005), but it predicted less depression in another study (Tan et al., 2005), and it was unrelated to negative affect in a third research study (Jordan et al., 1998). Although it is difficult to draw conclusions from this mixed evidence, which is based solely on cross-sectional studies, the link between religious coping and worse health outcomes among ethnic minorities (e.g., greater disability, pain, or psychological distress) suggest a possible negative effect of religious coping, or vice-versa, that health status determines religious coping. For example, ethnic minorities and other individuals with physical limitations might turn to prayer and faith as a means of coping (Jordan et al., 1998, p. 86). Supporting this hypothesis, in a longitudinal study of non-Latino Whites with rheumatoid arthritis, the relationship between religious coping and greater disability disappeared after controlling for earlier levels of disability (Smith, Wallston, Dwyer, & Dowdy, 1997). Alternatively, some authors suggest that prayer, if used exclusively without other more active forms of coping may be maladaptive (Jordan et al., 1998, p. 86), as it may prevent individuals from using other more adaptive (Edwards et al., 2005, p. 95) ways of coping and possibly result in waiting for symptoms to worsen before seeking health care. It is interesting that such conclusions focus solely on the prayer aspect of the findings, even though the observed associations in these studies were between disability, pain, and/or distress, and a composite scale of prayer and hoping.

In a study on Latinas with arthritis, religious coping was not related to pain or depression, although it was associated with greater psychological well-being, but the effect was modest (Abraído-Lanza, Vásquez, & Echeverría, 2004). Interestingly, in tests of a mediation model the effect of religious coping on psychological well-being was direct, that is, the relationship was not mediated by self-efficacy over pain or acceptance of illness. These results suggest that religious coping does not operate on psychological adjustment via beliefs concerning control over or acceptance of the illness. Two other important findings of that study warrant mention. First, a factor analysis indicated that religious items loaded on a distinct, religious coping factor. Second, religious coping was positively correlated with active but not with passive coping strategies, such as catastrophing. These findings run counter to traditional coping theory, which views religious coping as a passive method of dealing with stress (e.g., Carver et al., 1989; Lazarus & Folkman, 1984). These results also question conclusions in other studies described above (e.g., Jordan et al., 1998; Edwards et al., 2005) indicating that religious coping prevents individuals from using other "more adaptive" active coping strategies. Instead, the findings support the position that religious coping is an active means of managing stress (e.g., Pargament & Park,

1995). Similarly, qualitative studies of Hispanics indicate that prayer is an active form of seeking help (Guarnaccia et al., 1992).

In conclusion, research on ethnic minorities with chronic illness, and the impact (if any) of religiosity and religious coping on mental and physical health outcomes, provides a mixed picture. The most consistent evidence from these studies is that rates of religiosity and religious coping are higher among ethnic minorities relative to Whites. We should emphasize that, unlike studies of non-Latino Whites, this is a growing field. There is limited research in this area, and the mechanisms linking religiosity or coping to health have not been adequately explored. Longitudinal analyses are especially needed. The cross-sectional nature of many studies precludes addressing questions of causality, or the potential long-term effects of religiosity and other forms of coping on the mental and physical health of ethnic minorities with chronic illness.

Structural Explanations

Although the hypotheses discussed thus far tend to focus on individual-level models of the impact of religiosity on health, it is also important to consider broader structural explanations, including the impact of religious institutions on the health of ethnic minority populations. On the individual level, one of the most common methods for assessing the extent to which religious organizations promote health is to examine the association between religious involvement (e.g., participation in religious activities, such as church attendance) and a variety of health outcomes. A handful of community-based, epidemiologic studies of Latinos (predominantly Mexican Americans) provide evidence of the beneficial effects of religious involvement on health. In a large, three-generation community study of Mexican Americans, religious attendance showed positive cross-sectional relationships with mental health (i.e., greater life satisfaction) among older generations, and beneficial longitudinal effects in the youngest generation (i.e., lower depression), even after controlling for physical health (Levin, Markides, & Ray, 1996). The lack of a prospective relationship between measures of religious attendance and mental health may be due to the effects of functional disability, especially among older adults for whom physical limitations may prevent or restrict attendance to religious services (Levin & Markides, 1986; Markides, Levin, & Ray, 1987). Another cohort study on the effects of religious attendance on Hispanics' mortality (Hill, Angel, Ellison, & Angel, 2005) found that the rate of mortality was approximately one-third lower among respondents who reported attending church or religious services once per week, relative to those who never or almost never attend.

The association between health and religiosity in African Americans is stronger among Blacks than in Whites (Marks, Nesteruk, Swanson, Garrison, & Davis, 2005). Religious African Americans not only appear to live longer but also to benefit from having better mental health and to suffer from lower levels of psychological distress, including depression, low life satisfaction, substance abuse, and suicidal attempts (Ball, Armistead, & Austin, 2003). Recent evidence from the epidemiological and ethnographic literature reveals the protective religious effect on depressive symptoms and psychological distress among African Americans (Levin et al., 2005; Holt, 2005). By far, there is a more expansive literature on the role of religious institutions that provide essential resources to African Americans and immigrants in the U.S. We turn now to a review of this research.

The Role of Organized Churches

In recent years, there has been growing interest in the effects of religion and faith-based organizations on the mental health of minority groups in the U.S. This interest has been prompted by research efforts sponsored by federal, local and private agencies (e.g., the U.S. Bureau of Primary Health Care and the NIH, the RWJ foundation) aimed at launching partnerships between mainstream health services and religious and spiritual churches (Swanson, Crowther, Green, & Armstrong, 2004). As noted by Campbell (2007, pp. 213–234): *This shift reflects the recognition that churches and faith organizations may be well positioned to provide such services more efficiently and effectively than can some federally administered programs and agencies.* These research collaborations often materialize in community-based participatory projects and ecological-holistic programs that include both physical and spiritual dimensions, with professionals working with clergy and minority leaders (Ammerman, 2002; Yanek, Becker, Moy Gittelsohn, & Koffman, 2001). Certainly, church-based lay health education programs have an almost endless potential to effect social change related to minorities' mental and physical health (Peterson, Atwood, & Yates, 2002; Quinn & McNabb, 2001).

This section addresses the importance of organized churches, particularly the Black church, as a source of social and emotional support, specifically regarding the role of the clergy in providing informal mental counseling to parishioners. The importance of the Black church as a source of strength and spiritual support has long been recognized by the fields of advocacy, education, political activism, and mental health (Clay, Newlin, & Leeks, 2005; Lincoln & Mamiya, 1990). Throughout American history, Black churches played a pivotal role in the lives of African Americans via the provision of emotional and spiritual guidance, social and instrumental support, and political advocacy (Campbell, 2007; Crowther et al., 2002; Swanson et al., 2004). In the 1920s, Black churches offered important services, such as free clinics and access to health care and counseling to African Americans (Mays & Nicholson, 1933). Blank, Mahmood, Fox, & Guterbock (2002) noted that churches have continued providing de facto mental health deliveries principally in rural areas (see also Fox, Merwin, & Blank, 1995).

The Catholic Church, as well various Protestant churches, has also a long tradition in providing immigrants with both moral and spiritual support, as well as with material and financial help. Survey research and in-depth studies on the church's impact on immigrants' patterns of social incorporation have sparked a renewed interest in immigrants' social integration and mental health in the U.S. Studies among diverse immigrant groups, from Salvadorians to Taiwanese (Ebaugh & Saltzman Chafetz, 2000; Menjívar, 2000; Levitt, 1998; Kim, 1994) agree on the importance of the buffering effect against distress that churches provide to their followers, particularly among newer and less integrated immigrants (see Cadge, 2006). Overall, as Menjívar (2006) notes in the case of Salvadorians in the U.S., in absence of existing settlement organizations, churches play a unique role in providing material, practical, and emotional support to immigrants, as well as precious social capital resources.[3] Recent debates on immigration policy in the U.S. illustrate the political and advocacy roles of the Catholic Church in fighting for immigrants' rights. In March of 2006, a Senate Judiciary Committee voted against an earlier proposal by the House of Representatives to criminalize illegal immigrants and created an amendment that would prohibit federal prosecution of those who provided them with assistance, many of whom included priests and other leaders of churches serving immigrant communities. As on many other occasions, the Catholic Church has played a pivotal role in mobilizing grassroots movements to protect vulnerable immigrants and in supporting public outcries against these policies.

Clergy as Ad Hoc Mental Health Counselors

The literature on mental health among immigrant and minority groups consistently reports the reluctance of minority populations to access formal mental health services, partially due to their lack of familiarity with Western forms of healing, their cultural reliance on traditional healing forms, the importance of family and social support, and the taboo and stigma prevailing over mental health conditions (Bernstein, 2007; Viladrich, 2007a; Martínez Pincay & Guarnaccia, 2007; Wynaden et al., 2005; Blank et al., 2002; Tobin, 2000). A growing body of literature on immigrant groups in the U.S. reveals their underutilization of the mental health system and the preference of religious practices as surrogated mental health services, as in the case of Filipino Americans (Sanchez & Gaw, 2007).

Clergy are the most frequently sought source of help for psychological distress particularly among minority groups, including immigrants (Chalfant et al., 1990). A study on Kosovo Albanian refugees (Gozdziak, 2002) concludes that recently arrived refugees preferred religious services and sought one-on-one consultations with the imams, rather than with the mental health counselors available to them. Imams were trusted on the basis of sharing a similar religious faith, particularly during refugees' stressful period of social and individual accommodation to the recipient society. Gozdziak calls for the recognition of a *spiritual emergency* room as the legitimate space for addressing refugees' mental and emotional trauma, and as a counter-paradigm to clinical mental health services. The author finally notes that researchers tend to neglect the role of religion and spirituality as a source of emotional and cognitive support for immigrants, as well as a form of social and political mobilization for both community building and group identity.

In an in-depth study with 121 African American pastors, Young, Griffith, & Williams (2003) found that most pastors reported counseling clients with severe mental illness, suffering from similar conditions to those seen by secular mental health professionals. Researchers also found that clergy counseled individuals outside their own denominations and concluded that pastoral counseling represents a significant resource for those lacking access to needed mental health care. In agreement with these findings, Swanson et al. (2004, p. 84) notes that: *given that many church members may have their first professional contact with clergy who play a pivotal role in church-based programs, clergy represent important resources for needed collaboration in facilitating African Americans' use of health services.* On this line, a review of the literature on the provision of mental health services by clergy in African American communities (Taylor, Ellison, Chatters, Levin, & Lincoln, 2000) summarizes some of the most cited characteristics regarding pastors' involvement in the provision of mental health counseling. These include the clergy's versatility to play different roles and articulate the church's programs, as well as their importance as gatekeepers in providing referrals to mental health services. Ministers in Black churches counsel on a variety of personal problems including depression, marital and family issues, and alcohol and other forms of substance abuse (Taylor et al., 2003). Clergy has unique advantages in helping with personal problems, including affordability and access. In addition, they are the only professionals that most congregants will encounter through the lifetime, which make them even more relevant as personal counselors.[4] Unfortunately, and contrary to the well-documented role played by clergy and priests in healing, they are seldom considered partners in curing by the medical profession (Koenig, McCullough & Larson, 2001).

Despite the evidence presented above regarding the ubiquitous role of clergy as ad hoc spiritual counselors among minorities, the literature reveals a lack of systematic research on the specific services they provide. In a study that conceptualizes mental illness and referrals among Korean American clergymen, Kim-Goh (1993) found that those with psychological understanding of symptoms were more willing to refer their parish to psychological services than those holding religious conceptualizations. A content analysis of 44 articles from non-religious journals from 1980 and 1999 (Weaver, Flannelly, Flannelly, & Oppenheimer, 2003) revealed a paramount need for clergy's training and a demand for closer collaborations with the medical profession, particularly regarding sharing information about referral services. Blank et al. (2002) point out that a culture of distrust has pervasively obstructed a constructive dialogue between church leaders (particularly in the South of the US) and mental health professionals, which has precluded research and clinical collaborations. This is rooted in historical patterns (mostly due to racial and ethnic segregation), as well as in conceptual discrepancies regarding the nature and treatment of mental health conditions. In addition, as noted by Gee, Smucker, Chin, and Curling (2005) faith partnerships seem hampered by dissimilar goals, philosophies, and lack of resources. Whereas church leaders seem to be considered key players in the successful implementation of African American church-based health programs, there is no clear agreement on the clergy's role in service delivery and mental health counseling (Carter-Edwards, Jallah, Goldmon, Roberson, & Hoyo, 2006). Hopefully, as most of the reviewed literature suggests, slowly but steadily we are moving toward a better understanding on how minorities may seek different sources of help for the resolution of their mental, spiritual, and emotional needs.

Although the information on the role of organized churches in providing mental health counseling to migrant communities is not as vast as the literature on African Americans, the reviewed literature reveals similar trends in terms of the clergy's barriers to training, their limited referrals, and lack of collaboration with both mental health agencies and the medical profession. For example, in a study on a faith-based network in an ethnically diverse area, Dossett, Fuentes, Klap, and Wells (2005) found that although 69 percent of respondents felt that referrals to nonreligious counselors were appropriate, 50 percent were reluctant to collaborate with government agencies. Among the obstacles to providing direct mental health services and referrals, researchers found financial and staffing limitations, limited professional training, and reluctance to partner with government programs. In addition, partnerships between mental health professionals, researches, and minority groups encounter several barriers (Laborde, Brannock, Breland-Noble, & Parrish, 2007; Taylor et al., 2000). Typically, mental health researchers seek the assistance of community-faith groups to either recruit participants and/or implement their studies, thus resulting in communities' apprehension to trust researches and formal providers.

Summarizing the findings presented above, we conclude that further systematic research is needed on the overlapping nature of faith communities and formal mental health services. This includes conducting in-depth studies on the services provided by clergy, both regarding their professional counseling skills and their knowledge on mental health nosology. This information is not only critical for a more comprehensive understanding of the church's role in responding to minorities' mental health needs, but also for developing better models of service delivery including promoting enduring and meaningful partnerships with formal health care providers. As noted in this review, churches do more than taking care of individual issues, as they are a source of social support and spiritual comfort. Nonetheless, most clergy seem to have little training in mental health counseling and often deal with mental and social service problems that are beyond their areas of expertise (Ali, Milstein, & Marzuk, 2005). And this seems to be an issue not only in the U.S. but also in other countries. In a study of different faiths in London, Leavey, Loewenthal, & King (2007) found that clergy played a confined role in mental health counseling, which was neither recognized by central organizations nor by the medical profession. This lack of appreciation was also undermined by their own anxiety, fear of the unknown and stereotyped attitudes toward mental illness. We now turn to another case of informal provision of mental health services represented by folk healers in urban areas.

Folk Healing in the Urban Milieu

Although the field of religious healing would demand a chapter of its own, in this section we highlight its importance as a mental health resource for vulnerable minority groups in the U.S. The blooming market of religious healing in the U.S. in recent decades has conspicuously revealed the role of religion in American society on the one hand and the multiplicity of coexisting healing systems on the other, a fact that somehow mirrors America's cultural diversity. Popular folk healing practices have blossomed in the U.S. in recent decades, along with the holistic health movement (developed in the 1970s, and its successor the New Age movement), followed by the institutionalized field of complementary and alternative medicine (Baer, 2005; Barnes & Sered, 2005).

While the safety net for health services has become more unraveled in recent years, the burden of health care in the U.S has increasingly shifted to immigrant communities that serve the poor and the undocumented (see Lopez, 2005). In this context, folk health systems, rather than being diluted by globalization and the ubiquitous presence of western practices, are blossoming more than ever before. Folk healers of Latino origin, whose denominations range from *curanderos* to *herberos,* represent one case in point. The literature documents their role as informal counselors who fulfill the silent demand for mental health services among diverse groups of Latino immigrants in the U.S. (see Viladrich, 2006b, 2007b; Reiff, O'Connor, Kronenberg, Balick, & Lohr, 2003). In U.S. cities, these healers are mostly multidisciplinary practitioners who combine religious-healing practices rooted in folk-belief systems from the Americas (mostly Santeria and Spiritism), as well as with other psychic disciplines. As Singer & Garcia (1995) note, these religious-therapeutic movements, share a common belief in communication with and possession by an array of incorporeal spirits. Spiritism and Santeria, although related to different bodies of knowledge, remain as polyfunctional faiths, an issue supported by Harwood (1977a, 1977b). As Garrison (1977), Koss-Chioino (1992), and Singer and Garcia (1995) report, Spiritism and Santeria have an enormous potential for change and adaptability, also characterized by their importance as commoditized products representing the quintessential combination of the old and the new (see also Romberg, 2003; Singer & Garcia 1995; Singer & Borrero, 1984).

Recent research reveals the role of botánicas as the visible entry to the concealed world of Latino healers' practices in urban milieus, as they provide health care products or informal health services on their premises and refer their clients to informal and formal health care practitioners (Viladrich, 2006a,). Botánicas' presence works as material proof of the thriving economy of religious healing that serves a pan-ethnic population of Latino immigrants in many U.S. cities (Jones, Polk, Flores-Peña, & Evanchuk, 2001; Long, 2001). As part of an urban social network, they function as informal hubs for the dissemination of information about community resources. In fact, not only do they provide a physical and a social space for the exchange of information and resources, but they also support informal faith-healing networks on the basis of religious belonging.

To a certain extent, Latino healers are botánicas' ethnic gatekeepers that connect immigrants, like themselves, to alternative networks of care within a culturally meaningful explanatory model of disease and healing. Botánicas' clients are largely recruited among the uninsured, who are most likely to experience the psychological impact of grueling economic conditions, including unemployment, the loss of safety net services, access barriers to health care, discrimination, and so on. The effectiveness of practices that are cheap and highly available also attracts Latinos to the botánicas' doors. An ethnographic study on Latino healers in NYC (based on participant observation and in-depth interviews with 56 healers) examined their roles as holistic providers who deal with emotional and psychological problems beyond their patients' physical complaints. Healers combine natural and supernatural explanatory methods of treatment while searching for cost-effective solutions to ailments that belong to the *immigrant continuum* (Viladrich, 2007a). This term refers to the complex set of emotional and life-management issues brought by Latino immigrants to the consultation, ranging from stress-related conditions (e.g., *nervios* due to financial problems and undocumented status) to difficulties in coping with severe chronic ailments. This study shows that most healers in NYC follow diverse therapeutic methods, including referrals to professionals (e.g., psychotherapy, Western medicine), particularly when assessing their patients' problems as severe and as surpassing their own expertise.

As previously pointed out in the case of the clergy, healers state uneasy and contradictory relationships with biomedical providers in general and with mental health professionals in particular. While on the one hand, they acknowledge their own limited skills to deal with their patients' serious mental problems (e.g., clinical depression), on the other, they are critical of professionals' treatments, including the use (and abuse) of chemical substances, the limited reliance on verbal therapies, and the narrowed scientific criteria that disregards Latinos' spiritual and religious beliefs. In addition, and contrary to the clergy's role in organized churches, healers tend to keep a low profile for the purpose of avoiding being identified and prosecuted by either health inspectors or immigration authorities (Mautino, 1999). As in the case of religious healers in other countries, such as Uganda and Taiwan (see Teuton, Dowrick, & Bentall, 2007;

Lin, 2005), Latino healers neither feel understood nor accepted by organized medicine that usually considers them as either charlatans or as mentally disturbed individuals. As a result, and despite botánicas' visibility, Latino folk healers have mostly remained a hidden population in urban settings, as they mostly practice without medical license; therefore, they tend to conceal their identity to outsiders.

The case study on Latino healers' discussed above, provides us with a glimpse into the richness of healing traditions in the U.S. vis-à-vis the need to thoroughly address minorities' diverse mental health needs. Learning about what Latino healers do (and do not do) can lead us to further understand how they respond not just to individual pathologies but also to the political and social forces that place the blame on the most vulnerable of all (Castro & Singer, 2004; Farmer, 2003). If, according to the Latino healers in Viladrich's study, Latino immigrants are actually using botánicas and healers as subsidiaries of mental health services, policies oriented at providing affordable and meaningfully professional services are needed, including approaches to overcome language and financial barriers (Gomez-Beloz & Chavez, 2001). In addition, by tackling the medicalization of social experiences, we will be able to address the underlying factors under which the sufferers' pain is constructed. In this regard, we should question the ability of the biomedical model to account for the social causes that underscore Latinos' idioms of distress (Kleinman & Sung, 1979). In the end, policies that bridge Western and religious healing systems should be effective in overcoming the fear of retaliation that keep folk practitioners, as well as their patients, from sharing their mental health beliefs and practices with mainstream mental health service providers.

Nevertheless, we should be cautious when assessing the beneficial impact of folk healers on patients' physical and mental health ailments. The tendency of healers to consider their clients' emotional problems as normal indicators of stress could also prevent Latinos from seeking professional help when needed. Also, more attention should be paid to the extent to which religious healing systems (e.g. Santeria and Spiritism) disguise psychotic symptoms under the belief of spirit possession or intrusion. Spiritual beliefs associated with the interpretation of distress may result in the misdiagnosis of schizophrenia and of other psychotic illness. Finally, misunderstanding regarding practices of Santeria, often misconstrued as a cult related to witchcraft and Satanism, may actually discourage practitioners of these faiths from seeking formal health services in the U.S.

Conclusions and Directions for Future Research

This chapter merely touches upon the vast corpus of literature on some of the most researched areas regarding the influence of religion on the mental health of minorities in the U.S. In this section, we examine some of the lacunae of this research and suggest areas for future study. As noted in previous pages, churches play a unique role in mental counseling and spiritual guidance in a nonstigmatizing way (Campbell, 2007; Blank et al., 2002). Nevertheless, little is known on how to link the clergy's counseling endeavors with formal providers of care. In addition, and despite the rich literature on faith-based health programs, there has been little formative and evaluation research on the impact of churches on the mental health of minority groups, with most programs focusing on physical rather than on mental health outcomes (see Campbell, 2007, DeHaven, Hunter, Wilder, Walton, & Berry, 2004). There is also a lack of effective models guiding mental health researcher/minorities community partnerships (Swanson, 2004). In addition, policy initiatives aimed at increasing the appropriate use of mental health care should be built upon the (often informal) referral processes already in place by many religious organizations (see Harris, Edlund. & Larson, 2006). As examined earlier, although mental health professionals often count on religious providers to get referrals, they rarely reciprocate, and their limited understanding of the role of religion in healing may lead them to misinterpret their patients' mental problems.

More information on how formal and informal systems of care coexist, and even conflict, is necessary to further understand the unmet needs of minorities in the U.S. As discussed in this chapter, botánicas often work in opposition to the medical and mainstream religious institutions (Latorre, 2007), and fear and mistrust have made healers' practices even more secretive to strangers. Furthermore, there is limited research training in psychiatry, especially regarding diagnosis, etiology, and treatment of patients from different ethnic and cultural backgrounds (Laborde et al., 2007). In sum, the potential for forging collaborations among mental health providers, churches, and informal healing systems (see Ng, 2003) is crucial for a better understanding of minorities' help-seeking behaviors vis-à-vis the channels that meet their spiritual, mental and emotional needs. In this regard, the role of cultural psychiatry has become a growing force in promoting dialogue between psychiatry and religion, in the areas of immigrant and refugee health, trauma, and loss (Boehnlein, 2006). The role of lay health advisors and health brokers (Viladrich, 2007b; Blank et al., 2002; Jackson & Parks, 1997) in bridging different systems, from networks of faith-based organizations to informal webs of folk healing providers, is also a promising field for future research and advocacy. One of the enduring lessons drawn from faith-based participatory partnerships is the need to involve religious grassroots in the early phases of research implementation, toward building a shared planning agenda (Jackson & Reddick, 1999).

More attention should also be paid to the specific mental health needs of diverse ethnic populations in the U.S. For example, religious discrimination has become a salient problem among Muslim communities in the U.S. and Europe, particularly following the terrorist attacks on September 11th, 2001 (Youssef & Deane, 2006). Growing levels of *Islamophobia* have been affecting the physical and mental health of Muslim families and their children (Shendan, 2006), with perceived discrimination and social hostility having direct and indirect mental effects on those self-identified as Muslims (Laird, Amer, Barnett, & Barnes, 2007; Ali, Milstein, & Marzuk, 2005; Seebohm et al., 2005).[5] Regardless of the long-term history of Muslims in the U.S., there has been little research on their health problems and health-seeking behaviors, including reliance on divine healing (see Rasanayagam, 2006), and on the rising stressors that prompt many of their current mental health issues (see Haque, 2004; Morioka-Douglas et al., 2004). As in the case of Gozdiak's work (2002) reviewed earlier, a study by Ali et al. (2005) noted the pivotal role played by imams in meeting the counseling needs of the Muslim community, particularly in congregations where a majority of followers are Arab Americans.

Further quantitative and qualitative work is necessary on the barriers that keep minorities from accessing and using mental health services. As noted by Vega et al. (2007), the need for more anthropological and open-ended exploratory studies on the roles of religion, spirituality, and folk beliefs are critical for a better understanding of Hispanics' persistent mental health illness, in addition to clinical interventions at the family level. Even when minorities feel the need for help, lack of familiarity, fear, mistrust, and taboo may keep them away from seeking services, a pattern noticed in diverse minority and immigrant groups. In-depth cross-cultural studies on the meaning of religiosity and spirituality are needed from the point of view of non-Western theological frameworks, which may not be aligned with Judeo-Christian religions (see Traphagan, 2005; Fitzgerald, 2000). For example, the Hindu concept of karma has no parallel in Western models of thought, although it may have crucial implications for the well-being of immigrants from Asian and Chinese-based belief systems (see Hill & Pargament, 2003). As amply reported in the medical anthropological literature, many idioms of distress that characterize individual and social suffering, have neither conceptual representations in all cultures nor are directly translated into other languages (see Guarnaccia et al., 1992; Pilgrim & Bentall, 1999; Kleinman & Good, 1985). Among certain Latino populations, the notion of spirit is related to a tangible soul that can be "lost" in particular situations, as is reported in the vast literature on the intrinsic relationship between psychiatric symptoms and the culture-bound syndrome known as *soul loss* (Weller et al., 2002). Integrating indigenous understanding of religion and spiritual beliefs, including minorities' subjective experiences, is critical for improving clinical practice and for guaranteeing the success of prevention and intervention programs aimed at serving vulnerable minority groups in the U.S. (Lewis, Hankin, Reynolds, & Ogedegbe, 2007; D'Souza & George, 2006; Loue, Lane, Lloyd, & Loh, 1999).

In sum, we still have a long way to go in understanding the specific pathways that may link religiosity to the health of ethnic minorities and immigrants. Although there is a rich theoretical literature on the processes and mechanisms by which religiosity might affect mental and physical health, relative to ethnic majority groups, there has been less research on ethnic minority and immigrant populations. Additional studies on the behavioral, social, cognitive, psychological, and structural factors associated with religiosity among ethnically diverse groups could help validate existing theories and models, as well as identify areas of divergence. Future research should focus on the influence of structural and organizational religious factors on individual mental health outcomes, as well as on the processes responsible for their recurring correlations (Marks et al., 2005). Hopefully, a closer look at ecological models may lead to comprehensive frameworks able to grasp the overlapping and complementary effects of religion and spirituality at the individual, group, and institutional levels, both regarding their independent effects and interactions. These models have the potential to offer the most promising frameworks for our understanding of the pathways through which minorities' mental health status is influenced by the social, cultural, and physical environments (Gee & Payne-Sturges, 2004).

Notes

1. In the U.S., cohort studies such as the Alameda county study, found enduring associations between religious attendance and mortality, partly explained by participants' improved health practices, increased social contacts, and more stable marriages in combination with religious attendance (Strawbridge, Cohen, Shema, & Kaplan, 1997). Studies with samples of predominantly non-Hispanic Whites report similar trends (see Hummer, Rogers, Nam, & Ellison, 1999; Hill et al., 2005).
2. Hill et al. (2000) note that this polarization may lead to the duplication of concepts and measures and suggest finding commonalities by relying on the sacred as the common denominator of the religious and spiritual life. In their own words: *new measures developed under the rubric of spirituality may in fact represent old wine in new wineskins* (Hill & Pargament, 2003, p. 65).
3. As Menjívar (2000:6) suggests: *Immigrants are not only already familiar with the churches they come to join, but the church is perhaps one of the most supportive and welcoming institutions for immigrants, particularly for those who arrive to live in difficult circumstances. Institutionally, churches not only provide spiritual comfort to the immigrants but they also respond in a variety of ways o the needs of immigrants, offering the newcomers material and financial support, as well as legal counsel, access to medical care and housing, an even lobbying for less stringent immigration policies.*
4. As noted by Taylor (2000:75): *Distinct from other sources of professional assistance, clergy do not charge fees for their services or require insurance, co-payments, or completion of required forms.*
5. Seebohm et al. (2005:16) point out that Muslims communities in England are psychologically hurting from rising discrimination after September 11, 2001: "Muslims *en mass* have been portrayed in the national press as potential enemies, subject to focused stop and search activities by the police. Newspaper and verbal reports suggest Muslim women have been subjected to spitting, abuse and having their hijab torn from them."

References

Abraído-Lanza, A. F., Guier, C., & Revenson, T. A. (1996). Coping and social support resources among Latinas with arthritis. *Arthritis Care and Research, 9*(6), 501–508.

Abraído-Lanza, A. F., Vásquez, E., & Echeverría, S. E. (2004). *En las manos de Dios* [in God's Hands]: Religious and other forms of coping among Latinos with arthritis. *Journal of Consulting and Clinical Psychology, 72*(1), 91–102.

Ali, O. M., Milstein, G., & Marzuk, P. M. (2005). The imam's role in meeting the counseling needs of Muslim communities in the United States. *Psychiatric Services*, *56*(2), 133.

Ammerman, A. (2002). Process evaluation of the church-based PRAISE project: Partnership to reach African Americans to increase smart eating. In A. Steckler & L. Linnan (Eds.), *Process evaluation for public health interventions and research* (pp. 96–111). San Francisco, CA: Jossey-Bass Publishers.

Baer, H. A. (2005). Trends in religious healing and the integration of biomedicine and complementary and alternative medicine in the United States and around the globe: A review. *Medical Anthropology Quarterly*, *19*(4), 437–442.

Ball, J., Armistead, L., & Austin, B. (2003). The relationship between religiosity and adjustment among African-American, female, urban adolescents. *Journal of Adolescence*, *26*, 431–446.

Barnes, L. L., & Sered, S. S., (Eds.). (2005). *Religion and healing in America*. New York: Oxford University Press.

Bernstein, K. S. (2007). Mental health issues among urban Korean American immigrants. *Journal of Transcultural Nursing*, *18*(2), 175–180.

Blank, M. B., Mahmood, M., Fox, J. C., & Guterbock, T. (2002). Alternative mental health services: The role of the black church in the South. *American Journal of Public Health*, *92*(10), 1668–1672.

Boehnlein, J. K. (2006). Religion and spirituality in psychiatric care: Looking back, looking ahead. *Transcultural Psychiatry*, *43*(4), 634–651.

Buck, H. G. (2006). Spirituality: Concept analysis and model development. *Holistic Nursing Practice*, *20*(6), 288–292.

Cadge, W. (2006). Religious service attendance among immigrants. *American Behavioral Scientist 49*(11), 1574–1595.

Campbell, M. K., Hudson, M. A., Resnicow, K., Blakeney, N., Paxton, A. & Baskin, M. (2007). Church-based health promotion interventions: Evidence and lessons learned. *Annual Review of Public Health 28*, 213–234.

Carter-Edwards, L., Jallah, Y. B., Goldmon, M. V., Roberson, J. T. Jr., & Hoyo, C. (2006). Key attributes of health ministries in African American churches: An exploratory survey. *North Carolina Medical Journal*, *67*(5), 345–350.

Carver, C. S., Scheier, M. F., & Weintraub, J. K. (1989). Assessing coping strategies: A theoretically based approach. *Journal of Personality and Social Psychology*, *56*, 267–283.

Castro, A., & Singer, M. (Eds.). (2004). *Unhealthy health policy: A critical anthropological examination*. Walnut Creek, California: AltaMira Press.

Chalfant, H. P., Heller, P. L., Roberts, A., Briones, D., Aguirre-Hochbaum, S., Farr, W. (1990). The Clergy as a resource for those encountering psychological distress. *Review of Religious Research*, *31*(3), 305–313.

Chan, C. L., Ng, S. M., Ho, R. T., & Chow, A. Y. (2006). East meets West: Applying Eastern spirituality in clinical practice. *Journal of Clinical Nursing*, *15*(7), 822–832.

Chatters, L. M. (2000). Religion and health: Public health research and practice. *Annual Review of Public Health*, *21*, 335–367.

Clay, K. S., Newlin, K., & Leeks, K. (2005). Pastors' wives as partners: An appropriate model for church-based health promotion. Cancer Control. Suppl 2:111–115.

Connell, C., & Gibson, G. (1997). Racial, ethnic, and cultural differences in dementia caregiving: Review and analysis. *Gerontologist*, *37*, 355–364.

Crowther, M., Parker, M., Larimore, W., Achenbaum, A., & Koenig, H. (2002). Rowe and Kahn's model of successful aging revisited: Positive spirituality – the forgotten factor. *The Gerontologist*, *42*(5), 613–620.

DeHaven, M. J., Hunter, I. B., Wilder, L., Walton, J. W., & Berry, J. (2004). Health programs in faith-based organizations: Are they effective? *American Journal of Public Health*, *94*(6), 1030–1036.

Dossett, E., Fuentes, S., Klap, R., & Wells, K. (2005). Brief reports: Obstacles and opportunities in providing mental health services through a faith-based network in Los Angeles. *Psychiatric Services, 56*, 206–208.

D'Souza, R., & George, K. (2006). Spirituality, religion and psychiatry: Its application to clinical practice. *Australasian Psychiatry, 14*(4), 408–412.

Dull, V. T., & Skokan, L. A. (1995). A cognitive model of religion's influence on health. *Journal of Social Issues, 51*, 49–64.

Ebaugh, H. R., & Saltzman Chafetz, J. (2000). *Religion and the new immigrants: Continuities and adaptations in immigrant congregations.* Walnut Creek, California: Altamira Press.

Edwards, R. R., Moric, M., Husfeldt, B., Buvanendran, A., & Ivankovich, O. (2005). Ethnic similarities and differences in the chronic pain experience: A comparison of African American, Hispanic, and White patients, *Pain Medicine, 6*, 88–98.

Farmer, P. (2003). *Pathologies of power: Health, human rights, and the new war on the poor.* Berkeley: University of California Press.

Fetzer Institute/National Institute on Aging. (1999). Multidimensional measurement of religiousness/spirituality for use in health research: A report of the Fetzer Institute/National Institute on Aging Working Group. Kalamazoo, MI: John E. Fetzer Institute.

Fitzgerald, T. (2000). *The ideology of religious studies.* New York: Oxford University Press.

Foley, M. W., & Hoge, D. R. (2007). *Religion and the new immigrants.* USA: Oxford University Press.

Fowler, J. W. (1981). *Stages of faith: The psychology of human development and the quest for meaning.* San Francisco: Harper and Row.

Fox, J. C., Merwin, E. R., & Blank, M. B. (1995). De facto mental health services in the rural South. *Journal of Health Care for the Poor and Underserved 6*, 434–468.

Garrison, V. (1977). The "Puerto Rican syndrome" in psychiatry and *Espiritismo.* In V. Crapanzano & V. Garrison (Eds.), *Case studies in spirit possession* (pp. 383–448). New York: John Wiley.

Gee, G. C., & Payne-Sturges, D. C. (2004). Environmental health disparities: A framework integrating psychosocial and environmental concepts. *Environmental Health Perspectives, 112*(17), 1645–1653.

Gee, L., Smucker, D. R., Chin, M. H., & Curling, F. A. (2005). Partnering together? Relationships between faith-based community health centers and neighborhood congregations. *Southern Medical Journal, 98*(12), 1245–1250.

George, L. K., Ellison, C. G., & Larson, D. B. (2002). Explaining the relationships between religious involvement and health. *Psychological Inquiry, 13*, 190–200.

Gomez-Beloz, A., & Chavez, N. (2001). The botanica as a culturally appropriate health care option for Latinos. *The Journal of Alternative and Complementary Medicine, 7*(5), 537–546.

Gozdziak, E. (2002). Spiritual emergency room: The role of spirituality and religion in the resettlement of Kosovar Albanians. *Journal of Refugee Studies, 15*(2), 136–152.

Guarnaccia, P. J., Parka, P., Deschamps, A., & Milstein, G., & Argiles, N. (1992). Si Diós quiere: Hispanic families' experiences of caring for a seriously mentally ill family member. *Culture, Medicine & Psychiatry, 16*, 187–215.

Haque, A. (2004). Religion and mental health: The case of American Muslims. *Journal of Religion and Health, 43*(1), 45–58.

Harris, K. M., Edlund, M. J., & Larson, S. L. (2006). Religious involvement and the use of mental health care. *Health Services Research, 41*(2), 395–410.

Harwood, A. Puerto Rican Spiritism. (1977a). Part I – Description and analysis of an alternative psychotherapeutic approach. *Culture, Medicine and Psychiatry, 1*(1), 69–95.

Harwood, A. Puerto Rican Spiritism. (1977b). Part II – An institution with preventive and therapeutic functions in community psychiatry. *Culture, Medicine and Psychiatry, 1*(2), 135–153.

Hill, T. D., Angel, J. L., Ellison, C. G., & Angel, R. J. (2005). Religious attendance and mortality: An 8-year follow-up of older Mexican Americans. *Journals of Gerontology Series B-Psychological Sciences & Social Sciences, 60*(2), S102–109.

Hill, T. D., Ellison, C. G., Burdette, A. M., & Musick, M. A. (2007). Religious involvement and healthy lifestyles: Evidence from the survey of Texas adults. *Annals of Behavioral Medicine, 34*, 217–222.

Hill, P. C., & Pargament, K. I. (2003). Advances in the conceptualization and measurement of religion and spirituality. Implications for physical and mental health research. *American Psychologist, 58*(1), 64–74.

Hill, P. C., Pargament, K. I., Hood, R. W. Jr., McCullough, M. E., Swyers, J. P., Larson, D. B., & Zinnbauer, B. J. (2000). Conceptualizing religion and spirituality: Points of commonality, points of departure. *Journal for the Theory of Social Behaviour, 30*, 51–77.

Holt, C. L. (2005). Exploring religion-health mediators among African American parishioners. *Journal of Health Psychology, 10*(4), 511–527.

Holt, C. L., & McClure, S. M. (2006). Perceptions of the religion-health connection among African American church members. *Qualitative Health Research, 16*(2), 268–281.

Hummer, R. A., Rogers, R. G., Nam, Ch. B., & Ellison, Ch. G. (1999). Religious involvement and U.S. adult mortality. *Demography, 36*, 273–285.

Jackson, E. J. & Parks, C. P. (1997). Recruitment and training issues from selected lay health advisor programs among African Americans: A 20-year perspective. *Health Education & Behavior, 24*(4), 418–431.

Jackson, R. S., & Reddick, B. (1999). The African American church and university partnerships: Establishing lasting collaborations. *Health Education and Behavior, 26*(5), 663–674.

Jones, M. O., Polk, P. A., Flores-Peña, Y., & Evanchuk, R. J. (2001). Invisible hospitals: Botanicas in ethnic health care. In E. Brady (Ed.), *Healing logics. Culture and medicine in modern health belief systems* (pp. 39–87). Logan, UT: Utah State University Press.

Jordan, M., Lumley, M. A., & Leisen, J. C. C. (1998). The relationships of cognitive coping and pain control beliefs to pain and adjustment among African-American and Caucasian women with rheumatoid arthritis. *Arthritis Care & Research, 11*, 80–88.

Kahn, R. L., & Antonucci, T. C. (1980). Convoys over the life course: Attachment, roles, and social support. In P. B. Baltes & O. G. Brim (Eds.). *Life span development and behavior* (pp. 253–286). New York: Academic Press.

Kark, J., Shemi, G., Friedlander, Y., Martin, O., Manor, O., & Blondheim, S. H. (2006). Does religious observance promote health? Mortality in secular versus religious kibbutzim in Israel. *American Journal of Public Health, 86*(3), 341–346.

Kawachi, I., & Berkman, L. (2000). Social cohesion, social capital and health. In L. F. Berkman & I. Kawachi (Eds.). *Social epidemiology.* New York, NY: Oxford University Press.

Kim, J. H. (2002). *Religions in Asian America: Building faith communities* (Critical Perspectives on Asian Pacific Americans Series). AltaMira Press.

Kim, Young-Il. (1994). The correlation between religiosity and assimilation of first-generation Korean immigrants in the Chicago metropolitan region. Ph.D. diss., Loyola University of Chicago, Abstract in *Dissertation Abstracts International* 55–05A, 1388.

Kim-Goh, M. (1993). Conceptualization of mental illness among Korean-American clergymen and implications for mental health service delivery. *Community Mental Health Journal, 29*(5), 405–412.

King, S., Burgess, E. O., Akinyela, M., Counts-Spriggs, M., & Parker, N. (2005). "Your body is God's temple". The spiritualization of health beliefs in multigenerational African American families. *Research on Aging, 27*(4), 420–446.

Kleinman, A. (1980). *Patients and healers in the context of culture: An exploration of the borderland between anthropology, medicine, and psychiatry.* Berkeley: University of California Press.

Kleinman, A., & Good, B., (Eds.). (1985). *Culture and depression: Studies in the anthropology and cross-cultural psychiatry of affect and disorder.* Berkeley: University of California Press.

Kleinman, A., & Sung, L. U. (1979). Why do indigenous practitioners successfully heal? *Social Science and Medicine, 13*B(1), 7–26.

Koenig, H. G., McCullough, M. E., & Larson, D. B. (2001). *Handbook of religion and health*. New York: Oxford University Press.

Koenig, H. G., Pargament, K. I., & Nielsen, J. (1998). Religious coping and health status in medically ill hospitalized older adults. *Journal of Nervous and Mental Disease, 185*, 513–521.

Koss-Chioino, J. (1992). *Women as healers, women as patients: Mental health care and traditional healing in Puerto Rico*. Boulder, San Francisco, Oxford: Westview Press.

Laborde, D. J., Brannock, K., Breland-Noble, A., & Parrish, T. (2007). Pilot test of cooperative learning format for training mental health researchers and Black community leaders in partnership skills. *Journal of the National Medical Association, 99*(12), 1359–1368.

Laird, L. D., Amer, M. M., Barnett, E. D., & Barnes, L. L. (2007). Muslim patients and health disparities in the UK and the US. *Archives Of Disease In Childhood, 92*(10), 922–926.

Latorre, G. (2007). Book review. Botánica Los Angeles: Latino popular religious art in the City of Angeles. Patrick Arthur Polk, ed. Los Angeles: The Fowler museum of cultural history, 2004. *Museum Anthropology, 30*(1), 57–85.

Lazarus, R. S., & Folkman, S. (1984). *Stress, appraisal, and coping*. New York: Springer.

Leavey, G., Loewenthal, K., & King, M. (2007). Challenges to sanctuary: The clergy as a resource for mental health care in the community. *Social Science and Medicine, 65*(3), 548–559.

Levin, J. S. (1994). Religion and health: Is there an association, is it valid, and is it causal? *Social Science and Medicine, 38*, 1475–1482.

Levin, J., Chatters, L. M., Taylor, R. J. (2005). Religion, health and medicine in African Americans: Implications for physicians. *Journal of the National Medical Association, 97*(2), 237–249.

Levin, J. S., & Markides, K. S. (1986). Religious attendance and subjective health. *Journal for the Scientific Study of Religion, 25*, 31–40.

Levin, J. S., Markides, K. S., Ray, L. A. (1996). Religious attendance and psychological well-being in Mexican Americans: A panel analysis of three-generations data. *Gerontologist, 36*, 454–463.

Levitt, P. (1998). Local-level global religion: The case of U.S.-Dominican migration. *Journal for the Scientific Study of Religion, 37*, 74–89.

Lewis, L. M., Hankin, S., Reynolds, D., & Ogedegbe, G. (2007). African American spirituality: A process of honoring God, others, and self. *Journal of Holistic Nursing: Official Journal of the American Holistic Nurses' Association, 25*(1), 16–23.

Lin, F. S. (2005). Healers or patients: The shaman's roles and images in Taiwan. *Bulletin of the Institute of History and Philology Academia Sinica, 76*(Part 3), 511–568.

Lincoln, C. E., & Mamiya, L. H. (1990). *Black church in the African American experience*. Durham, NY: Duke University Press.

Loewenthal, K. (2007). *Religion, culture, and mental health*. Cambridge University Press.

Long, C. M. (2001). *Spiritual Merchants*. Knoxville, TN: The University of Tennessee Press.

Lopez, R. A. (2005). Use of alternative folk medicine by Mexican American Women. *Journal of Immigrant Health 7*(1), 23–31.

Loue, S., Lane, S. D., Lloyd, L. S., & Loh, L. (1999). Integrating Buddhism and HIV prevention in U.S. southeast Asian communities. *Journal of Health Care for the Poor & Underserved, 10*(1), 100–122.

Loue, S., & Sajatovic, M. (2006). Spirituality, coping, and HIV risk and prevention in a sample of severely mentally ill Puerto Rican women. *Journal of Urban Health, 83*(6), 1168–1182.

Markides, K. S., Levin, J. S., & Ray, L. A. (1987). Religion, aging, and life satisfaction: An eight-year, three-wave longitudinal study. *Gerontologist, 27*, 660–665.

Marks, L., Nesteruk, O., Swanson, M., Garrison, B., & Davis, T. (2005). Religion and health among African Americans. A qualitative examination. *Research on Aging, 27*(4), 447–474.

Martínez Pincay, I. G., & Guarnaccia, P. J. (2007). "It's like going through an earthquake": anthropological perspectives on depression among Latino immigrants. *Journal of Immigrant and Minority Health, 9,* 17–28.

Mautino, K. S. (1999). Faith versus the law: Traditional healers and immigration. *Journal of Immigrant Health, 1*(3), 125–131.

Mays, B., & Nicholson, J. (1933). *The Negro's church.* New York: Russell and Russell.

McIntosh, D. N., Silver, R. C., & Wortman, C. B. (1993). Religions' role in adjustment to a negative life event: Coping with the loss of a child. *Journal of Personality and Social Psychology, 65,* 812–821.

Mellins, C. A., & Ehrhardt, A. A. (1994). Acquired immunodeficiency syndrome: Sources of stress and coping. *Journal of Developmental and Behavioral Pediatrics, 15,* S54–S60.

Menjívar, C. (2000). Networks and religious communities among Salvadoran immigrants in San Francisco, Phoenix, and Washington, D.C. The Center for Comparative Immigration Studies. *Working Paper 25,* October.

Menjívar, C. (2006). Introduction – Public religion and immigration across national contexts. *American Behavioral Scientist, 49*(11), 1447–1454.

Morioka-Douglas, N., Sacks, T., and Yeo, G. (2004). Issues in caring for Afghan American elders: insights from literature and a focus group. *Journal of Cross-cultural Gerontology. 19,* 27–40.

Ng, H. Y. (2003). The "social" in social work practice – shamans and social workers. *International Social Work, 46*(3), 289–301.

Novy, D. M., Nelson, D. V., Hetzel, R. D., Squitieri, P., & Kennington, M. (1998). Coping with chronic pain: Sources of intrinsic and contextual variability. *Journal of Behavioral Medicine, 21,* 19–34.

Pargament, K. I. (1997). *The psychology of religion and coping: Theory, research, practice.* NY: Guilford Press.

Pargament, K. I., Koenig, H. G., & Perez, L. M. (2000). The many methods of religious coping: Development and initial validation of the RCOPE. *Journal of Clinical Psychology, 56,* 519–543.

Pargament, K. I., & Park, C. L. (1995). Merely a defense? The variety of religious means and ends. *Journal of Social Issues, 51,* 13–32.

Perez Foster, R. (2001). When immigration is trauma: Guidelines for the individual and family clinician. *American Journal of Orthopsychiatry, 71,* 153–170.

Peterson, J., Atwood, J. R., & Yates, B. (2002). Key elements for church-based health promotion programs: Outcome-based literature review. *Public Health Nursing, 19*(6), 401–411.

Pilgrim, D., & Bentall, R. (1999). The medicalization of misery: A critical realist analysis of the concept of depression. *Journal of Mental Health,* 8:261–274.

Rasanayagam, J. (2006). Healing with spirits and the formation of Muslim selfhood in post-Soviet Uzbekistan. *Journal of the Royal Anthropological Institute, 1*(12), 377–393.

Reiff, M., O'Connor, B., Kronenberg, F., Balick, M., & Lohr, P., (2003). Ethnomedicine in the urban environment: Dominican healers in New York City. *Human Organization, 61*(1), 12–26.

Romberg, R. (2003). *Witchcraft and welfare: Spiritual capital and the business of magic in modern Puerto Rico.* Austin: University of Texas Press.

Quinn, M. T., & McNabb, W. L. (2001). Training lay health educators to conduct a church-based weight-loss program for African American Women. *The Diabetes Educator, 27*(2), 231–238.

Sanchez, F., & Gaw, A. (2007). Mental health care of Filipino Americans. *Psychiatric Services, 58*(6), 810–815.

Seebohm, P., Henderson, P, Munn-Giddings, C. (2005). *Together we will change Community development, Mental health and Diversity.* London: The Sainsbury Centre for Mental Health.

Seeman, T. E., Dubin, L. F., & Seeman, M. (2003). Religiosity/spirituality and health: A critical review of the evidence for biological pathways. *American Psychologist, 58,* 53–63.

Seybold, K. S., & Hill, P. C. (2001). The role of religion and spirituality in mental and physical health. *Current Directions in Psychological Science, 10*(1), 21–24.

Sheridan, L. P. (2006). Islamophobia pre- and post-September 11th, 2001. *Interpersonal Violence, 21*(3), 317–336.

Shreve-Neiger, A. K., & Edelstein, B. A. (2004). Religion and anxiety: A critical review of the literature. *Clinical Psychology Review, 24*(4), 379–397.

Simoni, J. M., & Ortiz, M. Z. (2003). Mediational models of spirituality and depressive symptomatology among HIV-positive Puerto Rican women. *Cultural Diversity and Ethnic Minority Psychology, 9,* 3–15.

Singer, M., & Borrero, M. G. (1984). Indigenous treatment for alcoholism: The case of Puerto Rican spiritism. *Medical Anthropology, 8*(4), 246–273.

Singer, M., & Garcia, R. (1995). Becoming a Puerto Rican espirista: Live history of a female Healer. In C. S. Mc Clain (Ed.). *Women as healers: Cross-cultural perspectives.* New Brunswick, NJ: Rutgers University Press, pp. 157–185.

Smith, C. A., Wallston, K. A., Dwyer, K. A., & Dowdy, S. W. (1997). Beyond good and bad coping: A multidimensional examination of coping with pain in persons with rheumatoid arthritis. *Annals of Behavioral Medicine, 19,* 11–21.

Stanton, A. L., Revenson, T. A., & Tennen, H. (2007). Health Psychology: Psychological adjustment to chronic disease. *Annual Review of Psychology.* 58, 565–592.

Strawbridge, W. J., Cohen, R. D., Shema, S. J., & Kaplan, G. A. (1997). Frequent attendance at religious services and mortality over 28 years. *American Journal of Public Health, 87*(6), 957–961.

Strawbridge, W. J., Shema, S. J., Cohen, R. D., & Kaplan, G. A. (2001). Religious attendance increases survival by improving and maintaining good health behaviors, mental health, and social relationships. *Annals of Behavioral Medicine, 23,* 68–74.

Swanson, L., Crowther, M., Green, L., & Armstrong, T. (2004). African Americans, faith and health disparities. *American Research Perspectives, Spring/Summer,* 79–88.

Tan, G., Jensen, M. P., Thornby, J., & Anderson, K. O. (2005). Ethnicity, control appraisal, coping, and adjustment to chronic pain among Black and White Americans. *Pain Medicine, 6,* 18–28.

Taylor, R. J., Chatters, L. M., & Levin, J. S. (2003). *Religion in the lives of African Americans: Social, psychological, and health perspectives.* Thousand Oaks, CA: Sage.

Taylor, R. J., Ellison, C. G., Chatters, L. M., Levin, J. S., Lincoln, K. D. (2000). Mental health services in faith communities: The role of clergy in Black churches. *Social Work, 45*(1), 73–87.

Teuton, J., Dowrick, C., & Bentall, R. P. (2007). How healers manage the pluralistic healing context: The perspective of indigenous, religious and allopathic healers in relation to psychosis in Uganda. *Social Science & Medicine, 65*(6), 1260–73.

Thoresen, C. E., & Harris, A. H. S. (2002). Spirituality and health: What's the evidence and what's needed? *Annals of Behavioral Medicine, 24,* 3–13.

Tix, A. P., & Frazier, P. A. (1998). The use of religious coping during stressful life events: Main effects, moderation, and mediation. *Journal of Consulting and Clinical Psychology, 66,* 411–422.

Tobin, M. (2000). Developing mental health rehabilitation services in a culturally appropriate context: An action research project involving Arabic-speaking clients. *Australian Review, 23,* 177–178.

Traphagan, J. W. (2005). Multidimensional measurement of religiousness/spirituality for use in health research in cross-cultural perspective. *Research on Aging, 27*(4), 387–419.

Vega, W. A., Karno, M., Alegria, M., Alvidrez, J., Bernal, G., Escamilla, M., Escobar, J., Guarnaccia, P., Jenkins, J., Kopelowicz, A., Lagomasino, I. T., Lewis-Fernandez, R., Marin, R., Lopez, S., & Loue, S. (2007). Research issues for improving treatment of U.S. Hispanics with persistent mental disorders. *Psychiatric Services, 58,* 385–394.

Viladrich, A. (2006a). Botánicas in America's backyard: Uncovering the world of Latino immigrants' herb-healing practices. *Human Organization, 65*(4), 407–419.

Viladrich, A. (2006b). Beyond the supranatural: Latino healers treating Latino immigrants in New York City. *The Journal of Latino-Latin American Studies, 2*(1), 134–148.

Viladrich, A. (2007a). Between bellyaches and lucky charms: Revealing latinos' plant-healing knowledge and practices in New York City. In A. Pieroni, & I. Vandebroek (Eds.). *Traveling cultures and plants: The ethnobiology and ethnopharmacy of migrations* (Chapter 3, pp. 64–85). New York and Oxford: Berghahn Books.

Viladrich, A. (2007b). From *shrinks* to urban shamans: Argentine immigrants' therapeutic eclecticism in New York City. *Culture, Medicine and Psychiatry, 31,* 307–328.

Walters, K. L., & Simoni, J. M. (2002). Reconceptualizing native women's health: An "indigenist" stress-coping model. *American Journal of Public Health, 92*(4), 520–524.

Weaver, A. J., Flannelly, K. J., Flannelly, L. T., & Oppenheimer, J. E. (2003). Collaboration between clergy and mental health professionals: A review of professional health care journals from 1980 through 1999. *Counseling and Values, 47*(3), 162–171.

Weller, S. C., et al. (2002). Regional variations in Latino descriptions of *susto. Culture, Medicine and Psychiatry, 26,* 449–472.

Wills, T., & Filer Fagen, M. (2001). Social networks and social support. In A. Baum, T. A. Revenson, & J. E. Singer (Eds.), *Handbook of health psychology* (pp. 209–234). Mahwah, NJ: Lawrence Erlbaum.

Wynaden, D., Chapman, R., Orb, A., McGowan, S., Zeeman, Z., Yeak, S. H. (2005). Factors that influence Asian communities' access to mental health care. *International Journal of Mental Health Nursing, 14*(2), 88–95.

Yanek, L. R., Becker, D. M., Moy, T. F., Gittelsohn, J., & Koffman, D. M. (2001). Project joy: Faith based cardiovascular health promotion for African American women. *Public Health Reports, 116*(Suppl 1), 68–81.

Young, J. L., Griffith, E. E. H., & Williams, D. R. (2003). The integral role of pastoral counseling by African-American clergy in community mental health. *Psychiatric Services, 54,* 688–692.

Youssef, J., & Deane, F. P. (2006). Factors influencing mental-health help-seeking in Arabic-speaking communities in Sydney, Australia. *Mental Health, Religion & Culture, 9(1),* 43–66.

Zuñiga Rojas, D. (1999). Spiritual well-being and its influence on the holistic health of Hispanic women. In S. Torres (Ed.). *Hispanic voices: Hispanic health educators speak out* (pp. 213–229). New York, NY: NLN Press.

Chapter 9
Cultural Considerations Regarding Perspectives on Mental Illness and Healing

Declan T. Barry and Mark Beitel

"Transcultural psychiatry should begin at home"

(Murphy, 1977, pg. 169)

Introduction

In recent years, mental health professionals have increasingly recognized the role of cultural factors in the diagnosis and treatment of mental disorders (Lewis-Fernandez & Kleinman, 1995). The growing interest in examining cultural considerations pertaining to clinical practice in the U.S. is, in large part, driven by demographic changes. For example, racial and ethnic minority group members in 2006 were estimated to comprise 18.6% and 14.8% of the overall U.S. population, respectively (U.S. Census Bureau, 2007). Given the increased diversity of the U.S. population, it is no longer unusual for clinicians to treat patients from dissimilar cultural backgrounds (Bernal & Castro, 1994; Barry & Bullock, 2001). Thus, in their daily clinical practice, many providers become "culture brokers" (Abudabbeh, 1998; Barry, Elliott, & Evans, 2000) who treat individuals with a variety of cultural norms, including those related to perspectives on illness and healing.

Whether or not clinicians should attend to cultural differences, including those pertaining to illness and healing, is an important question. At first blush, this may appear to be a straightforward task; in practice, assessing cultural differences and crafting culturally informed interventions with patients from dissimilar cultural backgrounds require careful consideration, particularly since there is an absence of evidence-based treatment models involving cultural competence (Kleinman & Benson, 2006; Whitley, 2007). One clinical approach is to eschew or minimize addressing cultural differences and to focus instead on "common factors" such as therapeutic alliance. Given that there is scant research on evidence-based practices with racial/ethnic minority populations

D.T. Barry (✉)
Yale University School of Medicine, New Haven CT
e-mail: declan.barry@yale.edu

S. Loue, M. Sajatovic (eds.), *Determinants of Minority Mental Health and Wellness*, DOI 10.1007/978-0-387-75659-2_9,

(Chambless et al., 1996; Hall, 2001), proponents of empirically supported psychotherapies who do not adapt their treatment approach with individuals of racial/ethnic minority groups may be viewed as adopting such an "etic" or "universalist" approach (Triandis et al., 1993). Conversely, similar to researchers in "cultural psychology" who espouse that culture is critical in understanding human behavior (Hughes, 1996), some clinicians adopt an "emic" or culture-specific approach (Triandis et al., 1993). One manifestation of this approach in American psychology is the debate on racial/ethnicity matching in psychotherapy (the notion that, despite limited research support (see Shin et al., 2005), racial/ethnic minority patients fare better in treatment with providers from similar cultural backgrounds). A compromise position involves the "transcendist" approach (La Roche & Maxie, 2003), which espouses that cultural differences are important to assess and address and that clinicians, regardless of their racial/ethnic background are capable of developing cultural competence (Barry, 2007; Sue, 1998). In this chapter, we adopt a transcendist approach to explore cultural considerations regarding perspectives on mental illness and healing and offer practice recommendations for clinicians who work with patients of dissimilar cultural backgrounds.

Classification of Mental Illness in the U.S.: *DSM-IV-TR*

The *Diagnostic and Statistical Manual*, (*DSM-IV-TR*; American Psychiatric Association, 2000), the predominant U.S. psychiatric classification system employs a multiaxial approach to assess mental disorders (Axes I and II), general medical conditions (Axis III), psychosocial and environmental factors (Axis IV), and global functioning (Axis V). Since the third edition of the *Diagnostic and the Statistical Manual* (*DSM-III*; American Psychiatric Association, 1980), the *DSM* has de-emphasized theories of psychopathology as an organizing principle to group symptoms in favor of a biomedical approach (Mayes & Horwitz, 2005). The *DSM* classification system, however, is not "culture-free": it embraces a "Western medical approach" in which lay perspectives on illness and healing are ignored, and biomedical concepts and diagnosis are viewed as neutral and impersonal (Fabrega, 1996). As Hughes (1996), among others, has noted, the *DSM-IV* (American Psychiatric Association, 1994) can be considered to represent Eurocentric "cultural psychiatry." Some authors have argued that by disavowing the assessment of indigenous beliefs of illness such as culturally shared beliefs pertaining to the display of seemingly bizarre symptoms (e.g., seeing spirits), there is a tendency to over-diagnose psychotic-spectrum disorders in non-White individuals, including schizophrenia in Blacks (Fabrega, Mezzich, & Ulrich, 1988) and Hispanics (Jones, Gray, & Parson, 1983).

The multi-axial system of the *DSM-IV-TR* (American Psychiatric Association, 2000) does not systematically assess patients' strengths or expectations about wellness and treatment. The importance of considering preexisting skills and framing therapeutic interventions to augment these skills, particularly in men, has been noted previously (see Barry, 2007). Moreover, consideration of patients' strengths broadens clinicians' conceptualizations (Sabshin, 1989).

Given that many of the research studies supporting the classification systems employed in the *DSM-IV* (American Psychiatric Association, 1994) and *DSM-IV-TR* (American Psychiatric Association, 2000) were conducted by Western researchers on Western samples, some researchers have queried the extent to which these classifications have cross-cultural validity. Kleinman (1996), for example, argues that universality of the *DSM-IV* (American Psychiatric Association, 1994) disorders is limited to organic brain disorders, substance use disorders, schizophrenia, bipolar disorder, major depression, and specific anxiety disorders, including panic disorders, obsessive-compulsive disorders and certain phobias, and contends that the remainder of the adult psychiatric categories are peculiar to North America and Western Europe. In particular, Kleinman argues that eating disorders (particularly anorexia nervosa) and dissociative disorders (particularly dissociative identity disorder) may be viewed as bound to Western cultures. However, as noted in the *DSM-IV-TR* (American Psychiatric Association, 2000), there is growing evidence that eating disorders and dissociative disorders are evident in non-Western cultures. For example, Sierra et al. (2006) reported comparable levels of dissociative symptoms among psychiatric inpatients in the U.K., Spain, and Colombia. However, individuals living in individualist countries may be more at risk of depersonalization than those in collectivist countries (Sierra et al., 2006).

Although some authors have argued for the addition of a "cultural axis" (i.e., a separate diagnostic axis pertaining to cultural issues; e.g., Good & Good, 1986; Kleinman, 1996), the *DSM-IV-TR* (American Psychiatric Association, 2000), instead, includes sections related to capturing patients' cultural contexts, including a general introductory cultural statement, information concerning cultural considerations for the use of diagnostic categories and criteria, a listing of culture-bound syndromes, and a suggested outline for a cultural formulation. While the introductory cultural statement encourages readers to attend to the importance of culture in arriving at a diagnosis, the sections of the text concerning cultural considerations for the use of diagnostic categories and criteria provides readers with information concerning the cultural variation in the presentation of specific disorders. Appendix I of the *DSM-IV-TR* (American Psychiatric Association, 2000) includes a glossary of culture-bound syndromes and a suggested outline for a cultural formulation.

To our knowledge, there is a dearth of systematic prevalence data on culture-bound syndromes. Unlike *DSM-IV-TR* (American Psychiatric Association, 2000) sections pertaining to Axis I and II disorder that contain relatively clear-cut diagnostic criteria, descriptions of culture-bound syndromes are largely anecdotal and lack specificity. Many culture-bound syndromes are better characterized as causal explanations or illness attributions than syndromes or symptom clusters (Prince & Tcheng-Laroche, 1987). One early example of an empirical investigation in this area is the work of Westermeyer and Wintrob (1979a,b) who published a study of "folk" theories of mental illness in rural Laos. The first study examined criteria for diagnosing mental illness among *baa* (insane) individuals, their relatives, and neighbors. Socially dysfunctional *behavior*, rather than disturbed *thoughts*, or *affect*, emerged as the key diagnostic determinant. The second study dealt with theories of mental illness etiology in the same group. Nearly 60% of the etiology theories elicited were consistent with Western psychiatric views. One difference that emerged was that a familial history of mental illness was not offered as an explanation for baa by the participants.

More research is needed to specify the criteria of "culture-bound syndromes" and the extent to which they are bound or restricted to particular cultural groups. The cultural formulation emphasizes the assessment of patients' personal experience and includes consideration of their cultural identity and cultural explanations of presenting symptoms. The extent to which clinicians use the outline for a cultural formulation in their clinical practices is currently unknown.

Addressing Culture

Culture is complex and fluid and may be viewed as "the man-made part of the environment" that comprises accepted behaviors, beliefs, and institutions that exhibit great variability but which make sense to its members (Herskovits, 1948). Individuals use culture as a lens to filter information and to make sense of the world, other people, and themselves (Barry & Bullock, 2001). Culture may serve as a buffer to minimize human awareness of vulnerability (Solomon, Greenberg, & Pyszcynski, 1991) and may satiate our basic human need to belong (Baumeister & Leary, 1995). Although many writers emphasize the importance of culture, its usefulness as an explanatory concept in examining psychological phenomena resides in the investigator's ability to "unpackage" or deconstruct it (Poortinga, van de Vijver, Joe, & van de Koppel, 1987; Whiting, 1976). Mental health researchers have traditionally deconstructed culture by using two categorical variables – race and ethnicity. Whereas race was initially viewed as a biological classification based on shared, fixed, immutable inborn traits (e.g., skin color) that could predictably categorize individuals into mutually exclusive groups (Barry, 2007), ethnicity is typically used to assign group membership based on cultural, nationality, or linguistic factors (Betancourt & Lopez, 1993).

The Three-Factor Approach

While mental health researchers have traditionally employed race- and ethnicity-based categories as a proxy for culture, these constructs may have limited usefulness to clinicians. For example, while a patient's race/ethnicity-based demographic classification is unlikely to change over the course of treatment, the meaning attributed to group membership may. Problems with solely relying on categorical measures of culture, such as ethnicity and race, have prompted researchers to recommend that (similar to the notion of culture itself) the constructs of race and ethnicity should be deconstructed (Barry, 2007). Phinney (1996) delineated three dimensions of race/ethnicity: cultural values and norms; salience and meaning of ethnic or racial identity; and experiences associated with ethnic/racial minority status. Barry and colleagues (Barry & Beitel, 2006; Barry, Bernard, & Beitel, 2006; Barry, Elliott, & Evans, 2000; Barry & Garner, 2001) have outlined a three-factor model to better assist mental health clinicians and researchers in deconstructing the concept of culture. The three factors—acculturation, self-construal, and ethnic identity— are cultural variables that have been shown to be related to human psychosocial functioning among individuals of racial/ethnic minority status (Berry, 1980; Markus & Kitayama, 1991; Phinney, 1996; Singelis, Bond, Sharkey, & Lai, 1999).

Acculturation, self-construal, and *ethnic identity* provide mental health professionals who work with patients from diverse racial/ethnic backgrounds a dimensional approach to examining culture. This approach is predicated on the view that culture is dynamic and complex, and may provide a more individualized or differentiated measure of culture than categorical variables, such as race and ethnicity (Barry & Garner, 2001; Barry & Grilo, 2002). In doing so, clinicians may avoid the "fallacy of the assumption of a homogeneous cultural environment" (Huges, 1996, p. 299). These three factors allow researchers and clinicians to directly measure issues related to culture rather than inferring them in a post-hoc fashion based on findings related to race/ethnicity differences (Barry & Garner, 2001; Barry & Grilo, 2003). A brief overview of the three components follows.

Acculturation encompasses social interaction and communication styles that individuals adopt when interacting with individuals and groups from another culture (Barry & Garner, 2001). Acculturation comprises both competence and ease/comfort in communicating with racial/ethnic group peers and outgroup members. Communication difficulty arising from cultural differences between racial/ethnic minority patients and their providers has been associated with underutilization of and unwillingness to use health care services (Barry & Grilo, 2002; Ma, 1999). The process and outcome of acculturation may also influence how symptoms are expressed and, in turn, subsequent entry into or use of the mental health system (Aponte & Barnes, 1995). Berry's (1980) scheme may be used to classify socialization and communication patterns: *assimilation* for socialization and communication primarily with individuals from the majority culture, *separation* for socialization and communication primarily with ethnic/ racial peers, *integration* for socialization and communication with members of both minority and majority cultural groups, and *marginalization* for absence of socialization and communication with ethnic/racial minority peers or majority culture members.

Self-construal refers to two types of self-concept, independent and interdependent, which appear to be linked to the degree to which one's culture makes a distinction between the individual and the group (Markus & Kitayama, 1991). Variations in self-construal may influence recognition and reporting of psychiatric symptoms, communication styles, and use of mental health services (Lin & Cheung, 1999; Oetzel, 1998; Yeh, 1999). Independent self-construal refers to a self that is viewed as a separate, stable, autonomous, and bounded entity, whereas interdependent self-construal is described as flexible, variable, and guided by external factors such as roles, status, and relationships.

Americans of ethnic/racial minority status may differ from those of European descent in terms of the salience of their self-construals. For example, Asian Americans, unlike Americans of European descent, tend to have more salient interdependent rather than independent self-construals (Chung, 1992). However, clinicians should assess both self-construal dimensions for each patient and should not assume, for example, that White patients will necessarily have a more salient independent than interdependent self-construal. Differences in self-construal may influence how mental disorders are experienced; for example, Japanese individuals may be more prone to experience social phobia as a fear about embarrassing others ("taijin kyofusho"), while those with social phobia in the U.S. typically report a fear of personal embarrassment. However, both types of social anxiety exist in both countries (Kleinknecht, Dinnel, Kleinknecht, Hiruma, & Harada, 1997).

The third factor—*ethnic identity*—may be a more useful psychological construct than ethnicity (Phinney, 1996). Ethnic identity may be defined as the ethnic component of social identity, defined by Tajfel (1981) as: "that part of an individual's self-concept which derives from his knowledge of his membership of a social group (or groups) together with the value and emotional significance attached to that membership" (p. 255). Ethnic identity has been identified as an important cultural variable in examining psychosocial functioning and health care utilization among racial/ethnic minority group members (Brinson & Kottler, 1995; Pillay, 2005).

Alternatives to the Three-Factor Approach

Measures of culture that may be useful to clinicians have been reviewed elsewhere (Burlew, Bellow, & Lovett, 2000; Kohatsu & Richardson, 1996). For example, Burlew, and colleagues group nineteen cultural identity measures into one of four categories: identity formation, cultural connectedness, multicultural experiences, and multidimensional measures encompassing more than one category. Semi-structured culture-based clinical interviews may also be of use to clinicians who have a multicultural clientele: Ponterotto, Gretchen, and Chauhan (2001) review five, clinically oriented cultural assessment systems, including Washington (1994), Grieger and Ponterotto (1995), Dana (1998),

Jacobsen (1988), Berg-Cross and Takushi-Chinen (1995). Ponterotto and colleagues outline an integrated, multicultural clinical interview guide based, in part, on these assessment systems.

Mental Illness Models

Assessing patients' perception of the etiology and nature of their presenting symptoms and disorders may assist clinicians to arrive at valid diagnoses and to develop optimal treatment recommendations (Good & Good, 1986). Culture-based attributions regarding mental illness may influence help-seeking behaviors. For example, a study comparing Americans of Japanese and European descent found that the former were more likely to attribute mental illness to external, social factors, which in turn was associated with avoiding professional mental health services in favor of an individual problem-solving approach (Narikiyo & Kameoka, 1992). Traditional cultural beliefs regarding serious mental illness may also influence help-seeking behaviors on the part of family members. For example, family members of patients with schizophrenia attending a teaching hospital in India reported that mental illness was a function of spirits and often viewed traditional healers as the providers of choice (Banerjee & Roy, 1998). Thus, professional mental health services may not be used as front-line treatment. Campion and Bhugra (1997) found that 45% of Indian patients seeking psychiatric treatment had previously sought services from a religious healer (Banerjee & Roy, 1998). Individuals may also exhibit a "mixed models" approach, i.e., their beliefs about treatment or healing may seem contradictory or may appear discordant with their health-seeking behaviors. For example, Beckerlag (1994) found that in Swahili, Africa, some individuals combined prayer, home-cures, and biomedicine. More research is needed to examine how decision making regarding the prioritization of health-seeking behaviors occur and what factors are emphasized (e.g., efficacy beliefs, cost, effort). Diverse help-seeking behaviors is not unusual in the U.S.; patients often use a range of treatments (e.g., allopathic, complementary, alternative), especially for chronic medical conditions such as chronic pain (Barry & Beitel, 2008; Barry, Beitel, Joshi, Falcioni, & Schottenfeld, 2007). Thus, while providers may limit their interventions to evidence-based practices, patients may avail themselves of a smorgasbord of interventions.

Neurotic Disorders (Depression/Anxiety)

Despite the common occurrence of mood disorders (Kessler et al., 2005), their associated economic burden (Greenberg et al., 2003) and attenuation in quality of life (Angermeyer, Holzinger, Matschinger, & Stengler-Wenzke, 2002; Greenberg et al., 2003), the majority of individuals with mood disorders do not seek treatment (Kessler et al., 2005). Given that many people with anxiety and depression do not view their symptoms as "psychiatric" and may reject professional mental health treatments, it behooves providers to solicit patients' viewpoints and preferences in order to appropriately diagnose and develop a referral or treatment strategy that may be viewed as credible and effective (Kirkmayer, 2001).

A study of White, Black Caribbean, and South Asian older adults in the U.K. found that White participants' reports of the meaning of depression were closer to the Western biomedical model than their Black Caribbean and South Asian counterparts (Lawrence et al., 2006a). South Asian participants were more likely to view depression as a normal feeling associated with grief and sadness that originated from a deficiency in character, while both South Asian and Black Caribbean older adults were more likely to define depression in terms of worry and "troubles within the mind" (Lawrence et al., 2006a, p. 30). The Black Caribbean group was more likely to view prayer as an effective coping strategy, while South Asian and White groups were more likely to endorse family support (Lawrence et al., 2006b). Karasz and colleagues (2003) investigated cultural differences in illness representations, including depression (Karasz, Sacajiu, & Garcia, 2003; Karasz, 2005) and everyday fatigue (Karasz & McKinley, 2007). Some research has also examined mental illness representations of providers from different cultural backgrounds (see Morant, 2006).

Psychotic Disorders (Schizophrenia)

Schizophrenia occurs worldwide and incurs a tremendous global burden and financial cost (Rossler, Salize, van Os, & Riecher-Rossler, 2005; World Health Organization, 1979); lifetime prevalence rates range from 0.5% to 1.6% (Jablensky, 1995) with differences in methodology, observation times—in addition to true prevalence differences—accounting for much of the variability (Wittchen & Jacobi, 2005). The symptom presentation and course of schizophrenia appears to vary geographically with individuals in developing countries exhibiting a noticeably better prognosis than their counterparts in developed countries, despite limited health services (Jablensky et al., 1992). For example, 62.8% of individuals with schizophrenia in developing countries were estimated to have a remitting course with full remission compared to 36.8% in developed countries (Jablensky et al., 1992). Improved positive outcomes in developing countries have been attributed to better community support for patients with schizophrenia (Jenkins & Karno, 1992). Thus, despite the universality of schizophrenia, variability in symptom expression and prognosis suggest the importance of environmental or cultural factors. Furthermore, some subtypes of schizophrenia (e.g., disorganized) appear to decline as a function of urbanization in some but not all cultures (Lin, 1996).

Mental Health Models

Similar to the recent emergence of "positive psychology" in mainstream American academic clinical psychology (Seligman, 2002), research on culture-related mental health models is a nascent field of inquiry. A major challenge involves the operational definition of mental health in different cultural contexts. Increased clarity regarding operationalization will facilitate the further examination of determinants of mental health in cultural minority populations. The facet of mental health that has received the most attention from cross-cultural researchers is quality of life (QOL) (see Utsey, Bolden, Brown, & Chae, 2001 for a review), which has been defined variously as subjective well-being, role satisfaction, and level of functioning (Chambers & Kong, 1996; Croog, Levine, & Testa, 1986). Two measures of QOL that show promise in cross-cultural studies (see Utsey, Bolden, Brown, & Chae, 2001 for a review) are the Schedule for the Evaluation of Individual Quality of Life (SEIQOL) (Coen, O'Mahony, O'Boyle, & Joyce, 1993), which employs an open phenomenological format and the World Health Organization Quality of Life—100 (WHOQOL-100) (De Vries & Van Heck, 1997), which consists of 100 questions covering six domains.

Research on QOL in Western cultures has typically included variables pertaining to independent self-construal such as autonomy and personal happiness. While these facets of QOL may resonate in both Eastern and Western cultures, the structure and function of QOL in collectivist cultures may differ from individualist cultures. For example, it has been suggested that an assessment of beliefs regarding energetics (i.e., *chi, prana*), harmonics (balance, interdependence, social relationships), and temporality (circularity, fluidity) is important in the formulation of QOL in collectivist cultures (Saxena, 1994).

Mental Health Services Utilization

Epidemiological findings regarding significant differences in morbidity and mortality among racial and groups focused attention on health disparities (Hummer, Benjamins, & Rogers 2004), and this area has become a major priority for federal health research funding (NIH, 2002). Differences in access to effective mental health services across racial and ethnic groups (i.e., mental health disparities) have also garnered increased research attention (Barry, 2007). In 2001, the U.S. Department of Health and Human Services (DHHS) issued a supplement to the Surgeon General's report on mental health that underscored the role of race and ethnicity in accounting for several disparities in mental health care in the U.S., including limited access to effective mental health services for Americans of racial and ethnic minority descent compared with those of European descent. Community-based studies have found that among individuals meeting psychiatric diagnostic criteria, Whites are more likely than those from racial/ethnic minority groups to utilize mental health services (Cook, McGuire, & Miranda, 2007; Garland, Lau, Yeh, & McCabe, 2005; Vega et al., 1998; Wells, Klap, Koike, & Sherbourne, 2001). (Koroukian addresses disparities in service access and utilization in Chapter 7.) Whereas structural barriers to mental health treatment (e.g., lack of linguistically competent staff) are important (see Barry, 2007), culture-related factors may also account for the relatively lower utilization of mental health treatment among racial and ethnic minority groups, in comparison to Whites. As noted in the previous section, racial/ethnic minority patients who possess culture-based models of pathology and treatment that differ from allopathic or conventional models may be reluctant to engage in professional mental health services or may delay seeking such services.

Instead of seeking help from mental health professionals, racial/ethnic minority individuals may seek out traditional healers or religious leaders (Deva, 2002). (See Chapter 9 by Viladrich and Abraído Lanza, for an in-depth discussion of reliance on religious healers for the treatment of psychological disorders.) Reluctance to use mental health treatments may also be associated with their perceived lack of efficacy or credibility. For example, among college students in China, the perceived inefficacy of mental health services has been linked to infrequent use of mental health services (Boey, 1999). Similarly, in a study of East Asian immigrants in the U.S., 50% expressed strong unwillingness to utilize psychological services; greater assimilation was associated with increased willingness to use them (Barry & Grilo, 2002). A proclivity to seek "informal" help from family and friends among individuals of East Asian descent has also been associated with decreased service utilization (Morrisey, 1997; Okazaki, 2000).

Some racial/ethnic minority individuals may not seek professional mental health treatment because of concerns that they may be ostracized by peers within their communities (Cinnirella & Loewenthal, 1999). Although stigma about seeking psychiatric services appears common across racial/ethnic groups in the U.S., some research suggests that it may be more pervasive among non-White racial groups. For example, a recent study found that in comparison to White women with depression, immigrant African and Caribbean women report decreased desire for mental health treatment due to stigma (Nadeem et al., 2007).

Assessment of psychiatric disorders and subsequent treatment referrals are further complicated because *DSM-IV* (American Psychiatric Association, 1994) diagnostic categories and indigenous labels of subjective distress may not correspond well (Lin & Cheung, 1999). For example, while mood disorders and anxiety disorders are two of the most frequently occurring psychiatric disorders internationally (Weissman et al., 1996, 1997), the manner in which symptoms of these disorders are displayed, interpreted, and received socially may vary widely (Kirkmayer, 1989; Kirkmayer, Young, & Hayton, 1995) and may result in the under-recognition or misidentification of psychological distress. In non-Western countries, there is less of a tendency to separate "psychic" and "somatic" (Fabrega, 2001; Lauber & Rossler, 2007). The tendency to experience psychological distress somatically influences treatment seeking so that individuals are more likely to seek help in primary care rather than mental health settings (Al Krenawi, 2005; Ng, 1997) and may be associated with decreased stigma. For example, a recent study conducted in South India found that somatoform disorders carried less stigma than depressive disorders (Raguram & Weiss, 2004).

Conclusions and Recommendations

Mental health professionals routinely treat patients from diverse cultural backgrounds. Culture-based perspectives on illness and healing may influence perspectives on illness and healing as well as help-seeking behaviors. Rigorous scientific research, involving larger samples and reliable and valid measures, is needed to further examine culture-based models of mental illness and mental health and to determine the extent to which these models direct help-seeking behaviors and engagement in evidence-based mental health treatments among diverse cultural groups. Acculturation, self-construal, and ethnic identity measures may assist researchers to adequately conceptualize and assess the complex construct of culture in such research endeavors.

Key Points

- The *Diagnostic and Statistical Manual* (*DSM-IV-TR*; American Psychiatric Association, 2000) is not a "culture-free" classification system.
- Culture-based models of mental illness and mental health may influence patients' help-seeking behaviors and decision making about treatments.
- Increased understanding of acculturation, self-construal, and ethnic identity provide clinicians with potentially useful clinical information regarding self-definition and relatedness.

Practice Recommendations

1. Consider assessing patients' models of mental illness and mental health, including those that are culturally based.
2. Consider assessing multiple psychologically meaningful dimensions of culture.
3. Consider framing clinical interventions to emphasize patient strengths and/ or building skills and avoid focusing exclusively on weaknesses.
4. Given that patients may not share clinicians' treatment models, consider providing a concrete, convincing rationale for clinical interventions.

Research Recommendations

1. Consider using dimensional (e.g., ethnic identity) in addition to categorical (e.g., ethnicity) measures of culture.
2. Consider using methods from cultural and cross-cultural psychology (e.g., rigorous recruitment and data-collection methods) rather than relying exclusively on anthropological methods (e.g., participant observation).

3. Consider examining a variety of noncultural factors (e.g., age, household income, gender) in addition to measures of culture when conducting research on illness and healing among cultural groups; differences on measures of mental illness and healing across racial/ethnic groups should not automatically be attributed to cultural factors.
4. Consider investigating how individual symptoms or factors are organized in culture-related mental illness models and consider examining patient investment in a variety of treatment models, including allopathic, complementary, and alternative, as patients' views of medical treatment models may not be concordant with those of mental health researchers.

References

Abudabbeh, N. (1998). Counseling Arab-American families. In P. U. Gielen (Ed.), *The family and family therapy in international perspective* (pp. 115–126). Edizioni Lint Trieste.

Al-Krenawi, A. (2005). Mental health practice in Arab countries. *Current Opinions in Psychiatry, 18*(5), 560–564.

American Psychiatric Association (1980). *Diagnostic and statistical manual for mental disorders, 3rd edition.* Washington, DC: American Psychiatric Association.

American Psychiatric Association (1994). *Diagnostic and statistical manual for mental disorders* (4th ed.). Washington, DC: American Psychiatric Association.

American Psychiatric Association (2000). *Diagnostic and statistical manual for mental disorders* (4th ed.). *text revision.* Washington, DC: American Psychiatric Association.

Angermeyer, M. C., Holzinger, A., Matschinger, H., & Stengler-Wenzke, K. (2002). Depression and quality of life: Results of a follow-up study. *International Journal of Social Psychiatry, 48*(3), 189–199.

Aponte, J. F., & Barnes, J. M. (1995). Impact of acculturation and moderator variables on the intervention and treatment of ethnic groups. In J. F. Aponte, R. Y. Rivers, & J. Wohl (Eds.), *Psychological interventions and cultural diversity* (pp. 19–39). Boston: Allyn and Bacon.

Banerjee, G., & Roy, S. (1998). Determinants of help-seeking behaviour of families of schizophrenic patients attending a teaching hospital in India: An indigenous explanatory model. *International Journal of Social Psychiatry, 44*(3), 199.

Barry, D. T. (2007). Culture, ethnicity, race, and men's mental health. In J. E. Grant & M. N. Potenza (Eds.), *Textbook of men's mental health* (pp. 343–362). Washington, DC: American Psychiatric Publishing, Inc.

Barry, D. T., & Beitel, M. (2006). Sex role ideology among East Asian immigrants in the United States. *American Journal of Orthopsychiatry, 76*(4), 512–517.

Barry, D. T., Beitel, M., Joshi, D., Falcioni, J., & Schottenfeld, R.S. (2007, June). *Prevalence rates of chronic pain and interest in pain management among patients seeking MMT.* Paper presented at the Sixty-Ninth College on Problems of Drug Dependence International Conference, Quebec, Canada.

Barry, D. T., & Beitel, M. (2008). The scientific status of complementary and alternative medicines for mood disorders: A review. In S. Loue & M. Sajatovic (Eds.), *Diversity issues in the diagnosis, treatment, and research of mood disorders* (pp. 110–134). New York: Oxford University Press.

Barry, D. T., Bernard, M. J., & Beitel, M. (2006). Gender, sex role ideology, and self-esteem among East Asian immigrants in the United States. *Journal of Nervous and Mental Disease, 194*(9), 708–711.

Barry, D. T., & Bullock, W. A. (2001). Culturally creative psychotherapy with a Latino couple by an Anglo therapist. *Journal of Family Psychotherapy, 12*, 15–29.

Barry, D. T., Elliott, R., & Evans, E. M. (2000). Foreigners in a strange land: Self-construal and ethnic identity in male Arabic immigrants. *Journal of Immigrant and Minority Health*, *2*(3), 133–144.

Barry, D. T., & Garner, D. M. (2001). Eating concerns in East Asian immigrants. *Eating and Weight Disorders*, *6*, 90–98.

Barry, D. T., & Grilo, C. M. (2002). Cultural, psychological, and demographic correlates of willingness to use psychological services among East Asian immigrants. *Journal of Nervous and Mental Disease*, *190*, 32–39.

Barry, D. T., & Grilo, C. M. (2003). Cultural, self-esteem, and demographic correlates of perception of personal and group discrimination among East Asian immigrants. *American Journal of Orthopsychiatry*, *73*, 223–229.

Baumeister, R. F., & Leary, M. R. (1995). The need to belong: desire for interpersonal attachments as a fundamental human motivation. *Psychological Bulletin*, *117*(3), 497–529.

Beckerleg, S. (1994). Medical pluralism and Islam in Swahili communities in Kenya. *Medical Anthropology Quarterly*, *8*, 299–313.

Berg-Cross, L., & Chinen, R. T. (1995). Multicultural training models and the person-in-culture interview. In J. G. Ponterotto, J. M. Casas, L. A. Suzuki, & C. M. Alexander (Eds.), *Handbook of multicultural counseling* (pp. 333–356). Thousand Oaks: Sage.

Bernal, M. E., & Castro, F. G. (1994). Are clinical psychologists prepared for service and research with ethnic minorities? Report of a decade of progress. *American Psychologist*, *49*(9), 797–805.

Berry, J. W. (1980). Acculturation as varieties of adaptation. In A. Padilla (Ed.), *Acculturation: Theory, models, and some new findings* (pp. 9–25). Boulder, CO: Westview Press.

Betancourt, H., & Lopez, S. R. (1993). The study of culture, ethnicity, and race in American psychology. *American Psychologist*, *48*(6), 629–637.

Boey, K. W. (1999). Help-seeking preference of college students in urban China after the implementation of the"open-door" policy. *International Journal of Social Psychiatry*, *45*(2), 104.

Brinson, J. A., & Kottler, J. A. (1995). Minorities. *Journal of Mental Health Counseling*, *17*(4), 371–385.

Burlew, A. K., Bellow, S., & Lovett, M. (2000). Racial identity measures: A review and classification system. In R. H. Dana (Ed.), *Handbook of cross-cultural and multicultural personality assessment* (pp. 173–196). London: Lawrence Erlbaum Associates.

Campion, J., & Bhugra, D. (1997). Experiences of religious healing in psychiatric patients in South India. *Social Psychiatry and Psychiatric Epidemiology*, *32*(4), 215–221.

Chambers, J. W., & Kong, B. W. (1996). Assessing quality of life: Construction and validation of a scale. In R. L. Jones (Ed.), *Handbook of tests and measurements for black populations* (pp. 335–349). Hampton, VA: Cobb & Henry.

Chambless, D. L., Sanderson, W. C., Shoham, V., Bennett, S., Pope, K. S., Crits-Christoph, P., et al. (1996). An update on empirically validated therapies. *The Clinical Psychologist*, *49*, 5–18.

Chung, D. K. (1992). Asian cultural commonalities: A comparison with mainstream American culture. In S. Furuto, R. Biswas, D. K. Chung, & F. Ross-Sheriff (Eds.), *Social work practice with Asian Americans* (pp. 27–44). Newbury Park, CA: Sage.

Cinnirella, M., & Loewenthal, K. M. (1999). Religious and ethnic group influences on beliefs about mental illness: A qualitative interview study. *British Journal of Medical Psychology*, *72*(4), 505–524.

Coen, R., O'Mahony, D., O'Boyle, C., Joyce, C. R. B., Hiltbrunner, B., Walsh, J. B., et al. (1993). Measuring the quality of life of dementia patients using the schedule for the evaluation of individual quality of life. *Irish Journal of Psychology*, *14*(1), 154–163.

Cook, B. L., McGuire, T., & Miranda, J. (2007). Measuring trends in mental health care disparities, 2002–2004. *Psychiatric Services*, *58*, 1533–1540.

Croog, S. H., Levine, S., Testa, M. A., Brown, B., Bulpitt, C. J., Jenkins, C. D., et al. (1986). The effects of antihypertensive therapy on the quality of life. *New England Journal of Medicine*, *314*(26), 1657–1664.

Dana, R. H. (1998). *Understanding cultural identity in intervention and assessment.* Thousand Oaks: Sage Publications.

De Vries, J., & Van Heck, G. L. (1997). The World Health Organization Quality of Life Assessment Instrument (WHOQOL-100): validation study with the Dutch version. *European Journal of Psychological Assessment, 13*(3), 164–178.

Deva, M. (2002). Mental health and mental health care in Asia. *World Psychiatry, 1,* 118–120.

Fabrega, H., Jr. (1996). Cultural and historical foundations of psychiatric diagnosis. In J. E. Mezzich, A. Kleinman, H. Fabrega, Jr. & D. L. Parron (Eds.), *Culture and psychiatric diagnosis: A DSM-IV perspective* (pp. 3–14). Washington, DC: American Psychiatric Press.

Fabrega, H., Jr. (2001). Culture and history in psychiatric diagnosis and practice. *Psychiatric Clinics of North America, 24*(3), 391–405.

Fabrega, H., Jr., Mezzich, J., & Ulrich, R. F. (1988). Black-white differences in psychopathology in an urban psychiatric population. *Comprehensive Psychiatry, 29*(3), 285–297.

Garland, A. F., Lau, A. S., Yeh, M., & McCabe, K. (2005). Racial and ethnic differences in utilization of mental health services among high-risk youths. *American Journal of Psychiatry, 162,* 1336–1343.

Good, B. J., & Good, M. (1986). The cultural context of diagnosis and therapy: A view from medical anthropology. In M. Miranda (Ed.), *Mental health research and practice in minority communities* (pp. 1–27). Washington, DC: U.S. Department of Health and Human Services.

Greenberg, P. E., Kessler, R. C., Birnbaum, H. G., Leong, S. A., Lowe, S. W., Berglund, P. A., et al. (2003). The economic burden of depression in the United States: How did it change between 1990 and 2000? *Journal of Clinical Psychiatry, 64,* 1465–1476.

Grieger, I., & Ponterotto, J. G. (1995). A framework for assessment in multicultural counseling. In J. G. Ponterotto, J. M. Casas, L. A. Suzuki, & C. M. Alexander (Eds.), *Handbook of multicultural counseling* (pp. 357–374). Thousand Oaks: Sage.

Hall, G. C. (2001). Psychotherapy research with ethnic minorities: empirical, ethical, and conceptual issues. *Journal of Consulting and Clinical Psychology, 69*(3), 502–510.

Herskovits, M. J. (1948). *Man and his works: The science of cultural anthropology.* New York: AA Knopf.

Hughes, C. C. (1996). The culture-bound syndromes and psychiatric diagnosis. In J. Mezzich, A. Kleinman, H. Fabrega, Jr., & D. L. Parron (Eds.), *Culture and psychiatric diagnosis: A DSM-IV perspective* (pp. 289–307). Washington, DC: American Psychiatric Press, Inc.

Hummer, R. A., Benjamins, M., & Rogers, R. (2004). Race/ethnic disparities in health and mortality among the elderly: A documentation and examination of social factors. In N. Anderson, R. Bulatao & B. Cohen (Eds.), *Critical perspectives on racial and ethnic differences in health in late life* (pp. 53–94). Washington, DC: National Academies Press.

Jablensky, A. (1995). Schizophrenia: recent epidemiologic issues. *Epidemiologic Reviews, 17*(1), 10–20.

Jablensky, A., Sartorius, N., Ernberg, G., Anker, M., Korten, A., Cooper, J. E., et al. (1992). Schizophrenia: manifestations, incidence and course in different cultures. A World Health Organization ten-country study. *Psychological Medicine Monograph Supplement, 20,* 1–97.

Jacobsen, F. M. (1988). Ethnocultural assessment. In L. Comas-Diaz & E. E. H. Griffith (Eds.), *Clinical guidelines in cross-cultural mental health* (pp. 135–147). New York: Wiley.

Jenkins, J. H., & Karno, M. (1992). The meaning of expressed emotion: Theoretical issues raised by cross-cultural research. *The American Journal of Psychiatry, 149*(1), 9–21.

Jones, B. E., Gray, B. A., & Parson, E. B. (1983). Manic-depressive illness among poor urban Hispanics. *American Journal of Psychiatry, 140*(9), 1208–1210.

Karasz, A. (2005). Cultural differences in conceptual models of depression. *Social Science and Medicine, 60*(7), 1625–1635.

Karasz, A., & McKinley, P. S. (2007). Cultural differences in conceptual models of everyday fatigue: A vignette study. *Journal of Health Psychology, 12*(4), 613.

Karasz, A., Sacajiu, G., & Garcia, N. (2003). Conceptual models of psychological distress among low-income patients in an inner-city primary care clinic. *Journal of General Internal Medicine, 18*(6), 475–477.

Kessler, R. C., Demler, O., Frank, R. G., Olfson, M., Pincus, H. A., Walters, E. E., et al. (2005). Prevalence and treatment of mental disorders, 1990 to 2003. *New England Journal of Medicine, 352*(24), 2515–2523.

Kirmayer, L. J. (1989). Cultural variations in the response to psychiatric disorders and emotional distress. *Social Science and Medicine, 29*, 327–339.

Kirmayer, L. J. (2001). Cultural variations in the clinical presentation of depression and anxiety: Implications for diagnosis and treatment. *Journal of Clinical Psychiatry, 62*, 22–20.

Kirmayer, L. J., Young, A., & Hayton, B. C. (1995). The cultural context of anxiety disorders. *Psychiatric Clinics of North America, 18*, 503–521.

Kleinknecht, R. A., Dinnel, D. L., Kleinknecht, E. E., Hiruma, N., & Harada, N. (1997). Cultural factors in social anxiety: A comparison of social phobia symptoms and Taijin Kyofusho. *Journal of Anxiety Disorders, 11*(2), 157–177.

Kleinman, A. (1996). How is culture important for DSM-IV? In J. E. Mezzich, A. Kleinman, H. Fabrega, & D. L. Parron (Eds.), *Culture and psychiatric diagnosis: A DSM-IV perspective* (pp. 15–25). Washington, DC: American Psychiatric Press, Inc.

Kleinman, A., & Benson, P. (2006). Anthropology in the clinic: The problem of cultural competency and how to fix it. *Public Library of Science Medicine, 3*(10), e294.

Kohatsu, E. L., & Richardson, T. Q. (1996). Racial and ethnic identity assessment. In L. A. Suzuki, J. G. Ponterotto & P. J. Meller (Eds.), *Handbook of multicultural assessment: Clinical, psychological, and educational applications* (pp. 611–650). San Francisco: Jossey-Bass.

La Roche, M. J., & Maxie, A. (2003). Ten considerations in addressing cultural differences in psychotherapy. *Professional Psychology: Research and Practice, 34*, 180–186.

Lauber, C., & Rossler, W. (2007). Stigma towards people with mental illness in developing countries in Asia. *International Review of Psychiatry, 19*(2), 157–178.

Lawrence, V., Murray, J., Banerjee, S., Turner, S., Sangha, K., Byng, R., et al. (2006a). Concepts and causation of depression: A cross-cultural study of the beliefs of older adults. *The Gerontologist, 46*(1), 23–32.

Lawrence, V., Banerjee, S., Bhugra, D., Sangha, K., Turner, S., & Murray, J. (2006b). Coping with depression in later life: a qualitative study of help-seeking in three ethnic groups. *Psychological Medicine, 36*(10), 1375–1383.

Lewis-Fernandez, R., & Kleinman, A. (1995). Cultural psychiatry: Theoretical, clinical, and research issues. *Psychiatric Clinics of North America, 18*(3), 433–448.

Lin, K. M. (1996). Cultural influences on the diagnosis of psychotic and organic disorders. In J. E. Mezzich, A. Kleinman, H. Fabrega, Jr. & D. L. Parron (Eds.), *Culture and psychiatric diagnosis: A DSM-IV perspective* (pp. 49–62). Washington, DC: American Psychiatric Press, Inc.

Lin, K. M., & Cheung, F. (1999). Mental health issues for Asian Americans. *Psychiatric Services, 50*(6), 774–780.

Ma, G. X. (1999). Access to health care by Asian Americans. In G. X. Ma & G. Henderson (Eds.), *Ethnicity and health care: A sociocultural approach* (pp. 99–121). Springfield, IL: Charles C. Thomas.

Markus, H. R., & Kitayama, S. (1991). Culture and the self: Implications for cognition, emotion, and motivation. *Psychological Review, 98*(2), 224–253.

Mayes, R., & Horwitz, A. V. (2005). DSM-III and the revolution in the classification of mental illness. *Journal of the History of the Behavioral Sciences, 41*(3), 249–267.

Morant, N. (2006). Social representations and professional knowledge: The representation of mental illness among mental health practitioners. *British Journal of Social Psychology, 45*(4), 817–838.

Morrisey, M. (1997). The invisible minority: Counseling Asian Americans. *Counseling Today*, *40(4)*, 21–22.

Murphy, H. (1977). Transcultural psychiatry should begin at home. *Psychological Medicine*, *7*, 369–371.

Nadeem, E., Lange, J. M., Edge, D., Fongwa, M., Belin, T., & Miranda, J. (2007). Does stigma keep poor young immigrant and U.S.-Born Black and Latina women from seeking mental health care? *Psychiatric Services*, *58*(12), 1547–1554.

Narikiyo, T. A., & Kameoka, V. A. (1992). Attributions of mental illness and judgments about help seeking among Japanese-American and White American students. *Journal of Counseling Psychology*, *39*(3), 363–369.

National Institutes of Health. (2002). *National Institutes of Health strategic research plan and budget to reduce and ultimately eliminate health disparities, Volume 1, Fiscal Years 2002–2006*. Washington, DC: U.S. Dept of Health and Human Services.

Ng, C. H. (1997). The stigma of mental illness in Asian cultures. *Australian and New Zealand Journal of Psychiatry*, *31*(3), 382–390.

Oetzel, J. G. (1998). The effects of self-construals and ethnicity on self-reported conflict styles. *Communication Reports*, *11*(2), 133.

Okazaki, S. (2000). Treatment delay among Asian-American patients with severe mental illness. *American Journal of Orthopsychiatry*, *70*(1), 58–64.

Phinney, J. (1996). When we talk about ethnic groups, what do we mean. *American Psychologist*, *51*(9), 918–927.

Pillay, Y. (2005). Racial identity as a predictor of the psychological health of African American students at a predominantly White university. *Journal of Black Psychology*, *31*(1), 46.

Ponterotto, J. G., Gretchen, D., & Chauhan, R. V. (2001). Cultural identity and multicultural assessment. In J. G. Ponterotto, J. M. Casas, L. A. Suzuki, & C. M. Alexander (Eds.), *Handbook of multicultural assessment: Clinical, psychological, and educational applications* (pp. 67–99). Thousand Oaks: Sage.

Poortinga, Y. H., van de Vijver, F. J. R., Joe, R. C., & van de Koppel, J. M. H. (1987). Peeling the onion called culture: A synopsis. In C. Kagitcibasi (Ed.), *Growth and progress in cross-cultural psychology* (pp. 22–34). Berwyn, PA: Swets North American.

Prince, R., & Tcheng-Laroche, F. (1987). Culture-bound syndromes and international disease classifications. *Culture, Medicine and Psychiatry*, *11*(1), 3–19.

Raguram, R., & Weiss, M. (2004). Stigma and somatisation. *British Journal of Psychiatry*, *185*, 174; author reply 174–175.

Rossler, W., Joachim Salize, H., van Os, J., & Riecher-Rossler, A. (2005). Size of burden of schizophrenia and psychotic disorders. *European Neuropsychopharmacology*, *15*(4), 399–409.

Sabshin, M. (1989). Normality and the boundaries of psychopathology. *Journal of Personality Disorders*, *6*, 19–31.

Saxena, S. (1994). Quality of life assessments in cancer patients in India. In J. Orley & W. Kuyken (Eds.), *Cross cultural issues in quality life assessment: International perspectives* (pp. 99–107). Heidelberg, Germany: Springer-Verlag.

Seligman, M. E. P. (2002). Positive psychology, positive prevention, and positive therapy. In C. R. Snyder & S. J. Lopez (Eds.), *Handbook of positive psychology* (pp. 3–12). New York: Oxford University Press.

Shin, S. M., Chow, C., Camacho-Gonsalves, T., Levy, R. J., Allen, I. E., & Leff, H. S. (2005). A meta-analytic review of racial-ethnic matching for African American and Caucasian American clients and clinicians. *Journal of Counseling Psychology*, *52*(1), 45–56.

Sierra, M., Gomez, J., Molina, J. J., Luque, R., Munoz, J. F., & David, A. S. (2006). Depersonalization in psychiatric patients: A transcultural study. *Journal of Nervous and Mental Disease*, *194*(5), 356–361.

Singelis, T. M., Bond, M. H., Sharkey, W. F., & Lai, K. (1999). Unpackaging culture's influence on self-esteem and embarrassability: The role of self-construals. *Journal of Cross-Cultural Psychology*, *30*(3), 315.

Solomon, S., Greenberg, J., & Pyszczynski, T. (1991). A terror management theory of social behavior: the psychological functions of self-esteem and cultural worldviews. *Advances in Experimental Social Psychology, 24*, 93–159.

Sue, S. (1998). In search of cultural competence in psychotherapy and counseling. *American Psychologist, 53*, 440–448.

Tajfel, H. (1981). *Human groups and social categories: Studies in social psychology.* Cambridge, England: Cambridge University Press.

Triandis, H. C., McCusker, C., Betancourt, H., Iwao, S., Leung, K., Salazar, J. M., et al. (1993). An etic-emic analysis of individualism and collectivism. *Journal of Cross-Cultural Psychology, 24*(3), 366.

U. S. Census Bureau. (2007). *2006 American Community Survey.* Retrieved from http://factfinder.census.gov.

Utsey, S. O., Bolden, M. A., Brown, C. F., & Chae, M. H. (2001). Assessing quality of life in the context of culture. In J. G. Ponterotto, J. M. Casas, L. A. Suzuki, & C. M. Alexander (Eds.), *Handbook of multicultural counseling* (pp. 191–212). Thousand Oaks: Sage.

Vega, W. A., Kolody, B., Aguilar-Gaxiola, S., Alderete, E., Catalano, R., & Caraveo-Anduaga, J. (1998). Lifetime prevalence of DSM-III-R psychiatric disorders among urban and rural Mexican Americans in California. *Archives of General Psychiatry, 55*(9), 771.

Washington, E. D. (2001). Three steps to cultural awareness: A Wittgensteinian approach. In P. Pedersen & J. C. Carey (Eds.), *Multicultural counseling in schools: A practical handbook* (pp. 81–102). Needham heights, MA: Allyn & Bacon.

Weissman, M. M., Bland, R. C., Canino, G. J., Faravelli, C., Greenwald, S., Hwu, H. G., et al. (1997). The cross-national epidemiology of panic disorder. *Archives of General Psychiatry, 54*(4), 305–309.

Weissman, M. M., Bland, R. C., Canino, G. J., Faravelli, C., Greenwald, S., Hwu, H. G., et al. (1996). Cross-national epidemiology of major depression and bipolar disorder. *Journal of the American Medical Association, 276*(4), 293–299.

Wells, K., Klap, R., Koike, A., & Sherbourne, C. (2001). Ethnic disparities in unmet need for alcoholism, drug abuse, and mental health care. *American Journal of Psychiatry, 158*(12), 2027–2032.

Westermeyer, J., & Wintrob, R. (1979a). "Folk" criteria for the diagnosis of mental illness in rural Laos: on being insane in sane places. *American Journal of Psychiatry, 136*(6), 755–761.

Westermeyer, J., & Wintrob, R. (1979b). " Folk" explanations of mental illness in rural Laos. *American Journal of Psychiatry, 136*(7), 901–905.

Whiting, B. B. (1976). The problem of the packaged variable. In K. F. Riegel & J. A. Meecham (Eds.), *The developing individual in a changing world* (pp. 303–309). New York: Hawthorne.

Whitley, R. (2007). Cultural competence, evidence-based medicine, and evidence-based practices. *Psychiatric Services, 58*(12), 1588–1590.

Wittchen, H. U., & Jacobi, F. (2005). Size and burden of mental disorders in Europe—a critical review and appraisal of 27 studies. *European Neuropsychopharmacology, 15*(4), 357–376.

World Health Organization. (1979). *Schizophrenia: An international follow-up study.* Chichester, England and New York: Wiley.

Yeh, C. J. (1999). Invisibility and self-construal in African American men: Implications for training and practice. *Counseling Psychologist, 27*(6), 810–819.

Chapter 10
Gender and Minority Mental Health: The Case of Body Image

Laura Simonelli and Leslie J. Heinberg

Introduction

Differing prevalence rates amongst mental illnesses has led to significant research interest in examining the impact of sex and gender on psychiatric illness and psychosocial quality of life. A number of prevalent psychiatric illnesses have differing prevalence rates when examined by sex. Autism, Attention Deficit with Hyperactivity Disorder, Substance Abuse and Antisocial Personality Disorder are more common in men. Major Depression and Agoraphobia with Panic are more common in women. Eating disorders are the most gendered disorders described in the *Diagnostic and Statistical Manual of Mental Disorders, fourth edition* (*DSM-IV;* American Psychiatric Association, 2004). Eight to nine times as many girls and women experience anorexia nervosa and bulimia nervosa than boys and men. Beyond this, body image dissatisfaction is also much higher in girls and women as compared to boys and men. These sex differences become apparent in elementary school, persist throughout the life span, and have been found across numerous ethnic groups within the U.S. and in cross-cultural studies.

This chapter will briefly review the concept of gender and will use body image as a case study to examine how gender differences can cut across demographic groups and interact with factors such as ethnicity. We will attempt to bring a larger life span perspective to this review. However, it should be noted that the vast majority of the literature has focused on adolescent and young, college-aged adults. We will begin this case study with an in-depth definition of body image and its subcomponents and review its important relationship to psychosocial functioning (such as self-esteem, depression, and eating disorders) and health (such as dieting and exercise behaviors and obesity). Next, we will explore the literature on gender differences for majority populations followed by the

L.J. Heinberg (✉)
Cleveland Clinic Lerner College of Medicine of Case Western Reserve University,
Cleveland, OH
e-mail: heinbel@ccf.org

S. Loue, M. Sajatovic (eds.), *Determinants of Minority Mental Health and Wellness*, DOI 10.1007/978-0-387-75659-2_10,
© Springer Science+Business Media, LLC 2009

relatively more recent investigations among various minority groups. Most of this work has been conducted in the United States, but gender and ethnic differences from a more global perspective will be included. The limited work examining the interaction between gender and ethnicity will also be reviewed. Finally, we will review the impact body image may have in explaining the etiology and maintenance of eating disorders and obesity among women and minorities. We will conclude this chapter with a summary of the findings, future directions for research, and the larger clinical implications of body image for gender and minority mental health.

Gender Versus Sex Differences

It is important to delineate between sex differences and gender differences on body image (or any other psychosocial variable for that matter). In a 2000 Institute of Medicine (IOM) report – *Exploring the Biological Contributions to Human Health: Does Sex Matter?* – the expert committee recommended that the term sex should be used as a classification (i.e., male or female) according to the reproductive organs and functions as derived by an individual's chromosomal makeup (IOM, 2001). In contrast, gender is the recommended term when distinguishing between men and women of a society as they take part in their respective social roles. Thus, an individuals' gender, although not independent of their sex, develops through sociocultural norms and experiences (IOM, 2001). This report explains that the term gender should be used to refer to a person's own representation of the self as male or female, as well as how that person is responded to by others based upon their gender representation. Unfortunately, the larger literature often confuses the two terms or uses them interchangeably. In the context of this chapter, however, we will use the term gender where appropriate and identify body image as an ideal case study for *gender* differences because of the very important influence of sociocultural norms and experiences.

Body Image

Body image is a multifaceted, multidimensional concept that embodies one's perceptions, attitudes, and behaviors in relation to one's appearance, weight, and shape (Heinberg & Thompson, 2006). Body image is best conceptualized as a continuum model, where body image disturbance ranges from none to severe, with most individuals experiencing mild-to-moderate concern or dissatisfaction (Thompson, Heinberg, Altabe, & Tantleff-Dunn, 1999). Nonetheless, researchers have identified individual differences that often place people at greater risk for dealing with more extreme body image disturbance (Thompson, Heinberg, Altabe, & Tantleff-Dunn, 1999). Body image disturbance has important implications for an individual's mental health, including reduced self-esteem, mood disturbance, and disordered eating. On the other hand, a realistic perception of one's body image, especially if one is overweight, may influence healthy dieting behavior, exercise, and prevention of obesity and obesity-related health problems (Heinberg, Thompson, & Matzon, 2001).

Historical Context

Historically, the status of body image ideals has varied. Body image ideals do not only differ across genders, but also change somewhat dramatically over time. As a result, certain body types are more, or less, desirable at different points in time. Early signs of beauty were more likely to be related to biological indicators of reproductive capability (e.g., Venus of Willendorf, circa 24,000–22,000 BC). However, for more modern societies, aesthetic ideals of feminine beauty and male strength relate more to cultural influences than biological ones (Fallon, 1990). Indeed there is no biological advantage to standards of beauty such as bound feet in women or decorative tattooing in men. Centuries ago, beauty ideals were communicated in art (e.g., Botticelli's Venus). However, because of the glorified and rarefied nature of art, it has been suggested that these ideals were considered other-worldly and unattainable rather than societal expectations as ideals are today (Thompson et al., 1999).

Briefly, in Westernized societies between the 15th and 18th century, an overweight body shape was considered to be sexually appealing and attractive for women. The ideal woman was matronly and plump (Thompson et al., 1999). By the 19th century, however, the hourglass ideal became fashionable epitomized by corsets and even bustles. In the early 20th century, thinness began to be valued as seen by the "Gibson Girl" or by small-breasted flappers. As a result, women began dieting and wearing binding garments, leading to the first concern by physicians related to eating disorders (Fallon, 1990). This ideal was relatively short-lived, however, with the replacement of a voluptuous, leggy ideal during World War II (e.g., Betty Grable), and an idealization of curvaceousness during the 1950s (e.g., Marilyn Monroe). This trend in ideals was discarded in the 1960s with the onset of angular, thin models such as Twiggy. Although there have been alterations in ideals related to breast size and athleticism in the intervening years, the thin ideal of beauty for women has persisted in Westernized societies for the past 40 years. Ironically, as the thin ideal has increased, so has the weight of the average woman (Thompson et al., 1999).

Examination of ideals in men is more complicated than in women. Unlike women where there is a relatively universal thin ideal, male body image may be more complex with numerous ideals such as "heroin chic," "metro-sexual," and "body-builder" noted (Warren & Hildebrand, 2006). Other researchers have examined the influence of having a more mature physique in adolescent boys, facial dominance, and attributes such as ambition and financial success (Corson & Andersen, 2002).

The shifting trends in the thin ideal, as well as pressure to achieve that ideal has been well documented through archival research of print media marketed to women (Andersen & DiDomenico, 1992; Garner, Garfinkel, Schwartz, & Thompson, 1980; Wiseman et al., 1992). The shift from a curvaceous ideal to a slimmer one has been demonstrated by examining the decreasing size of Playboy models, Miss America contestants, magazine models, ballerinas, and mannequins (Garner et al., 1980; Rintala & Mustajoki, 1992; Wiseman, Gray, Mosimann, & Ahrens, 1992). Similar studies have also noted an increase in the number of articles on diet and exercise in popular teen girl's and women's magazines (Nemeroff, Stein, Diehl, & Smilack, 1994).

Comparable trends were demonstrated by examining the two most popular men's fashion magazines, *GQ* and *Esquire* (Petrie et al., 1996). Article and advertisement content and male models' body sizes were assessed during the period 1960–1992. Linear trend analyses revealed that, like women's magazines, the number of messages concerning physical activity and health have increased over time. However, in contrast to print media aimed at female audiences, messages concerning weight and physical attractiveness have declined since the late 1970s and measurements of male models' body sizes have not changed significantly since the 1960s (Petrie et al., 1996). Although pressures for thinness may be absent for men, the increasing pressure to be involved in fitness activity may lead to unhealthy body changing practices (e.g., crash dieting, steroid use; Petrie et al., 1996). Similarly, the influence of media consumption on straight and gay males' body image (Duggan & McCreary, 2004) has been examined. This study found that consumption of muscle and fitness magazines was positively related to body dissatisfaction in both gay and straight males, but pornography exposure was only related to physique anxiety in gay men. Such pressures may be present for boys at far younger ages. Pope and colleagues (1999) examined popular action figure toys across 30 years. Progressive enlargements in chest and bicep size were found for toys like GI Joe, as well as Star Wars figure toys.

In 1985, Rodin and her colleagues coined the term "normative discontent" to describe the pervasive dissatisfaction with body image experiences by girls and women. Over 20 years, little has changed. Indeed it is hard to conceptualize body image as a "disturbance" when endorsed by the majority of females. Sadly, many body image researchers conclude that anxiety, dissatisfaction, and disregard for weight, shape, and appearance is a normal part of the female experience (Thompson et al., 1999). However, the next section of the chapter will focus on the psychosocial correlates of body image and why a better understanding of body image is essential for evaluation of mental health.

Body Image and Mental Health

Clinicians and researchers have focused on the concept of body image dissatisfaction due to its strong connection with self-esteem, depression, eating disordered behavior, problematic dieting, and other risky health behaviors (Heinberg & Thompson, 2006). In addition, there is often comorbidity among depressive disorders and eating disorders, and body image factors have been identified as predictive of these mental health disorders and their correlates, including low self-esteem (Santos, Richards, & Bleckley, 2007). Conversely, overweight or obese individuals with body image satisfaction may be less motivated for exercise, thus potentially missing out on exercise benefits including improved self-esteem (MacDonald & Thompson, 1992), improved mood (Smith et al., 2007; Johnson & Krueger, 2007; Landers & Arent, 2007), and decreases in stress (Landers & Arent, 2007). In general, the construct of body image remains useful in predicting the development, maintenance and severity of a wide variety of mental health concerns, in addition to influencing health behaviors. A number of psychosocial factors related to body image dissatisfaction will be discussed in the following sections.

Self-Esteem

Self-esteem involves one's orientation (positive or negative) toward the self, or an overall evaluation of one's worth or value. Self-esteem results from personal and environmental influences. Higher self-esteem is linked to life satisfaction, happiness, healthy behavioral practices, perceived efficacy, and adjustment, while lower self-esteem is associated with depression, anxiety, and eating disorders among other psychiatric disorders (Michaels, Barr, Roosa, & Knight, 2007; Swenson & Prelow, 2005). Body image plays an integral role in the development of self-esteem. More often, one's subjective ratings of attractiveness, rather than objective ones, are found to be significantly associated with self-esteem (Feingold, 1992). Body image dissatisfaction and overvaluation of weight, shape, and appearance are frequently linked to problems with self-esteem in women with eating disorders (Geller et al., 1998; Hrabosky, Masheb, White, & Grilo, 2007). In addition, self-esteem is often an important predictor of eating disordered behavior; for example, women with eating disorders often associate weight loss with self-worth and feelings of mastery (Jarry & Kossert., 2007).

Depression

Depression is a widespread mental health problem commonly influenced by low self-esteem and poor body image. Historically, there has been an interest in examining the relationship between body image and depression. A number of researchers found a positive correlation between these two domains (Heinberg, Thompson, & Stormer, 1995; Wood, Becker, & Thompson, 1996). In recognition of this relationship, the Beck Depression Inventory, one of the most widely used screening measures for depression, includes an item on body image disturbance (Beck, Steer, & Brown, 1996).

Some recent work suggests that the relationship between depression and body image may be more complex. In a study of 650 fifth graders and their parents, children with greater body image discrepancy (actual vs. ideal) reported greater internalizing problems and more negative affect (Gilliland et al., 2007). However, while children with high discrepancy scores also reported higher levels of positive affect compared to children with lower discrepancy scores, parents who reported high child discrepancies reported greater negative affect in their children when compared to parents with lower child discrepancies (Gilliland et al., 2007).

Moreover, there has been some interest in examining the relationship between alexithymia and body image. Alexithymia involves various cognitive and affective features including trouble identifying and describing feelings and having difficulty distinguishing emotions from physical sensations (Sifneos, 1973). The concept of alexithymia originated in relation to psychosomatic illnesses, but investigators have now demonstrated connections with body image, depression, and eating disorders (Carano et al., 2006; De Berardis et al., 2007). For example, De Barardis and colleagues (2007) found alexithymics were more prone to body checking behaviors and higher body dissatisfaction and were at greater risk for the development of eating disorders than non-alexithymics. Similarly, among a sample of binge eating disorder patients, others have found alexithymia was associated with great eating disorder severity, as well as higher rates of body dissatisfaction and depressive symptoms (Carano et al., 2006). So, over time, our understanding of the relationships between body image and depression has become more complex, but the door is open for new research to identify mechanisms important for prevention and treatment of depression linked with body image concerns.

Eating Disorders

There is persistent evidence to support body image disturbance as a required criterion for the diagnosis of anorexia nervosa (AN) and bulimia nervosa (BN) (APA, 1994; Kovacs & Palmer, 2004; Perez & Joiner, 2003). Nonetheless, the field of eating disorder research would benefit from an operationalization of the body image construct as phrases such as "undue influence of body weight or shape on self-evaluation" (anorexia nervosa) and "self-evaluation is unduly influenced by body weight and shape" (bulimia nervosa) are subjective and hard to define (Thompson, 2004; Thompson et al., 1999).

Body image dissatisfaction has been proposed as a consistent risk factor for eating disorders through several mechanisms. Body image dissatisfaction may be directly related to eating disorders, but it has also been proposed that body image dissatisfaction may trigger an increased desire to achieve a thin ideal leading to dieting behaviors, which often increase risk for eating pathology (Haines & Sztainer, 2006; Stice, 2002). In addition, body dissatisfaction is thought to contribute to negative affect, which may lead to binging and compensatory purging behaviors (Stice, 2001). Body image may also serve a maintaining role. Higher levels of body image disturbance are associated with (1) poorer response to treatment and (2) higher rates of relapse (Rosen, 1990). Indeed, compared to other variables, body image dissatisfaction has been demonstrated to be the most important prognostic factor in weight gain and weight maintenance at follow-up (Keel, Dooer, Franko, Jackson, & Herzog, 2005; Rosen, 1990) or treatment non-response (Hilbert et al., 2007). In several prospective studies of anorexia nervosa treatment response, greater perceptual and subjective body image dissatisfaction at the beginning of inpatient treatment predicted greater attrition and less weight gain (Keel et al., 2005). Similarly, greater satisfaction with emaciated appearance predicted poorer weight gain and greater likelihood of relapse (Fairburn et al., 1993).

While there is a myriad of research exploring the role of body image in anorexia and bulimia nervosa, it is becoming increasingly recognized as influential in binge eating disorder (BED) as well. For instance, body dissatisfaction is an identified predictor of binge eating, and this may be mediated by dieting behavior leading to increased hunger, negative affect, and/or self-esteem (Haines & Neumark-Sztainer, 2006). Among BED patients, shape and weight overvaluation appear to be unrelated to body mass index but strongly linked to eating-related pathology, depression, and low self-esteem (Hrabosky, Masheb, White, & Grilo, 2007).

Body Image and Health Behaviors

Dieting Behavior

In addition to its connection with eating disorders, body image dissatisfaction has been linked to chronic dieting (Gingras, Fitzpatrick & McCarger, 2004), dieting behavior in adolescents (Borresen & Rosenvinge, 2003), and intent to use weight loss products regardless of knowledge of their harmful effects (Whisenhunt, Williamson, Netemeyer, & Andrews, 2003). In addition, in females, body dissatisfaction and concerns about weight throughout middle childhood are found to be consistent over time, systematically related to weight status, and predictive of dietary restraint, eating attitudes, and the likelihood of dieting at age 9 (Krahnstoever Davison, Markey & Birch, 2003).

Dieting behavior is becoming increasingly more common among younger populations, with reports up to 56% of girls and 39% of boys engaging in dieting behavior to try to lose weight (Haines & Neumark-Sztainer, 2006). Dieting behavior is of concern because it appears to be linked to the development of both obesity and eating disorders (Haines & Neumark-Sztainer, 2006). Furthermore, one impetus behind dieting behavior seems to be pressure to achieve an ideal body image (thinness for females and muscularity and leanness for males) (Haines & Neumark-Sztainer, 2006; Stice, 2000).

Exercise Behavior

Body image is increasingly recognized as an important predictor of health behaviors. Some research has indicated that to some extent body dissatisfaction may benefit average to above-average weight individuals by motivating healthy behaviors, such as exercise; however, the evidence is mixed (Haines & Neumark-Sztainer, 2006; Heinberg, Thompson, & Matzon, 2001; Neumark-Sztainer, Paxton, & Hannan, 2006). For instance, body dissatisfaction was not a predictor of regular exercise in older adults ages 50–98 (Schuler et al., 2004), but a desire to look like media figures was a predictor of adolescent boys' and girls' physical activity (Taveras et al., 2004).

Exercise participation has been considered a risk for eating-related pathology, particularly when considering athleticism, but it has also been viewed as a protective factor for obesity and other health problems (Lipsey, Barton, Hulley, & Hill, 2006). The direction of influence is largely based on one's perception of and feelings related to body weight and shape (Lipsey et al., 2006). In a sample of 260 female exercisers, Lipsey and colleagues (2006) found that commitment to exercise, but not frequency or duration of exercise, was related to weight and mood regulation in women with more eating disorder psychopathology (Lipsey et al., 2006). Similarly, others have found physical activity has been linked to enhanced psychological well-being, which is related to body image (Kim & Kim, 2007; Lutz, 2007; Stubbe, de Moor, Boomsma, & de Geus, 2007).

Exercise has been shown to relate to enhanced body image across all ages and among males and females, but there were some differences in effect sizes across study designs (Hausenblas & Fallen, 2006). For example, when examining experimental versus control group studies and single group studies, the influence of exercise on body image was stronger among women compared to men, and among adolescents compared to college students and adults; however, when examining correlational studies, there were larger effect sizes for men compared to women and college students and adults compared to adolescents. Other research has suggested variable findings for the relationship between exercise and body image. In a sample of 144 female college students, Slater and Tiggeman (2006) found that women who exercise at a gym had significantly higher drive for thinness, but also saw themselves as more overweight than women who do not exercise, though there were no group differences in BMI. In addition, women who participated in organized sports and women who spent more time engaged in physical activity reported higher body image dissatisfaction (Slater & Tiggeman, 2006). These findings may reflect that some level of body image dissatisfaction may motivate exercise behavior (Heinberg, Thompson, & Matzon, 2001), or it is possible the gym atmosphere or the nature of organized sports contribute to body image concerns (Slater & Tiggeman, 2006).

Obesity

Problems with the rise of overweight and obese individuals have become a greater concern over the past few decades. For example, 15% of youth aged

6–19 are overweight (Ogden, Flegal, Carroll,& Johnson, 2002). Among adults aged 20–74, rates of obesity have been steadily increasing from 15% in the late 1970s to 32.9% in 2003 to 2004 (Center for Disease Control, 2007).

Being overweight may be another risk factor for body image concerns. Thompson and colleagues (2007) studied 325 adolescent females and found that overweight and at risk for overweight girls reported greater body dissatisfaction and dieting behavior then average weight girls (Thompson et al., 2007). In addition, overweight and at risk for overweight girls reported more negative comments from peers and attributions about appearance, and friends influenced body image for overweight and at risk for overweight girls but not average weight girls (Thompson et al., 2007). Additional research might examine if overweight and at risk for overweight girls may benefit from developing coping skills for handling negative appearance-related remarks, as well as learning healthy weight management strategies.

Body image may play an important role in the maintenance of obesity, but the positive versus negative quality of the role remains unclear. Some degree of body image disturbance had been associated with engaging in helpful lifestyle change that may aid obesity, such as diet and exercise (Cash, 1994; Heinberg, Haythornthwaite, Rosofsky, McCarron, & Clarke, 2000; MacDonald & Thompson, 1992; Striegel-Moore, Wilfley, Caldwell, Needham, & Brownell, 1996). Other studies, however, indicate the negative influence of body image suggesting that it may lead to greater unhealthy dieting behaviors and weight gain (van den Berg & Neumark Sztainer, 2007; Whisenhunt et al., 2003).

There appear to be several factors that influence help-seeking behavior in obese individuals. In a study of 120 overweight (BMI > 25) females (58% African American), Annunziato and Lowe (2007) found that when seeking help for weight control was examined as a continuous variable, concern about body weight and shape, as well as obesity-related knowledge and psychological distress, were associated with greater help seeking. In addition, sociodemographic variables, including gender, appear to influence help-seeking behavior for overcoming obesity. For example, men are less likely to participate in weight control efforts than women (Wardle et al., 2004; Wolfe & Smith, 2002).

The impact and relevance of body image on mental and physical health is broad. Again, much of this research has primarily been conducted with White female samples, but consideration of minority populations including those from distinct ethnic and cultural backgrounds, as well as men, would be valuable.

Body Image, Minority Populations, and Gender

Overview of Body Image in Minority Populations

A number of studies have evaluated racial/ethnic differences (Freedman, Carter, Sbrocco & Gray, 2004; Perez & Joiner, 2003) or lack thereof (Shaw, Ramirez,

Trost, Randall, & Stice, 2004) in body dissatisfaction in women. In general, studies demonstrate differences in body image ideals and severity of body dissatisfaction (BD), with ethnicities that endorse a broader range of acceptable body types also endorsing greater body size satisfaction. Specific assessment of ethnicity rather than the use of gross categories should be included in future studies as almost all published work utilizes very broad categories of ethnicities lumped into an over-arching label (e.g., considering "Asian" or "Latino" rather than country of origin; Tsai, Curbow, & Heinberg, 2003; Yates, Edman, & Aruguete, 2004).

Unfortunately, very little work has examined male body image and eating disorder pathology in minority populations. Rather, the extant literature has focused almost exclusively on White, college-aged males (Heinberg & Thompson, 2006), with a small body of work on African American men (Heinberg et al., 2000; Pulvers et al., 2004), and there are no published studies specifically examining eating disorders in Latino men.

The changes in body image dissatisfaction are also important to examine from both a historical and cross-cultural perspective. Of particular interest was the recent publication of a cross-sectional study examining body image from 1983 to 2001 (Cash, Morrow, Hrabosky, & Perry, 2004). Significant changes in the body image of college-aged men and women occurred over the 19-year period. Non-Black (predominantly White) women evidenced a worsening body image from the 1980s to mid-1990s. Conversely, Black women generally did not evince these changes. More recent non-Black and Black cohorts, however, reported a more favorable body image in spite of the population becoming heavier over time (Cash et al., 2004). In contrast to earlier findings, men's body image was remarkably stable over time. Although it was not particularly positive, 43% of men were dissatisfied with their mid torso, 52% with their weight, and 43% overall.

An important gender difference relates to the interaction between gender and sexual orientation. Sexual orientation has been consistently identified as a significant gender-specific risk factor for both body image dissatisfaction and eating disturbance in men (Andersen, 1999; Boroughs & Thompson, 2002; Strong, Williamson, Netemeyer, & Geer, 2000). In contrast, homosexuality as a general risk factor for psychiatric illness has been consistently empirically rejected (Russell & Keel, 2002). In a population-based study, 27.8% of homosexual male adolescents reported body image dissatisfaction compared to 12% of heterosexual male teens (French, Story, Remafedi, Resnick, & Blum, 1996). Among adult men diagnosed with eating disorders, 10–42% self-identify as homosexual or bisexual (Carlat, Camargo & Herzog, 1997; Russell & Keel, 2002). This is significantly higher than the base rate of homosexuality amongst men (~6%; Seidman & Rieder, 1994). Further, gay men score significantly higher on eating disorder screening measures suggesting higher sub-threshold disorders (Siever, 1994; Williamson & Hartly, 1998). Bingeing and purging symptomatology may be particularly relevant for homosexual males with lifetime prevalence rates 2.5× higher than heterosexual men (French et al., 1996).

Gender Comparative Studies

Because body image represents a normative discontent for women, and because eating disorders are significantly more common in girls and women than boys and men (approximately 1 in 9 patients with eating disorders are male, American Psychiatric Association, 1994), significant interest has focused on the role of gender in the development and maintenance of body image dissatisfaction. A number of feminist theories have been advanced including those investigating a "culture of thinness," weight as a power or control issue, and anxieties about female appearance and achievement (Gilbert & Thompson, 1996). A number of studies have also examined the influence of sex role orientation. A 1997 meta-analysis (Murnen & Smolak) found a small positive relationship between femininity and eating problems and a negative relationship between masculinity and eating disturbances.

The influence of sex role orientation has been seen as potentially explanatory for why male homosexuality may contribute an inordinate risk for eating disorder. The most commonly accepted theory is that body image disturbance (BID) plays a critical role in making homosexual men vulnerable to eating disorders (Hospers & Jansen, 2005). However, other studies suggest that femininity is the relevant risk factor for both heterosexual women and homosexual men, whereas masculinity confers a protective effect (Hospers & Jansen, 2005; Meyer, Blissett, & Oldfield, 2001). These studies, however, have focused almost exclusively on self-identified gay, White men.

A positive change in research direction is recent work examining the relationships and influences of body image on mental and physical health outcomes in males, in addition to females, and comparing gender. Some research has suggested that gender differences – females reporting twice the rates of depression by adolescence – may be partially accounted for by risk factors such as pressure to be thin, body dissatisfaction, and dieting and bulimic symptoms (Stice & Bearman, 2001); however, much of this research does not include male comparison groups. Recently, Shea and Pritchard (2007) found that in a sample of 196 male and 263 female college students, women were more likely than men to report drive for thinness, bulimia, and body dissatisfaction. In addition, they found that gender was the primary predictor of drive for thinness and body dissatisfaction, though other factors such as self-esteem, perfectionism, stress and coping style were also influential (Shea & Pritchard, 2007). This study was cross-sectional; therefore, prospective replication is warranted to draw causal conclusions.

Other research has indicated that body image concerns among males may be more prevalent than previously thought, but the mechanism for concerns may differ by gender. For example, in a one-year longitudinal study of body image in adolescents, internalization of a muscular ideal was predictive of body dissatisfaction in males, while body dissatisfaction in female adolescents was predicted by BMI, conversations about appearance with friends, and social comparison tendencies (Carlson Jones, 2004). Furthermore, Santos and colleagues (2007) examined 202 (101 males, 101 females) high school students and found that 23% met criteria for depression and 12% met criteria for eating disorders. When comparing males and females they found no differences in overall disordered eating symptomatology. Upon further examination, they found females were more likely to report dieting behavior, but there were no differences in frequencies of bulimic or oral control behaviors. The authors also found that depressive and eating disorder symptoms were equally comorbid among males and females, and they concluded that adolescent males and females are quite similar regarding comorbid depression and disordered eating behaviors (Santos et al., 2007).

A good portion of body image research has examined the influence of media exposure. Exposure to thin-ideal media images has been linked to self-esteem, derogatory self-evaluations, anger, depression, negative mood, and poor body image (Harrison, Taylor, & Marske, 2006). Again, most of these studies have explored these relationships in female samples, and those comparing male and female samples have found inconsistent evidence of gender differences. Recently the connection between ideal media images and self-evaluation in males has been explored. For example, Hobza and colleagues (2007) found that body esteem, both physical condition and attractiveness, were lower in males who viewed ideal physical image versus those who viewed neutral images; however, state self-esteem was unrelated (Hobza, Walker, Yakushko, & Peugh, 2007).

Gender differences in the relationship between body comparison with media influences and body dissatisfaction have also been suggested (van den Berg, Paxton, Keery, Wall, Guo, & Neumark-Sztainer, 2007). In a study of high school and college students, media body comparison partially or fully mediated relationships between self-esteem, depressive mood, friends dieting, and body dissatisfaction in females (n = 1,386), while media body comparison did not influence body dissatisfaction in males (n = 1,130); however, gender was not examined as a moderator (van den Berg et al., 2007). The authors suggest that males may be more influenced by admired sport figures and peers than traditional media. While media body comparison influences differed among males and females, both genders reported significant relationships between BMI and self-esteem with body dissatisfaction; however, depressive mood appears to be more influential in males than females regarding body dissatisfaction (van den Berg et al., 2007).

Conversely, body dissatisfaction also influences mood and self-esteem, and this pattern may be consistent for both genders at various developmental stages. In a prospective study of adolescents, Paxton, Neumark-Sztainer, Hannan, & Eisenberg (2007) examined the role of body dissatisfaction in the development of depression and low self-esteem. A sample of 440 early-adolescent females 366 early-adolescent males, 946 mid-adolescent females and 764 mid-adolescent males were followed over 5 years (Paxton et al., 2007). Body dissatisfaction at baseline was predictive of depressive mood and low self-esteem at follow-up, after controlling for mood and self-esteem at baseline, ethnicity, socio-economic status, and BMI, in early adolescent girls and mid-adolescent boys. These findings suggest body image concerns are relevant to both males and females but at different stages of development (Paxton et al., 2007); however, future research should examine such relationships while considering the stability of body image dissatisfaction over time.

In addition to media exposure influences on body dissatisfaction and mental health, others have explored its relationship with eating behavior. In a study of 373 subjects (72% White), 222 females were exposed to images of attractive females with long, slender, and lean bodies and 151 males were exposed to images of attractive young men with low body fat and large, well-defined muscles in the chest, arms, and abdomen. After exposure to images, participants completed follow-up questionnaires in a room where food was presented and offered. Among participants who viewed slides with or without body-relevant text, males with a high discrepancy between actual versus ideal body image demonstrated increased eating behavior, while high-discrepancy females demonstrated decreased eating behavior relative to participants who viewed no slides or slides with incongruent text. The authors concluded that males with higher self-discrepancies, who believe larger more muscular bodies are preferable would be more motivated to increase eating in front of peers; on the other hand, high self-discrepancies females believing a thinner body type is desirable will be motivated to eat less in front of peers (Harrison et al., 2006).

For males, the dissatisfaction with muscularity has been linked to decreased self-esteem, depression, anxiety, and appearance orientation (Gray & Ginsberg, 2007; McCreary, Hildebrandt, Heinberg, Boroughs, & Thompson, 2007). On the other hand, body image dissatisfaction regarding muscularity does not appear to be as relevant or impactful on female mental health. Muscular dysmorphia – an extreme need for muscularity despite being objectively more muscular than the average male – has been identified within the realm of body dysmorphia (Pope, Gruber, Choi, Olivardia, & Phillips, 1997). This disorder is thought to lead to extreme anxiety and shame leading to reduced social, recreational, and occupational functioning (Pope et al., 1997). Factors contributing to muscular dysmorphia include media influences, negative affect, body dissatisfaction, low self-esteem, and perfectionism, and muscle dysmorphia is often comorbid with mood and anxiety disorders, such as obsessive compulsive disorder, and eating disorders (McCreary et al., 2007; Olivardia).

The extreme need for muscularity in males may be problematic for health, if the use of anabolic steroids or excessive exercise is prompted. Anabolic-androgenic steroids (AAS) are frequently taken with fat-burning supplements, thyroid hormones, analgesics, prohormones, or other ancillary drugs to prevent side effects such as breast enlargement, and yet AAS and these substances pose dangers, including psychiatric and physical complications (McCreary et al., 2007). For example, depression, anxiety, aggression, and psychosis have been noted, as have cardiovascular, endocrine, and musculoskeletal system harm (Bahrke, 2007; McCreary et al., 2007). Muscle dysmorphia also lends itself to excessive exercise training and body building, which can be detrimental, if it leads to overtraining or functional impairments in other life areas due to disproportionate amounts of time (e.g. up to 5 hours per day) being dedicated to exercise (Olivardia, 2007).

Gender differences have also been noted concerning body image and exercise behavior. Markland and Ingledew (2007) examined autonomous motivation for exercise in a sample of 50 male and 48 female adolescents. Among males, exercise autonomy was predicted by both body mass and body size discrepancies, while among females, exercise autonomy was predicted by body size discrepancies alone (Markland & Ingledew, 2007). For males a desire to either be less bulky/overweight or more bulky/muscular was related to less autonomous motivation to exercise, while among females this relationship only held for wanting to be less bulky/overweight. These distinctions may be related to sociocultural expectations for an ideal slender female but a neither too thin nor too large muscular male ideal (Markland & Ingledew, 2007).

Body image dissatisfaction has been noted as a predictor of lower levels of physical activity among both male and female adolescents, after controlling for other demographic variables (Neumark-Sztainer et al., 2006). However, when body mass index is also considered, this relationship remained significant among girls, but not among boys, suggesting that the association between body image satisfaction and physical activity may differ by gender (Neumark-Sztainer et al., 2006).

Body image gender differences also appear to be influential regarding cosmetic surgery. For instance, cosmetic surgery is nine times more common among females than males (Sarwer & Magee, 2006). This may be related to women's greater acceptance of appearance enhancing tools, or it could be due to the greater evolutionary emphasis placed on physical appearance for females versus males (Sarwer & Magee, 2006). Nonetheless, the number of men seeking cosmetic surgery has dramatically increased over the past decade. Approximately 10% of males have procedures including rhinoplasty, hair transplantation, and liposuction, though body shape and contouring procedures such as abdomininoplasty are also on the rise (Sarwer, Crerand, & Gibbons, 2007). Although research is limited, body image dissatisfaction, including body dysmorphia, muscle dysmorphia, and eating disorders are likely contributing psychological characteristics among some of those seeking cosmetic surgery (Sarwer et al., 2007).

More recent research is exploring body image gender differences in other psychosocial domains, including sexual functioning and satisfaction. For instance in a study of 105 males, sexual efficacy and attractiveness were positively associated with self-esteem and mediated the negative relationship between drive for muscles and self-esteem (Filiault, 2007). In addition, drive for thinness was negatively related to self-esteem but not linked with sexual indices. Filiault (2007) suggests that the ideal of male muscularity may have a greater impact on sexuality than thinness, which is often related to sexual indices in females. In females, low body dissatisfaction is related to high sexual assertiveness and sexual esteem, low sexual anxiety, and fewer sexual problems, and positive body image has been linked to higher sexual functioning, after controlling for BMI and exercise levels (Weaver & Byers, 2006).

As a whole, body image research has expanded both its exploration of unique concerns in men and women, while also considering its relevance to additional indices of mental and physical health and functioning.

Ethnicity Comparative Studies

In addition to individual differences and gender differences, a number of ethnic and cultural differences have been noted in the body image literature. As we have previously noted, body image is largely influenced by sociocultural factors, and body image development occurs within a cultural context that defines the cultural standards of attractiveness, body weight, and body shape (Heinberg, 1996). As these cultural ideals vary, so too does body image dissatisfaction. Differences in body image satisfaction, dieting behavior, obesity and eating disordered behaviors between Whites and ethnic minorities have been shown across the life span (Contento, Basch, & Zybert, 2003; Heinberg et al., 2000; Marcus, Bromberger, Wei, Brown, & Kravitz, 2007; Sanchez-Johnsen et al., 2004; White, Kohlmaier, Varnado-Sullivan, & Williamson, 2003). These differences have largely been explained as due to cultural differences in ideal body shape and size.

For example, African American women have been shown to have a broader window of acceptable weight/shape and size than White women (Thompson et al., 1999). Further, African Americans describing themselves as normal weight are considerably heavier than Whites describing themselves as within the normal weight range (Heinberg et al., 2000). African Americans also differ from Whites in the belief that weight is infinitely changeable and easy to modify (Thompson et al., 1999). More recent studies have demonstrated that Asians may be at greater risk for body image disturbance than Whites, although Asian populations tend to be of lower weight (Wardle, Haase, & Steptoe, 2006). These differences may be more pronounced in native Asian populations than Asian American ones (Tsai, Curbow, & Heinberg, 2003). Latina adolescent girls may also be at higher risk for body image dissatisfaction and overweight concerns (Robinson, Chang, Haydel, & Killen, 2001; Vander Wal, & Thomas, 2004), although others have found Latina adolescents to be similar to non-Hispanic White girls (Erickson & Gerstle, 2007).

With regards to male body image, African American males (adolescents and adults) have a greater preference for a larger body shape and overall greater body image satisfaction than White males (Ricciardelli, McCabe, Williams, & Thompson, 2007). Latino males appear to have body image that is relatively similar to non-Hispanic Whites whereas the findings for Asian males is largely inconsistent, with some studies showing greater concerns than Whites and others showing the two ethnic groups as equivocal or with Asians having fewer body image concerns (Ricciardelli et al., 2007). Finally, the very limited literature on Native American males suggests worse body image in this group compared to White men (Ricciardelli et al., 2007).

The literature on body image in minority populations, particularly men, and the interaction between gender and ethnicity is still in its infancy, particularly when compared to the very large literature on White women. The topic is ripe for investigation, and a number of potentially interesting topics are starting to be examined. For example, a history of hurtful racial teasing was recently found to be associated with eating and body image disturbance, whereas acculturation was not (Sahi Iyer & Haslam, 2003).

Interaction Between Gender and Ethnicity

Though the literature is small, interactions between gender and ethnicity and body image and its correlates have been examined. Paxton, Eisenberg, and Neumark-Sztainer (2006) found that baseline body dissatisfaction, BMI, socio-economic status (SES), ethnicity, friends dieting and teasing, self-esteem, and depression were predictors of body dissatisfaction at a five-year follow-up in early and mid-adolescent girls and boys but that the profile of these predictors varied by sample (Paxton, et al., 2006). For instance, being African American predicted a lower increase in body dissatisfaction in mid-adolescence but not early adolescence. Concerning additional subcultural variables, lower SES was predictive of body dissatisfaction in early adolescent males and mid-adolescent females.

Similarly, in another study, Paxton et al. (2006) found body image dissatisfaction predicted depression and low self-esteem in early adolescent girls and mid-adolescent boys, and ethnic background predicted depressive mood and self-esteem in boys but not girls. Specifically, in boys, being African American was related to higher self-esteem, while being Hispanic was predictive of higher levels of depressed mood, but these relationships did not exist among females. Nonetheless, other research indicates depression in African American teens is higher, if they live among non-Hispanic White Americans than African Americans (Wight, Aneshensel, Botticello, & Sepulveda, 2005). Together these studies suggest gender, ethnic, and cultural factors, as well as developmental stages, are relevant to body image and mental health.

As previously noted, the Western ideal of a muscular body type for males is linked to views that strength, physical fitness, and athletic success are preferable for the male gender role (Gray & Ginsberg, 2007). However, recent research investigating body image among Pacific Islanders has suggested that this male body ideal may be emerging in other ethnicities and cultures as well (Ricciardelli et al., 2007). Ricciardelli and colleagues (2007) performed a qualitative analysis of attitudes and behaviors associated with food, eating, physical activity, and body image in 24 Indigenous Fijian, 24 Indo-Fijian, and 24 Tongan males, aged 13–20. The authors found that a muscular ideal – larger body size and muscles and greater physical strength – and body change strategies to achieve this ideal were common themes in narratives in males across all three cultures. In addition, participants reported pursuit of this ideal primarily in relation to fitness and athletic performance goals and, less commonly, the sample mentioned goals related to physical appearance. Strategies to attain a more muscular appearance were consistent with those used in Western cultures, including eating more/less food depending on need for weight gain/loss, eating healthier foods, and exercise, most specifically weight training (Cafri et al., 2005; Ricciardelli, McCabe, & Ridge, 2006; Ricciardelli et al., 2007).

The research exploring gender and ethnic interactions in relation to body image is only recent. Notwithstanding, there are many areas to expand upon, including greater inclusion of additional ethnic groups, teasing apart ethnic versus cultural influences, and understanding the role of development stages in these relationships. Better understanding will also be essential for matching the best interventions to subgroups to prevent and treat body image and problematic behaviors associated with body image disturbance.

Impact on ED and Obesity for Women and Minorities

As the previous review has suggested, differing rates of body image dissatisfaction and differing body image ideals may result in ethnic, as well as gender differences in problematic behavior. African American women have consistently been shown to have a lower risk of body image disturbance (Heinberg et al., 2000; Thompson et al., 1999). While this has been offered as a potential explanation of lower rates of anorexia and bulimia nervosa (i.e., positive body image is a protective factor), the wider range of acceptable weights may also put African American women at greater risk for obesity or difficulty with engaging in healthy lifestyle change behaviors (Heinberg, Thompson, & Matzon, 2001). While less is known about minority men, it may be that cultures that value greater muscularity in men may also be at greater risk for problematic behaviors such as steroid use or obligatory exercise. As previously mentioned, the differing ideals within the gay male community may explain greater body image and eating disorders, and more recent work suggests that this also holds true for minority gay men (Heinberg, Pike & Loue, in press). However, much more work needs to be done to understand the protective and risk aspects of body image in men and women of all cultures.

Conclusions

As we began this chapter, we noted that eating disorders are the most gendered disorders described in the *DSM-IV*, and body image disturbance differs significantly between men and women, as well as across different ethnic and cultural groups. Given the relationship between body image and a number of psychosocial factors reviewed including self-esteem, depression, eating disordered behaviors, dieting, exercise, and obesity, a better understanding of these gender differences is essential. This chapter included a brief review of the historical context of body image ideals and some differences noted between the genders, between different ethnicities or cultural groups, and the very limited literature looking at the interaction between the two.

Although differences in body image may be protective against some mental health problems (e.g., anorexia nervosa being less prevalent in African American women possibly because of a broader range of acceptable weights), these same differences may make subgroups more susceptible to other problems (e.g., obesity). Further, although a lack of thin ideal may explain the much lower rates of eating disorders in men, a muscular ideal in men may lead to greater risk of obligatory exercise, muscle dysmorphia, and use of substances such as anabolic steroids.

Future Directions and Clinical Implications

As noted, there are many areas within gender, ethnicity, and body image that require further research, analysis, and understanding. Although, of late there has been improvement, the vast majority of our knowledge on body image and its correlates are based upon White women. Not only have minorities and men been underrepresented but sexual minorities have also been largely understudied. Relatively elemental research expanding upon these subgroups would greatly broaden and enrich our understanding of body image. A starting point might be developing body image measures that are appropriate for use with these subgroups as their body image ideals may vary. In addition, since some inconsistencies remain regarding gender and body image, and their relationships to mental health, research should explore other possible mechanisms for these differences, aside from media and drive for thinness versus muscularity.

Related to the mental health correlates of body image, research identifying mechanisms of depression and eating disorders as they relate to body image concerns (i.e. alexithymia) has important implications for prevention and treatment. Further, although it is well established that body image is highly relevant in the development and maintenance of eating disorders, better definitions and treatments for body image disturbance among eating disordered populations is lacking. This is particularly true of the most common eating disturbance, binge eating disorder.

With regards to weight management, some preliminary work suggests the importance of help-seeking behavior. Gender differences have been noted, which suggests the importance of message matching for health promotion (Annunziato & Lowe, 2007). However, research into ethnic and cultural differences in help-seeking behaviors is also warranted. Overall body image research would benefit from an understanding of gender and ethnic interactions in a broader range of ethnic groups, as well as having studies that distinguish ethnic versus cultural influences.

As discussed, overweight and obese individuals are at greater risk for body image disturbance and, in turn, the negative psychosocial sequelae associated with it. Future research should examine whether overweight and at-risk-for-overweight children would benefit from learning coping skills for handling negative appearance-related remarks or teasing. Further, how can we treat those who are obese or overweight in youth without engendering greater body image distress? That is, we would benefit from knowing what the risks and benefits of learning healthy weight management strategies in childhood/adolescence are.

Innovative treatment strategies described in the recent literature are generating significant interest. These forays are ripe for further development and expansion across gender and ethnicities. For example, McVey and colleagues (2004) conducted a six-session school-based intervention in middle-school aged girls to improve body image, self-esteem, and eating behaviors. At post-intervention, body image, self-esteem, and dieting attitudes were reduced. However, at 6 and 12 months, the intervention group did not differ from controls on body image and self-esteem, although reductions in disturbed eating attitudes and behaviors were maintained. Wade, Davidson, and O'Dea (2003) compared a school-based media literacy program to a self-esteem enhancement group and a control group, finding that the media literacy had improved scores on weight concern versus the control group at post-intervention. However, there were no differential group effects on shape concern, dietary restriction, or body dissatisfaction. Conversely, a one-year diet and physical activity intervention with adolescents was related to improvements in body image satisfaction among girls who lost weight or maintained weight had (Huang Norman, Zabinski, Calfas, & Patrick, 2007). In addition, the inclusion of body image and self-esteem education and treatment tailoring around these concerns may have helped reduce any negative psychological impact of the intervention (Huang et al., 2007).

In an innovative Internet-based study, a professionally moderated Internet chat-room reduced eating pathology and heightened self-esteem among college-aged women at risk for developing eating disorders (Zabinski, Wilfley, Calfas, Winzelberg, & Taylor, 2004). Other research indicates the importance of exercise in improving body image distress. A meta-analysis of exercise interventions suggests that exercise can have a positive influence on body image (Hausenblas & Follen, 2006). Other work demonstrates that a combination of aerobic, anaerobic, and strength training may be more beneficial for improving body image when compared to aerobic exercise alone or no exercise (Henry et al., 2006). Whether the effects of this combination exercise on body image are related to changes in fitness level, increased self-efficacy, or/and improvements in self-esteem is in need of further investigation, though there is a clear relationship between a combination exercise program and psychological and physical health enhancement. In addition, research exploring the influence of combination exercise programs in males and across cultures and age groups are needed. Thus, exercise interventions may be promising treatments for body image disturbance, which may in turn impact depression, obesity, and eating disorders. Nonetheless, concerns about excessive exercise and preoccupation with weight argue for the careful development and monitoring of such interventions. As this review has suggested, the body image intervention literature is relatively new and identifying what interventions work for which individuals has yet to occur.

Body image has been shown to be important in mental health and in a variety of health behaviors. Given its salience, our lack of understanding of body image in non-White, female populations is of great concern. The changing demographics of Western societies are not yet reflected within the body image literature. Overall, future research on body image would benefit from considering ethnic/cultural and gender differences, including sexual minorities. In addition, these should be explored across the life span, as developmental stages appear to be important in the relationships between body image and health. Understanding the complex nature of gender, cultural, and developmental influences on the role of body image in both mental illness (e.g. depression; eating disorders), as well as in health promotion and disease prevention (exercise; obesity) will be invaluable in order to address the public health needs of our increasingly diverse population.

References

American Psychiatric Association (1994). *Diagnostic and statistical manual for mental disorders* (4th ed.). Washington: American Psychiatric Association.

Andersen, A. (1999). Eating disorders in gay males. *Psychiatric Annals, 29*(4), 206–212.

Andersen, A. E., & DiDomenico, L. (1992). Diet vs. Shape content of popular male and female magazines: A dose-response relationship to the incidence of eating disorders. *International Journal of Eating Disorders, 11*(3), 283–287.

Annunziato, R. A., & Lowe, M. R. (2007). Taking action to lose weight: Towards an understanding of individual differences. *Eating Behavior, 8*(2), 185–194.

Bahrke, M. S. (2007). Muscle enhancing substances and strategies. In J. K. Thompson & G. Cafri (Eds.), *The muscular ideal: Psychological, social, and medical perspectives* (pp. 141–160). Washington, DC: American Psychological Association.

Beck, A. T., Steer, R. A., & Brown, G. K. (1996). *Manual for Beck Depression Inventory-II.* San Antonio, Texas: Psychological Corporation.

Boroughs, M., & Thompson, J. K. (2002). Exercise status and sexual orientation as moderators of body image disturbance and eating disorders in males. *International Journal of Eating Disorders, 31*(3), 307–311.

Borresen, R., & Rosenvinge, J. H. (2003). Body dissatisfaction and dieting in 4,952 Norwegian children aged 11–15 years: Less evidence for gender and age differences. *Eating and Weight Disorders, 8*, 238–241.

Cafri, G., Thompson, J. K., Ricciardelli, L. A., McCabe, M. P., Smolak, L., Yesalis, C. (2005). Pursuit of the muscular idea: Physical and psychological consequences and putative risk factors. *Clinical Psychology Review, 25*(2), 215–239.

Carano, A., De Berardis, D., Gambi, F., DiPaolo, C., Campanella, D., Pelusi, L., et al. (2006). Alexithymia and body image in adult outpatients with binge eating disorder. *International Journal of Eating Disorders, 39*(4), 332–340.

Carlat, D. J., Camargo, C. A., & Herzog, D. B. (1997). Eating disorders in males: A report of 135 patients. *American Journal of Psychiatry, 154*, 1127–1132.

Cash, T. F. (1994). Body image and weight changes in a multisite comprehensive very-low-calorie diet program. *Behavior Therapy, 25*, 239–254.

Center for Disease Control & Prevention. (2007). Introduction. *Overweight and Obesity.* January 15, 2008. Available at http://www.cdc.gov/nccdphp/dnpa/obesity/index.htm

Cash, T. F., Morrow, J. A., Hrabosky, J. I., & Perry, A. A. (2004). How has body image changed? A cross-sectional investigation of college women and men from 1983 to 2001. *Journal of Consulting and Clinical Psychology, 72*(6), 1081–1089.

Contento, I. R., Basch, C., & Zybert, P. (2003). Body image, weight and food choices of Latina women and their young children. *Journal of Nutrition, Education and Behavior, 35*(5), 236–248.

De Berardis, D., Carano, A., Gambi, F., Campanella, D., Giannetti, P., Ceci, A., et al. (2007). Alexithymia and its relationships with body checking and body image in a non-clinical female sample. *Eating Disorders, 8*, 296–304.

Duggan, S. J., & McCreary, D. R. (2004). Body image, eating disorders, and the drive for muscularity in gay and heterosexual men: The influence of media images. *Journal of Homosexuality, 47*(3/4), 45–58.

Erickson, S. J., & Gerstle, M. (2007). Investigation of ethnic differences in body image between Hispanic/biethnic-Hispanic and non-Hispanic White preadolescent girls. *Body Image, 4(1)*, 69–78.

Fairburn, C. G., Peveler, R. C., Jones, R., Hope, R. A., & Doll, H. A. (1993). Predictors of 12-month outcome in bulimia nervosa and the influence of attitudes to shape and weight. *Journal of Consulting and Clinical Psychology, 61*, 686–698.

Fallon, A. E. (1990). Culture in the mirror: Sociocultural determinants of body image. In T. F. Cash & T. Pruzinsky (Eds.). *Body images: Development, deviance and change* (pp. 80–109). New York: Guilford Press.

Feingold, A. (1992). Good-looking people are not what we think. *Psychological Bulletin, 111*(2), 304–341.

Filiault, S. M. (2007). Measuring up in the bedroom: Muscle, thinness and men's sex lives. *International Journal of Men's Health, 6*(2), 127–142.

Freedman, R. E., Carter, M. M., Sbrocco, T., & Gray, J. J. (2004). Ethnic differences in preferences for female weight and waist-to-hip ration: A comparison of African-American and White American college and community samples. *Eating Behaviors, 5*(3), 191–198.

French, S. A., Story, M., Remafedi, G., Resnick, M. D., & Blum, R. W. (1996). Sexual orientation and prevalence of body dissatisfaction and eating disordered behaviors: A population-based study of adolescents. *International Journal of Eating Disorders, 19*(2), 119–126.

Garner, D. M., Garfinkel, P. E., Schwartz, D., & Thompson, M. (1980). Cultural expectations of thinness in women. *Psychological Reports, 47*, 483–491.

Geller, J., Johnson, C., Madsen, K., Goldner, E., Remick, R., & Birmingham, C. L. (1998). Shape-and weight-based self-esteem and the eating disorders. *International Journal of Eating Disorders, 24*(3), 285–298.

Gilbert, S., & Thompson, J. K. (1996). Feminist explanations of the development of eating disorders: Common themes, research findings and methodological issues. *Clinical Psychology: Science and Practice, 3*, 183–202.

Gilliland, M. J., Windle, M., Grunbaum, J. A., Yancey, A., Hoelscher, D., Tortolero, S. R., et al. (2007). Body image and children's mental health related behaviors: Results from the Healthy Passages Study. *Journal of Pediatric Psychology, 32*(1), 30–41.

Gingras, J., Fitzpatrick, J., & McCargar, L. (2004). Body image of chronic dieters: Lowered appearance evaluation and body satisfaction. *Journal of the American Dietetic Association, 104*(10), 1589–1592.

Goldfein, J. A., Walsh, B. T., & Midlarsky, E. (2000). Influence of shape and weight on self-evaluation in bulimia nervosa. *International Journal of Eating Disorders, 27*(4), 435–445.

Gray, J. J., & Ginsberg, R. L. (2007). Muscle dissatisfaction: An overview of psychological and cultural research and theory. In J. K. Thompson & G. Cafri (Eds.). *The muscular ideal: Psychological, social and medical perspectives* (pp. 15–40). Washington, DC: American Psychological Association.

Haines, J., & Neumark-Sztainer, D. (2006). Prevention of obesity and eating disorders: A consideration of shared risk factors. *Health Education Research Theory and Practice, 21*(6), 770–782.

Harrison, K., Taylor, L. D., & Marske, A. L. (2006). Women's and men's eating behavior following exposure to ideal-body images and text. *Communication Research, 33*(6), 507–529.

Hausenblas, H. A., & Fallon, E. A. (2006). Exercise and body image: A meta-analysis. *Psychology and Health, 21*(1), 33–47.

Heinberg, L. J. (1996). Theories of body image: Perceptual, developmental and Sociocultural factors. In J. K. Thompson (Ed.), *Body image, eating disorders, and obesity: an integrative guide to assessment and treatment* (pp. 27–48). Washington, DC: American Psychological Association.

Heinberg, L. J., Haythornthwaite, J. A., Rosofsky, W., McCarron, P., & Clarke, A. (2000). Body image and weight loss maintenance in elderly African-American hypertensives. *American Journal of Health Behavior, 24*(3), 163–173.

Heinberg, L. J., Pike, E., & Loue, S. (in press). Body image and eating disturbance in minority men who have sex with men: Preliminary observations. *Journal of Homosexuality.*

Heinberg, L. J. & Thompson, J. K. (2006). Body image. In S. Wonderlich, J. E. Mitchell, M. deZwaan, & H. Steiger (Eds.), *Annual review of eating disorders: Part 2 – 2006* (pp. 81–96). Oxford, UK: Radcliffe Publishing, Ltd.

Heinberg, L. J., Thompson, J. K., & Matzon, J. L. (2001). Body image dissatisfaction as a motivator for healthy lifestyle change: is some distress beneficial? In R. H. Striegel-Moore & L. Smolak (Eds.). Eating disorders: Innovative directions in research and practice (pp. 215–232). Washington, DC: American Psychological Association.

Heinberg; L. J., Thompson J. K., & Stormer, S. (1995). Development and validation of the Sociocultural attitudes towards appearance questionnaire (SATAQ). *International Journal of Eating Disorders, 17*, 81–89.

Henry, R. N., Anshel, M. H., & Michael, T. (2006). Effects of aerobics and circuit training on fitness and body image among women. *Journal of Sports Behavior, 29*(4), 281–303.

Hilbert, A., Saelens, B. E., Stein, R. I., Mockus, D. S., Welch, R. R., Matt, G. E., et al. (2007). Pretreatment and process predictors of outcome in interpersonal and cognitive behavioral psychotherapy for binge eating disorder. *Journal of Consulting and Clinical Psychology, 75*(4), 645–651.

Hobza, C. L., Walker, K. E., Yakushko, O., & Peugh, J. L. (2007). What about men? Social comparison and the effects of media images on body and self-esteem. *Psychology of Men and Masculinity, 8*(3), 161–172.

Hospers, H. J., & Jansen, A. (2005). Why homosexuality is a risk factor for eating disorders in males. *Journal of Social and Clinical Psychology, 24*, 1188–1201.

Hrabosky, J. I., Masheb, R. M., White, M. A., & Grilo, C. M. (2007). Overvaluation of shape and weight in binge eating disorder. *Journal of Consulting and Clinical Psychology, 75*(1), 175–180.

Huang, J. S., Norman, G. J., Zabinski, M. F., Calfas, K., & Patrick, K. (2007). Body image and self-esteem among adolescents undergoing an intervention targeting dietary and physical activity behaviors. *Journal of Adolescent Health, 40*, 245–251.

Institute of Medicine. (2001). *Exploring the biological contributions to human health: Does sex matter?* Washington, DC: National Academy Press.

Jarry, J. L., & Kossert, A. L. (2007). Self-esteem threat combined with exposure to thin media images leads to body image compensatory self-enhancement. *Body Image, 4*, 39–50.

Johnson, W., & Krueger, R. F. (2007). The psychological benefits of vigorous exercise: A study of discordant MZ twin pairs. *Twin Research and Human Genetics, 10*(2), 275–283.

Keel, P. K., Dorer, D. J., Franko, D. L., Jackson, S. C., & Herzog, D. B. (2005). Postremission predictors of relapse in women with eating disorders. *American Journal of Psychiatry, 162*(12), 2263–2268.

Kim, S., & Kim, J. (2007). Mood after various brief exercise and sport modes: Aerobics, hip-hop dancing, ice skating and body conditioning. *Perceptual and Motor Skills, 104*(3, Pt2), 1265–1270.

Krahnstoever-Davison, K., Markey, C. N., & Birch, L. L. (2003). A longitudinal examination of patterns in girls' weight concerns and body dissatisfaction from age 5 to 9 years. *International Journal of Eating Disorders, 33*(3), 320–332.

Landers, D. M., & Arent, S. M. (2007). Physical activity and mental health. In G. Tanenbaum & R. C. Eklund (Eds.), *Handbook of sport psychology* (3rd ed., pp. 469–491). Hoboken, New Jersey: John Wiley & Sons, Inc.

Lipsey, Z., Barton, S. B., Hulley, A., & Hill, A. J. (2006). "After a workout." Beliefs about exercise, eating and appearance in female exercisers with and without eating disorder features. *Psychology of Sports and Exercise, 7*, 425–436.

Lutz, R. B. (2007). Physical activity, exercise and mental health. In J. H. Lake & D. Spiegel (Eds.), *Complementary and alternative treatments in mental health* care (pp. 301–320). Washington, DC: American Psychiatric Publishing, Inc.

McDonald, K., & Thompson, J. K. (1992). Eating disturbance, body image dissatisfaction and reasons for exercising: Gender differences and correlational findings. *International Journal of Eating Disorders, 11*, 289–292.

Marcus, M. D., Bromberger, J. T., Wei, H., Brown, C., & Kravitz, H. M. (2007). Prevalence and selected correlates of eating disorder symptoms among a multiethnic community sample of midlife women. *Annals of Behavioral Medicine, 33*, 269–277.

Markland, D., & Ingledew, D. K. (2007). The relationships between body mass and body image and relative autonomy for exercise among adolescent males and females. *Psychology of Sport and Exercise, 8*, 836–853.

Masheb, R. M., & Grilo, C. M. (2003). The nature of body image disturbance in patients with binge eating disorders. *International Journal of Eating Disorders, 33*(3), 333–341.

McCreary, D. R., Hildenbrandt, T. B., Heinberg, L. J., Boroughs, M., & Thompson, J. K. (2007). A review of body image influences on men's fitness goals and supplement use. *American Journal of Men's Health, 1*(4), 307–316.

Meyer, C., Blissett, J., & Oldfield, C. (2001). Sexual orientation and eating psychopathology: The role of masculinity and femininity. *International Journal of Eating Disorders, 29*, 314–318.

Michaels, M. L., Barr, A., Roosa, M. W., & Knight, G. P. (2007). Self-esteem: Assessing measurement equivalence in a multiethnic sample of youth. *Journal of Early Adolescence, 27*(3), 269–295.

Murnen, S. K., & Smolak, L. (1997). Femininity, masculinity and disordered eating: A meta-analytic review. *International Journal of Eating Disorders, 22*, 231–242.

Nemeroff, C. J., Stein, R. I., Diehl, N. S., & Smilack, K. M. (1994). From the Cleavers to the Clintons: Role choices and body orientation as reflected in magazine article content. *International Journal of Eating Disorders, 16*, 167–176.

Neumark-Sztainer, D., Paxton, S. J., Hannan, P. J., Haines, J., & Story, M. (2006). Does body satisfaction matter? Five-year longitudinal associations between body satisfaction and health behaviors in adolescent females and males. *Journal of Adolescent Health, 39*, 244–251.

O'Brien, K. O., Venn, B. J., Perry, T., Green, T. J., Aitken, W., Bradshaw, A., et al. (2007). Reasons for wanting to lose weight: Different strokes for different folks. *Eating Behaviors, 8*, 132–135.

Ogden, C. L., Flegal, K. M., Carroll, M. D., & Johnson, C. L. (2002). Prevalence and trends in overweight among US children and adolescent, 1999–2000. *Journal of the American Medical Association, 288*, 1728–1732.

Olivardia, R. (2007). Muscle dysmorphia: Characteristics, assessment and treatment. In J. K. Thompson & G. Cafri (Eds.), *The muscular ideal: Psychological, social and medical perspectives* (pp. 123–129). Washington, DC: American Psychological Association.

Paxton, S. J., Eisenberg, M. E., & Neumark-Sztainer, D. (2006). Prospective predictors of body dissatisfaction in adolescent girls and boys: a five-year longitudinal study. *Developmental Psychology, 42*(5), 888–899.

Paxton, S. J., Neumark-Sztainer, D., Hannan, P. J., & Eisenberg, M. E. (2007). Body dissatisfaction prospectively predicts depressive mood and low self-esteem in adolescent girls and boys. *Journal of Clinical Child and Adolescent Psychology, 35*(4), 539–549.

Perez, M. & Joiner, T. E. (2003). Body image dissatisfaction and disordered eating in black and white women. *International Journal of Eating Disorders, 33*, 342–350.

Petrie, T. A., Austin, L. J., Crowley, B. J., Helmcaup, A., Johnson, C. E., Lester, R., et al. (1996). Sociocultural expectations of attractiveness for males. *Sex Roles, 35*, 581–601.

Pope, H. G., Gruber, A. J., Choi, P., Olivardia, R., & Phillips, K. A. (1997). Muscle dysmorphia: An under recognized form of body dysmorphic disorder. *Psychosomatics, 38*, 548–557.

Pope Jr., H. G., Olivardia, R., Gruber, A., & Borowiecki, J. (1999). Evolving ideals of male body image as seen through action toys. *International Journal of Eating Disorder, 26*, 65–72.

Pulvers, K. M., Lee, R. E., Kaur, H., Mayo, M. S., Fitzgibbon, M. L., Jeffries, S. K., et al. (2004). Development of a culturally relevant body image instrument among urban African Americans. *Obesity Research, 12*, 1641–1651.

Rabkin, J., Charles, E., & Kass, F. (1983). Hypertension and DSM-III depression and psychiatric outpatients. *American Journal of Psychiatry, 140*, 1072–1074.

Ricciardelli, L. A., McCabe, M. P., Mavoa, H., Fotu, K., Goundar, R., Schultz, J., et al. (2007). The pursuit of muscularity among adolescent boys in Fiji and Tonga. *Body Image, 4*, 361–371.

Ricciardelli, L. A., McCabe, M. P., & Ridge, D. (2006). The construction of the adolescent male body through sports. *Journal of Health Psychology, 11*, 577–587.

Ricciardelli, L. A., McCabe, M. P., Williams, R. J., & Thompson, J. K. (2007). The role of ethnicity and culture in body image and disordered eating among males. *Clinical Psychology Review, 27*, 582–606.

Rintala, M., & Mustajoki, P. (1992). Could mannequins menstruate? *British Medical Journal, 305*, 1575–1576.

Robinson, T. N., Chang, J. Y., Haydel, K. F., & Killen, J. D. (2001). Overweight concerns and body dissatisfaction among third-grade children: The impacts of ethnicity and socio-economic status. *Journal of Pediatrics, 138*, 181–187.

Rodin, J., Silberstein, L. R., & Striegel-Moore, R. H. (1985). Women and weight: A normative discontent. In T. B. Sonderegger (Ed.), *Psychology and gender: Nebraska symposium on motivation. 1984* (pp. 267–307). Lincoln, Nebraska: University of Nebraska Press.

Ruffolo, J. S., Phillips, K. A., Menard, W., Fay, C., & Weisberg, R. B. (2006). Comorbidity of body dysmorphic disorder and eating disorders: severity of psychopathology and body image disturbance. *International Journal of Eating Disorders, 39*(1), 11–19.

Russell, C. J., & Keel, P. K. (2002). Homosexuality as a specific risk factor for eating disorders in men. *International Journal of Eating Disorders, 31*, 300–306.

Sacco, W. P., Wells, K. J., Friedman, A., Matthew, R., Perez, S., & Vaughan, C. (2007). Adherence, body mass index and depression in adults with Type 2 Diabetes: The mediational role of diabetes symptoms and self-efficacy. *Health Psychology, 24*(4), 493–700.

Sahi Iyer, D. & Haslam, N. (2003). Body image and eating disturbance among South Asian-American women: The role of racial teasing. *International Journal of Eating Disorders, 34*, 142–147.

Sanchez-Johnsen, L. A., Fitzgibbon, M. L., Martinovich, Z., Stolley, M. R., Dyer, A. R., & Van Horn, L. (2004). Ethnic differences in correlates of obesity between Latin-American and black women. *Obesity Research, 12*, 652–660.

Santos, M., Richards, C. S., & Bleckley, M. K. (2007). Comorbidity between depression and disordered eating in adolescents. *Eating Behaviors, 8*, 440–449.

Sarwer, D. B., Crerand, C. E., & Gibbons, L. M. (2007). Cosmetic procedures to enhance body shape and muscularity. In J. K. Thompson & G. Cafri (Eds.), *The muscular ideal: Psychological, social and medical perspectives* (pp. 183–198). Washington, DC: American Psychological Association.

Sarwer, D. B., & Magee, L. (2006). Physical appearance and society. In D. B. Sarwer, T. Pruzinsky, T Cash, R. M. Goldwyn, J. A. Persing & L. A. Whitaker (Eds.), *Psychological aspects of reconstructive and cosmetic plastic surgery: Clinical, empirical, and ethical perspectives*. Philadelphia: Lippincott Williams & Wilkins.

Schuler, P. B., Broxon-Hutcherson, A.,Philipp S. F., Ryan, S., Isosaari, R. M., & Robinson, D. (2004). Body-shape perceptions in older adults and motivations for exercise. *Perceptual and Motor Skills, 98*, 1251–1260.

Seidman, S. N., & Rieder, R. O. (1994). A review of sexual behavior in the United States. *American Journal of Psychiatry, 151*(3), 330–341

Seiver, M. D. (1994). Sexual orientation and gender as factors in socioculturally acquired vulnerability to body dissatisfaction and eating disorders. *Journal of Consulting and Clinical Psychology, 62*, 252–260.

Shea, M. E., & Pritchard, M. E. (2007). Is self-esteem the primary predictor of disordered eating. *Personality and Individual Differences, 42*, 1527–1537.

Shaw, H., Ramirez, L., Trost, A., Randall, P., & Stice, E. (2004). Body image and eating disturbances across ethnic groups: More similarities than differences. *Psychology of Addictive Behaviors, 18*(1), 12–18.

Sifneos, P. E. (1973). The prevalence of alexithymic characteristics in psychosomatic patient. *Psychotherapy and Psychosomatics, 22*, 255–262.

Slater, A., & Tiggeman, M. (2006). The contribution of physical activity and media use during childhood and adolescence to adult women's body image. *Journal of Health Psychology, 11*(4), 553–565.

Smith, P. J., Blumenthal, J. A., Babyak, M. A., Georgiades, A., Hinderliter, A., & Sherwood, A. (2007). Effects of exercise and weight loss on depressive symptoms among men and women with hypertension. *Journal of Psychosomatic Research, 63*, 463–469.

Stice, E. (2001). A prospective test of the dual-pathway model of bulimic pathology: Mediating effects of dieting and negative affect. *Journal of Abnormal Psychology, 110*, 124–135.

Stice, E. (1994). Review of the evidence for a sociocultural model of bulimia nervosa and an exploration of the mechanisms of action. *Clinical Psychology Review, 14*, 633–661.

Stice, E. (2002). Risk and maintenance factor for eating pathology: A meta-analytic review. *Psychological Bulletin, 128*, 825–848.

Stice, E., & Bearman, S. (2001). Body image and eating disturbances prospectively predict increase in depressive symptoms in adolescent girls: A growth curve analysis. *Developmental Psychology, 37*, 597–607.

Striegel-Moore, R. H., Franko, D. L., Thompson, D., Barton, B., Schreiber, G. B., & Daniels, S. R. (2004). Changes in weight and body image over time in women with eating disorders. *International Journal of Eating Disorders, 36*, 315–327.

Strong, S. M., Williamson, D. A., Netemeyer, R. G., & Geer, J. H. (2000). Eating disorder symptoms and concerns about body differ as a function of gender and sexual orientation. *Journal of Social and Clinical Psychology, 19*, 240–255.

Stubbe, J. H., deMoor, M. H. M., Boomsma, D. I., & deGeus, E. J. C. (2007). The association between exercise participation and well-being: A co-twin study. *Preventive Medicine: An International Journal Devoted to Practice and Theory, 44*(2), 148–152.

Taveras, E. M., Rifas-Shiman, S. L., Field, A. E., Frazier, A. L., Colditz, G. A., & Gillman, M. W. (2004). The influence of wanting to look like media figures on adolescent physical activity. *Journal of Adolescent Health, 35*, 41–50.

Taylor, G. J., Bagby, R. M., & Parker, J. D. A. (1997). *Disorders of affect regulation: Alexithymia in medical and psychiatric illness.* New York: Cambridge University Press.

Thompson, J. K., Heinberg, L. J., Altabe, M. N., & Tantleff-Dunn, S. (1999). *Exacting beauty: Theory, assessment and treatment of body image disturbance.* Washington, DC: American Psychological Association.

Thompson, J. K., Shroff, H., Herbozo, S., Cafri, G., Rodriguez, J., & Rodriguez, M. (2007). Relations among multiple peer influences, body dissatisfaction, eating disturbance and self-esteem: A comparison of average weight, at risk of overweight and overweight adolescent girls. *Journal of Pediatric Psychology, 32*(1), 24–29.

Tsai, G., Curbow, B., & Heinberg, J. L. (2003). Sociocultural and developmental influences on body dissatisfaction and disordered eating attitudes and behaviors of Asian women. *The Journal of Nervous and Mental Disease, 191*, 309–318.

van den Berg, P., & Neumark-Sztainer, D. (2007). Fat'n happy 5 years later: Is it bad for overweight girls to like their bodies? *Journal of Adolescent Health, 41*, 415–417.

van den Berg, P., Paxton, S. J., Keery, H., Wall, M., Guo, J., & Neumark-Sztainer, D. (2007). Body dissatisfaction and body comparison with media images in males and females. *Body Image, 4*, 257–268.

Vander Wal, J. S., & Thompson, N. (2004). Predictors of body image dissatisfaction and disturbed eating attitudes and behaviors in African American and Hispanic girls. *Eating Behaviors, 5*, 291–301.

Wardle, J., Haase, A., & Steptoe, A. (2006). Body image and weight control in young adults: International comparisons in university students from 22 countries. *International Journal of Obesity, 30*, 644–651.

Wardle, J., Haase, A., Steptoe, A., Nillapun, M., Jonwutiwes, K., & Bellisle, F. (2004). Gender differences in food choices: the contribution of health beliefs and dieting. *Annals of Behavioral Medicine, 27*(2), 107–116.

Warren, M., & Hildebrand, T. (2006). Proceedings from the Male Special Interest Group. International Conference for Eating Disorders, Barcelona, Spain.

Weaver, A. D., & Byers, E. S. (2006). The relationships among body image, body mass index, exercise and sexual functioning in heterosexual women. *Psychology of Women Quarterly, 30*, 333–339.

Whisenhunt, B. L., Williamson, D. A., Netemeyer, R. G., & Andrews, C. (2003). Health risks, past usage and intention to use weight loss products in normal weight women with high and low body dysphoria. *Eating and Weight Disorders, 8*, 114–123.

White, M. A., Kohlmaier, J. R., Varnado-Sullivan, P., & Williamson, D. A. (2003). Racial/ethnic differences in weight concerns: Protective and risk factors for the development of eating disorders and obesity among adolescent females. *Eating and Weight Disorders, 8*, 20–25.

Wight, R. G., Aneshensel, C. S., Botticello, A. L., & Sepulveda, J. E. (2005). A multilevel analysis of ethnic variation in depressive symptoms among adolescents in the United States. *Social Science in Medicine, 60*, 2073–2084.

Williamson, I., & Hartley, P. (1998). British research into the increased vulnerability of young gay men to eating disturbance and body dissatisfaction. *European Eating Disorders Review, 6, 160–170.*

Wiseman, C. V., Gray, J. J., Mosimann, J. E., & Ahrens, A. H. (1992). Cultural expectations of thinness in women: An update. *International Journal of Eating Disorders, 11*, 85–89.

Wolfe, B. L., & Smith, J. E. (2002). Different strokes for different folks: Why overweight men do not seek weight loss treatment. *Eating Disorders: Journal of Treatment and Prevention, 10*(2), 115–124.

Wood, C., Becker, J., & Thompson, J. K. (1996). Body image dissatisfaction in preadolescent children. *Journal of Applied Developmental Psychology, 17*, 85–100

Yates, A., Edman, J., & Aruguete, M. (2004). Ethnic differences in BMI and body/self-dissatisfaction among White, Asian subgroups, Pacific Islanders and African-Americans. *Journal of Adolescent Health, 34*(4), 300–307.

Zabinski, M. F., Wilfley, D. E., Calfas, K. J., Winzelberg, A. J., & Taylor, C. B. (2004). An interactive psychoeducational intervention for women at risk of developing an eating disorder. *Journal of Consulting and Clinical Psychology, 72*(5), 914–919.

Chapter 11
Family Determinants of Minority Mental Health and Wellness

Stevan Weine and Saif Siddiqui

This chapter considers the possible determinants of families concerning mental health and wellness in ethnic minorities. First, it describes key characteristics of families that may be determinants based upon family therapy theory and practice knowledge. Next, it reviews summary descriptions of families of several U.S. minority groups, including African Americans, Native Americans, Latino Americans, Asian Americans, and Muslim Americans, with an emphasis on possible pertinent family determinants. It then provides a selective review of family determinants associated with key areas of minority mental health and wellness based upon research evidence. Further conceptual and research work on family determinants and minority mental health and wellness is needed. It should attend to the multidimensional complexities of family determinants and aim at developing new family-focused services for mental health promotion and treatment amongst ethnic minority families.

What Is a Family?

The family is a universal idea about groups of persons that is defined distinctly in different cultures. For example, in some cultures all family members are connected by blood relationships, as in parents and their offspring. Other cultures define family as a group of people that live together in a household. This distinction, which has been referred to as the dilemma of "family of origin" versus "family of choice" is one of many family-related cultural issues that bear upon mental health and wellness in ethnic minority families.

The family may differ not only by culture but also with respect to economic, social, and medical conditions. Many ethnic minority families either have at one time or still do live in or near poverty. Migration is a key factor, given that a significant proportion of ethnic minority families have experienced migration in

S. Weine (✉)
University of Illinois, Psychiatric Institute, Chicago, IL
e-mail: smweine@uic.edu

S. Loue, M. Sajatovic (eds.), *Determinants of Minority Mental Health and Wellness*, DOI 10.1007/978-0-387-75659-2_11,
© Springer Science+Business Media, LLC 2009

current or prior generations. Lastly, some families have a member with a physical or mental illness that requires specialized care. (Note: We are not necessarily implying that ethnic minority families differ in rates of illnesses but that their family behaviors in relation to illnesses are likely to vary significantly.) It is important to ask how these social, economic, and medical conditions should be considered in relation to family determinants.

It is also important to understand that the family is a group that interacts with other systems. According to Bronfenbrenner's ecological theory of child development, which frames this entire volume, the family is regarded as a "micro-system" for the developing child (Bronfenbrenner, 1986). This micro-system may initially consist only of parents and siblings in a home. Over developmental time the family as a system expands to incorporate other individuals, groups, and organizations that directly interact with the child. What then are we to make of the fact that minority families, in comparison with nonminority families, are likely to have different patterns of interaction with these other systems? For example, some ethnic minority families may experience barriers to accessing organizations stemming from discrimination or mistrust. These interactions then become associated with the family, although they are not necessarily intrinsic properties of the family. How should these interactions be regarded with respect to possible family determinants of mental health and wellness?

We are not in a position to propose definitive answers for any of these questions. Rather we are drawing attention to them because they are important issues that must be considered as we look at particular family characteristics that may be functioning as determinants of minority mental health and wellness. We also cannot overlook the possibility that ethnic minority families may differ from families of the dominant group in part due to the tendency for these multidimensional interactions to be regarded as attributes of the family per se. Negative change in representation and self-perception of the family may have its own adverse consequences upon family members; families are regarded or may come to regard themselves as not "measuring up" to what families are expected to be in a given society.

We should take note of how these dimensions are being viewed by family therapists and researchers as they address the issue of possible family determinants such as family structure and family support. What family determinants are universal or culture-specific? What other social and economic conditions are at play? What impact do beliefs about the family have?

Learning About Families

Knowledge about the mental health issues of ethnic minority families in the U.S. increased beginning in the 1980s in part through the efforts of family therapists. Many family therapists were coming into contact with more diversity in their clinical practices and finding the need to expand the theory and practice of their field in ways that embraced cultural diversity. Some leaders in the field attempted to reenvision family therapy through a multicultural lens (McGoldrick, 1998a). This included a focus on the interrelated key issues of gender, race, class, religion, and ethnicity, as well as broad conceptualizations regarding the family in relation to communities, institutions, and society.

At times, the multicultural family approach has expressed suspicion of the *DSM-IV-TR* psychiatric diagnostic manual because of the manual's perceived inadequacies regarding understanding ethnic minorities:

> families of color, families of the poor, and immigrant families, whose norms and values are different from those within our naming scheme, remain peripheralized, invalidated, and pathologized as deficient or dysfunctional – or worse, invisible within our society.
> (McGoldrick, 1998a, p. 6).

The role of family therapy, as seen by some multicultural family therapists, was to offer care that provided families with validation, understanding, and healing, given their unique cultural experiences. To achieve this, family therapists relied upon clinical intuition and accumulated therapeutic experience, thus building a body of practice knowledge concerning ethnic minority families. Although this literature has identified family characteristics that may be determinants of mental illness in ethnic families, this literature has tended not to extend those understandings into the system of psychiatric diagnoses which was at times perceived as antithetical to family therapy's central aims. Family therapists leaned more in the direction of identifying the resources and strengths that lie in ethnic minority families and in helping to navigate the vicissitudes of family life (McGoldrick, Giordano, & Garcia-Preto, 2005). In doing so, they may have overlooked the possibility that vulnerability to some forms of mental illness amongst some family members, including due to cultural, social, economic, and biological risks, may be different among some ethnic minorities compared with the majority.

Psychiatric researchers, on the other hand, have approached the issue of family determinants by conducting mental health research on families that, in general, has tried to understand the causes or consequences of mental illness. Families have been investigated using various research methods, including quantitative, qualitative, and mixed methods (Greenstein, 2006). The first most important thing to notice about research on families of ethnic minorities is how little research there really is. Most of the limited research that exists regarding family determinants has been conducted with White Anglo Saxon subjects. The deficiency of research knowledge on ethnic minority families applies to the issue of family determinants of mental health and wellness, although there has been some growth in this area in the past decade, due in part to the Family Research Consortium of the U.S. National Institute of Mental Health (see http://www. semel.ucla.edu/frc4/). Even so, the focus on global family determinants, such as family support, cannot begin to get at the variability of the meanings and experiences of family characteristics both amongst and between diverse ethnic groups.

Both family-focused clinicians and researchers have relied upon theory to understand ethnic minority families. There are many different types of family theories which seek to explain families. These include, but are not limited to, family systems theory, family ecological theory, and communication theories (Boss, Doherty, LaRossa, Schumm, & Steinmetz, 1993). These theories offer very different perspectives upon families, varying according to scope and to level of abstraction. In recent years, family theorists have begun to focus more on ethnic minority families. They have attempted to modify the ways that families are theorized so as to adequately understand the unique cultural and social processes that may characterize a family's experiences of a particular ethnic reality. Further progress in learning about the roles of family determinants depends in part upon growth in theories.

Key Characteristics of Ethnic Minority Families That Are Potential Determinants

In this section, we introduce several characteristics of families that have been described in the family therapy literature and that could be possible family determinants of mental health or wellness. These include both (1) characteristics that may be considered universal and those that are more culture-specific; (2) characteristics that are more intrinsic to families and those that are a part of families' responses to external conditions. When we speak of mental health or wellness, we consider that the affected person may be any family member, regardless of age. We are fairly open in considering any type of mental health issue that has support in the family therapy literature, including specific mental disorders and behavioral problems, as well as indicators of mental health. However, mental health is clearly less often addressed in the professional and scientific literatures than mental disorders. We do not delve into the issue of culture-specific disorders, as it is beyond the scope of this paper. In this section, we also do not consider whether or not the characteristics have research support, which will be taken up in a subsequent section of this chapter.

Family Structure

In Western societies, the nuclear family has, in the post World War II era, been regarded as the ideal family structure. It consists of a breadwinner father, a homemaker mother, and several children, all living together in one home and largely self-sufficient. Over the past several decades the prevalence of nuclear families in the U.S. has declined from 40% (1970) to 24% (2000) of households (Williams, Sawyer, & Wahlstrom, 2005). Simultaneously, there has been a growth of other family forms including single-parent families, blended families, binuclear families, same sex families, and child-free couples. These evolutions in family structure have been determined by many factors, including social class, work, religion, sexual preference, and ethnicity.

As family therapists began to see more culturally diverse clients, they became more familiar with the extended family configuration, which is very common amongst many ethnic minorities. Family therapists have tended to find strengths in this type of family structure, such as family solidarity and support (McGoldrick, Giordano, & Garcia-Preto, 2005). They regarded these extended family networks as both adaptive responses to migration and other adversities and expressions of priority cultural values. From encounters with diverse families, it was also learned that the extended family can vary significantly across ethnic lines and within ethnic groups, as will be discussed later.

The extended family structure is not without difficulties. First, culturally based preferences, stated or unstated, that U.S. families should be nuclear families, may complicate families' interactions with schools, clinics, and other institutions, as well as families' views and expectations of themselves. Secondly, families that are in cultural transition due to recent immigration may be experiencing a transformation from a more extended family system to a more nuclear family system. Lastly, in families of migration, especially forced migration, the extended family may become a transnational family with family members living in multiple global settings, diminishing contact and increasing reliance on telecommunications and air travel.

The idea of family structure as applied to ethnic minority families has also been highlighted by Salvador Minuchin's structural family therapy (Minuchin, Montalvo, Guerney, Rosman, & Schumer, 1967). This approach emphasized the family as a system which performs certain functions through subsystems (e.g. parental) and which requires clarity and boundaries in order to maximize effectiveness. Family structures may be changed as a consequence of adverse experiences, such as poverty or violence. One key question is how well families that do not fit the nuclear family paradigm are able to adapt and to devise alternative effective structures and functional strategies. For example, how does a mother in a single-parent family effectively carry out parenting functions meant to be performed by two parents? This is an important concern regarding some ethnic minority families, as a higher percentage of children in Black families, compared to non-Hispanic White children, are living with single-parent families (Pollard & O'Hare, 1999). The suggestion is that single-parent families may be exposed to more stressors than two parent families and that this could impact children's mental health, unless single-parent families were able to effectively manage this stress.

Another important dimension regarding family structure in ethnic minority families concerns beliefs about how families should be organized in terms of roles. One prominent example in the family therapy literature concerns gender roles (McGoldrick, Giordano, & Garcia-Preto, 2005). Families in patriarchal cultures are likely to present women with roles that are more rigid, have less authority and power within the family, and have less access to the world outside the family. Upon immigration to a new society these families may experience new opportunities but also additional strains when they are exposed to more egalitarian values and lifestyles of the dominant culture in the receiving society. In this instance, beliefs about gender roles in the family may impact the mental health consequences of family members. Some will argue that resolution of the problem requires the restoration of patriarchal order, whereas others will claim that greater egalitarianism within the family would benefit the mental health of all family members (McGoldrick, 1998b).

Family Support

Family support is regarded as encompassing both the tangible and emotional assistance that families provide to their members. Tangible family support is composed of task-focusing and pragmatic assistance. Emotional support is garnered when family members provide assistance by showing and expressing concern, care, and reassurance. Ethnic families from ethnic minority groups have been observed to excel at providing family support to family members as this often reflects a prime cultural value. However, as families experience cultural transition and become heavily burdened by work or financial matters, they may find themselves less available to provide the family support that their culture expresses. One issue concerning ethnic families is that persons offering high levels of support in the family may be viewed as "co-dependent," which is the controversial term used in the recovery movement to describe a problematic behavior that in effect rewards a family member's negative behaviors.

Family support has another meaning in the particular context of families that are caring for a member with a physical or mental illness or disability. In this sense, family support is defined as "the assistance given to families to cope with the extra stresses that accompany caring for a child with emotional disabilities" (U.S. Department of Health and Human Services, 1999, Chapter 3). In the past several decades, when the tendency amongst mental health professionals was less to blame families with an ill member, and more to recognize their role as caregivers, the focus has been on providing family support that was designed to fit the priorities, needs, meanings, and strengths of the family. Family support aims to strengthen the roles of the caregivers, who are most often adults or parents (Weissbourd & Kagan, 1989). Family support services encompass the provision of information, tangible assistance, emotional support, and psycho-social counseling, and the facilitation of communication. Ethnic minority families coping with a physically or mentally ill family member may experience additional problems with family support due to discrimination that they experience as a consequence of ethnic, racial, religious, gender, or age factors. They may also experience stigma regarding mental health or health problems, or help seeking, in different ways than the majority population. Diverse families may also have very different expectations of what they need from service organizations, including high levels of mistrust (U.S. Department of Health and Human

Services, 2001). All these factors call for different strategies for providing family support services for ethnic minorities.

For the purposes of this discussion, family support also encompasses family advocacy regarding mental illness. Beginning in the 1970s, families with members who had a mental illness began to organize and to try to lobby for changes in services, research, training, and policy regarding mental illness. Their efforts have had a significant impact upon services for the mentally ill. However, in the U.S., family advocacy for mental illness has been much more of a focus for White middle class families rather than for ethnic minority families (Newbigging & Mckeown, 2007).

Familism

Familism is a term used to describe an approach to social experience that places the family above individual interests (Sabogal, Marín, Otero-Sabogal, Marín, & Perez-Stable, 1987). It may be reflected in shared living arrangements with multiple family members, including parents, children, grandparents, aunts/ uncles, and cousins. It may also take the form of a strong sense of obligation to the family as a whole and its members. Familism may reflect shared cultural practices of certain ethnic minorities, especially Latinos (Zambrana, 1995). Some regard it as a consequence of the social experience of migration. When ethnic minority families come to the U.S., they are often put in a position of having to rely much more upon the family until they are able to make connections to the broader community and institutions. Familism has been regarded by family therapists as a benefit that the family provides to its members. Familism means that the family supports and protects each of its members for life, as long as that person does not leave the family. The same sense of obligation may also be extended to cousins or other distant relations, which is sometimes difficult for mainstream organizations or providers to understand or to take into account (Zayas & Palleja, 1988).

Emotional Expression

Emotional expression may vary significantly amongst culturally diverse families. Families of some ethnic minorities favor emotional expressions, whereas others do not encourage it. Some ethnic groups may be distinct from one another in how families may avoid expression of certain topics, whereas other topics can be counted on to set off emotional fireworks in the family. Topics likely to be contested include sexuality, illness, trauma, loss, disability, and death.

The issue of emotional expression became a focus for mental health research on the family. Expressed emotion is a research term used to indicate the quantity and quality of emotions displayed in the family setting. Expressed emotions have been the focus of research that links family behaviors with the relapse of severe mental illness, as will be discussed in a later section. The research finding that families with higher expressed emotions have been shown to be more likely to lead to relapse of psychiatric conditions (depression and schizophrenia) informs therapeutic work in family therapy practice. One focus of this work with families of mentally ill persons is on containing high expressed emotions, which is characterized as hostility, emotional overinvolvement, and critical comments. Family therapists are aware that there may be important cultural differences in high expressed emotions such that what appears negative in one ethnic group may be positive in another (McGoldrick, Giordano, & Garcia-Preto, 2005).

Family Beliefs

According to Bell, Watson, and Wright (1996, p. 41), a belief is "the truth of a subjective reality that influences bio-psychosocial-spiritual structure and functioning." These authors focus on the family's core beliefs that shape how we approach the world. They are especially interested in beliefs that concern the family itself and illness in the family. This includes family beliefs regarding such issues as how the family names symptoms, what they believe is the cause of the illness, and what they believe is a helpful solution. Family beliefs may be "facilitative" or "constraining." Facilitative beliefs help to find solutions, whereas constraining beliefs present obstacles to flexibility, learning, and problem solving. The issue of family beliefs has not yet been the focus of much research. However, family therapy work with diverse cultural groups demonstrates the impact that different belief systems regarding health and illness (physical and mental) have upon individual and family behavior. This includes interactions with service providers, who have reported difficulties providing health and mental health services to culturally diverse families. Family beliefs also include beliefs of family members in God. Religious faith is a strong component of many ethnic families, providing spiritual fulfillment, emotional support, and community connection (McGoldrick, Giordano, & Garcia-Preto, 2005).

Family Economic Status

Overall, compared with White families, ethnic minorities in the U.S. are more likely to be living in poverty (Department of Human and Health Services, 1999). Of course, this does not mean that all ethnic minority families are poverty stricken. But family therapists working with ethnic minority families are on notice for the many different ways that economic status may impact families. Economic status affects family life in many ways, including housing, education, work, leisure, health, and stability. Worsening economy can lead to increased family conflict and violence, separation and divorce, and alcohol and substance abuse. Family therapists have warned of the importance of not mistaking the impact of adverse economic conditions upon families for an expression of culture (McGoldrick, Giordano, & Garcia-Preto, 2005).

Migrants and Refugees

The current era is one of the greatest migration waves in the history of the U.S., which of course, is a nation founded by immigrants. Legal immigration to the U.S. grew from 2.5 million in the 1950s to 4.5 million in the 1970s, and 7.3 million in the 1980s to about 10 million in the 1990s. Since 2000, legal immigrants to the U.S. number approximately 1,000,000 per year. Over 12% of the U.S. population are immigrants and over 20% of children are immigrants (Urban Institute, 2006). Latinos constitute 12.5% of the U.S. population, Asians nearly 4%, and Blacks from the Caribbean region also 4%.

Due to the adversity that immigrants are exposed to, mental health professionals have sometimes expected them to have higher rates of mental health disorders. This assumption was also supported by clinicians drawing conclusions based upon clinical sub-samples. Studies conducted on larger unbiased samples show that immigrants actually have better mental health than U.S. born persons (Vega et al., 1998). However, the longer they are exposed to life in the U.S., the more they resemble U.S. born persons with regards to types and rates of mental health disorders.

Migrants who come as refugees present a special set of conditions and vulnerability to certain mental disorders. According to the 1951 United Nations Convention Relating to the Status of Refugees, a refugee is a person who, "owing to a well-founded fear of being persecuted for reasons of race, religion, nationality, membership of a particular social group, or political opinion, is outside the country of their nationality, and is unable to or, owing to such fear, is unwilling to avail him/herself of the protection of that country" (United Nations High Commission on Refugees, 2002). These characteristics make refugees distinct from illegal immigrants, economic migrants, environmental migrants, labor migrants, and immigrants. Refugees are forced to flee their homes, communities, and loved ones without knowing where they will end up. Prior to or during flight they very often endure extreme traumatic experiences, including siege, combat, torture, atrocities, rape, witnessing violence, fear for their lives, hunger, lack of adequate shelter, separation from loved ones, and destruction and loss of property. The U.S. has admitted 2 million refugees since 1980. After a falloff in refugee admissions following September 11, 2001, the U.S. admitted 54,000 in 2005 and 41,000 in 2006. Refugees enter the U.S. either as part of legally approved refugee programs, or with some legal migration documents (e.g. student visas), or undocumented.

Refugee trauma is a construct used by mental health and human rights professionals to explain the damaging impact of the refugee experience on individual, family, and community mental health. With the advent of the Posttraumatic Stress Disorder (PTSD) diagnosis in the 1980 *DSM III*, refugee trauma was viewed primarily through the lens of traumatic stress theory. There was a burgeoning of scientific literature that documented traumatic stress symptoms and the PTSD diagnosis in multiple refugee populations displaced through the Vietnam War and the killing fields of Pol Pot in Cambodia (Freidman & Jaronson, 1994). (For a further discussion of the impact of migration on mental health, see Loue's chapter on migration.)

Family is a key issue in thinking about both refugees and refugee trauma. Families that experience political violence may have lost a family member in an armed conflict. Most, but not all, refugees come as families in some configuration. They carry with them family beliefs, rituals, and histories, and live within established patterns of family structure and functioning, all of which have profound implications for their experiences as refugees and their coping with refugee trauma (Weine, 1999). Loss and separation from family members is known to worsen mental health problems. Family resiliency is often cited as an important variable but is in need of greater understanding (Weine, 2008).

Family Conflict, Disruption, Trauma, and Loss

Families may impact the mental health of their members through adverse events within the family. Marital conflict, separation, or divorce may have a deleterious impact upon youth. Divorce rates are lower amongst several ethnic minority groups, including Mexican Americans and Black Caribbean immigrants, in comparison with Whites (Frisbie & Bean, 1995; Williams et al., 2007). Family members may experience trauma due to their exposure to a traumatic event that was brought from the outside upon their families. For example, a family member may be a soldier, a survivor of torture, or a civilian who was raped. Migrants and refugees may experience losses, which may be viewed as a type of ambiguous loss in that there is a discordance between physical absence/presence and psychological absence/presence (Boss, 2002; Falicov, 2004). Trauma in the family, such as domestic abuse or child abuse, may also occur because one family member may do harm to another family member through verbal, physical, or sexual abuse. The loss of a family member can be devastating to the remaining members and to the family as a whole. These types of events can happen in any family. One important question regarding ethnic minority families is whether some of these events are more or less likely to occur in ethnic minority families. If they do happen, are they more or less likely to result in symptoms or disorders?

Summary Descriptions of Families of Ethnic Minority Groups

Ethnicity, according to McGoldrick, "refers to a group's commonality of ancestry and history, through which people have evolved shared values and customs over the centuries" (McGoldrick, Giordano, & Garcia-Preto, 2005, p. 2). McGoldrick emphasized how ethnicity shapes identity, which in turn shapes values, tastes, habits, relationships, and lives.

A families' experience of ethnicity, in turn, is impacted by multiple factors, including social and economic conditions, migration, and religion. One of the most important social realities facing ethnic families is their status as minorities. A minority group is a collectivity within a given society that is regarded as having a lower social status. Minority groups in the U.S. include, but are not limited to, African Americans, Native Americans, Hispanics, Asian Americans, and Muslim Americans.

One of the achievements of family therapy has been to develop specific understandings of the families of ethnic minority groups. However, in the effort to focus on problems in need of therapeutic intervention, one of the unintended consequences of this effort may be to emphasize certain perceived negative characteristics of ethnic minorities. Another pitfall, about which the family therapy literature is highly conscious, is the tendency to reify certain group level characteristics without adequately appreciating in-group variability or cultural interaction.

In the following section, we reflect upon some, but certainly not all, of these descriptions of families of ethnic minorities, with a focus on identifying some of the characteristics of ethnic minorities that could be family determinants, as well as drawing out some of the social, economic, cultural, and historical contexts that make each group unique.

African American Families

The 2006 U.S. Census Bureau American Community Survey reports that over 39 million people identify themselves as "Black or African American," representing over 13% of the U.S. population. Although the racial designation of Black also includes African families who came to the U.S. as immigrants or refugees (Kamya, 2005), these groups will not be discussed in this brief overview. African American families share the historical trauma of violent removal from Africa and subsequent legacy of racist discrimination and oppression.

Economic studies show significant disparities between African American and non-Hispanic White families. Twenty-seven percent of African American families earn below the federal poverty level in comparison with 10% of non-Hispanic White families (Staveteig & Wigton, 2000). McKinnon's landmark report on the Black population in America revealed that African Americans averaged only 66% of the income of Whites ($30,439 vs. $45,904). The report

also showed that African Americans have a comparatively higher unemployment rate. They also have a substantially lower average life expectancy when
compared to other race populations and a higher rate of death due to AIDS and
homicide (Hines & Boyd-Franklin, 2005).

Despite these adversities, other research describes how certain family characteristics unique to African Americans contribute to what was described by
Billingsley (1968, p. 88) as an "amazing ability to survive in the face of impos-
sible conditions." The literature identifies strong kinship bonds as one of the
core characteristics of African American families. Studies by Arias (2002) and
Nobles (2004) traced these strong kinship bonds to their African heritage:

> where various tribes shared 'commonalities' (e.g. worldview) that were broader than
> bloodlines. In contrast to the European premise 'I think, therefore I am,' the prevailing
> African philosophy is 'We are, therefore I am.' In effect, individuals owed their
> existence to the tribe
>
> (Hines & Boyd-Franklin, 2005, p. 88).

Nobles (2004) interpreted this to mean that individuals owed their existence to
the tribe. During the slave trade, families were frequently torn apart as members
were sold to different plantations. Kinship bonds that went beyond traditional "blood" relations were critical to the survival of African American in
such cruel situations. Extensive and resilient kinship networks remain important to African Americans coping with present day hardships (Hines & Boyd-
Franklin, 2005).

Consequently, as documented by White (2004), there can be a large number
and wide variety of people (uncles, aunts, preachers, boyfriends, "big mamas,"
and others) involved in the functioning of an African American home. A broad
network of family support has been found to be vital in the case of single-parent
households, particularly when considering the potentially higher level of
stressors single-parent families can be exposed to. In 1997, 55% of African
American families were single-parent households (Staveteig & Wigton, 2000).
Adolescent single-mothers who have the support of kin are more likely to avoid
becoming dependent on welfare (Hill, 1993). Research has also shown that the
children of teenage mothers with the support of kin are more likely to achieve
healthy development when compared to the children of teenage mothers who
are without the support of relatives (Hill, 1993).

African American families also exhibit role flexibility which serves as a protective factor against stressors. Hines and Boyd-Franklin (2005) explain that in
times of crisis such as separation, illness, hospitalization, and death, it is common
for a child to be informally adopted by another member of the extended family.
Often, a grandparent or an uncle will informally adopt the child when the parent
is incapable of nurturing or caring for the child. While role flexibility allows for
multiple sources of support and assistance, it can also become a significant burden
for family networks. Hill notes that there is a growing gap for African Americans
between the cultural obligation of extending help to family members in need and
the economic ability to adequately do so (Hines & Boyd-Franklin, 2005).

Other important characteristics of African American families are the three-generation system, a strong spiritual orientation, and the strength of women. The "three-generation system" refers to the supportive role that grandmothers often play in African American families (Hines & Boyd-Franklin, 2005). A robust spirituality, likely a vestige of traditional African life, is common in African American families. Churches and other religious institutions play central roles in the functioning of many African American families as they can offer an extensive support system for adults and youth. A study by Boyd-Franklin in 2003 found that African American women, compared to men, are more often employed and are more likely to be working outside the home (Boyd-Franklin, 2003). (Viladrich and Abraído-Lanza examine the role of religion and spirituality with respect to minority mental health and wellness in Chapter 9 of this volume.)

Native American Families

It is commonly believed that the term "Native American" refers to one homogenous group of indigenous people. However, this is an inaccurate representation, as "Native American" encompasses a wide variety of cultures, languages, and traditions. There are over 560 tribes in the United States that are federally recognized – many of which are sovereign nations through treaties and by law – and have unique cultures in their own right. Of course one characteristic they share is massive historical traumas (Tafoya & Vecchio, 2005). This overview allows us only to draw out a few features of families that have been identified across Native American cultures.

Compared to African American families, the proportion of two-parent households is twice as large; 50% of Native American families were found to be two-parent households in 1997 (Staveteig & Wigton, 2000). This reflects the idea Red Horse described that family represents the "cornerstone for social and emotional well-being of individuals and communities" (as cited in Sutton & Nose, 2000, p. 45).

The literature reveals that Native American cultures are based on an extended family network. However, there are some differences that may distinguish Native American traditions from other ethnic groups. In their writings on Native American families, Sutton and Nose (2005) explained that the primary identifying familial link is not that of child and parent but of child and grandparent. In this system, biological parents will often assume a parental role over the children of their siblings (Tafoya, 1989). Linguistically, cousins are included in the words for brothers and sisters.

Another distinguishing factor of Native American families is the manner in which they approach relatives-by-marriage. Sutton and Nose noted that most Native American cultures do not have an exclusive term for "in-law" relations that are forged through marriage (Sutton & Nose, 2005). Members inducted by marriage are regarded equivalent to members linked by blood.

Native American tradition has a very high regard for members who give the most to their family, tribe, and community. Selfless generosity is a virtue in Native American culture that earns great respect. In everyday life, family members are supposed to constantly share material goods and necessities with members of their extended family unit. On certain special occasions and events (such as childbirth, marriage, or death), it is customary for family members to give many gifts to each other to mark the event. This can prove problematic for Native Americans in the context of capitalist society as they may find themselves sacrificing their independently earned financial or material resources for other members of their family or community.

Economic data demonstrate that Native Americans, along with Hispanics and African Americans, have poverty rates that are three times greater than non-Hispanic Whites. Data from the year 1996 show that 54% of Native Americans were in the low-income category (Staveteig & Wigton, 2000). Compared to African Americans, two-parent Native American families are twice as likely to be poor (below the federal poverty level) compared to African Americans and three times as likely compared to Asian families (Staveteig & Wigton, 2000). Economic hardship puts great stress upon all aspects of family life.

Native American culture has been described as acknowledging and identifying a bond between man and nature. Harmony with natural forces is a way of life, and it binds an individual not only to his or her blood relatives, the forebear's tribe, mankind, but also to Mother Nature, forging a "universal family." All life-forces are valuable and interdependent. As such, animals and plants as well as such inanimate entities as mountains and water can be sacred members of this universal family. And as with any human family member there exists a real and active relationship that a person should strive to maintain.

Latino American Families

The 40 million Latinos living in the U.S. are the largest and fastest growing ethnic minority (Garcia-Preto, 2005). The cultural designation of "Latino" or "Hispanic" encompasses a wide variety of national and cultural groups, distinguished by unique historical origins and traditions. The largest Latino groups in the U.S. are Mexicans, Puerto Ricans, and Cubans. Dominicans, Brazilians, and Central Americans are growing at fast rates.

The family therapy literature indicates that a high value attached to family unity is one of the major characteristics of Latinos (Garcia-Preto, 2005). The family is considered more important than the individual. According to data from the Urban Institute, 58% of Hispanic families are two-parent families, which is the second highest percentage of two-parent families among the ethnic minority groups discussed in this section (Staveteig & Winston, 2000). There is an obligation to the family and the family offers protection and care to individuals that stay within the system. "The expectation is that when a person is having problems, others will help, especially those in stable positions" (Garcia-Preto, 2005,

p. 162). The centrality of the family in Hispanic culture and its elevation above the individual is referred to as "familism." The family provides economic support, emotional support, and security as long as members of the family respect the system of familism. Leaving the system would amount to surrendering the benefits of familism, which could lead to a great deal of insecurity and anxiety (Garcia-Preto, 2005).

In Latino families, there is a practice of handing children over to extended members of the family in times of crisis. This practice has been referred to as *hijos de crianza*. The practice is not viewed as neglectful but is a provision that protects the children and allows the family to deal with a crisis at hand. Studies of the Latino population have also identified the practice referred to as *compadrazco* or godparent-hood. This "ritual kinship," designates relatives to assume parental responsibilities for a youth such as economic assistance, guidance, and discipline (Garcia-Preto, 2005).

The extended family, including non-blood relatives, enters into all aspects of an individual's life. Garcia-Preto (2005) explained that this can mean frequent dinners with the entire family. Problems and crises are brought to the family to be addressed and resolved. Although many Latino families are organized as a patriarchy, there is a tendency amongst younger families to assume a more egalitarian approach to gender roles in the family. Latino families that survived political violence in their home countries and fled to the U.S. may exhibit trauma-related symptoms or family difficulties

While all Latino ethnic groups share the traditions of family collectivism and strong bonds with the extended family, there is some variation in family organization between different groups. For example, Mexican families place emphasis on parent-child lifelong connectedness. The husband-wife bond is often secondary to the parent-child relationship and respect for parental authority. Garcia-Preto (2005) described that certain dyads such as the mother-eldest child relationship dyad, may be especially strong.

Economic data from the Urban Institute suggest that, economically, the state of the Hispanic population is comparable to that of African Americans and Native Americans. Sixty-one percent of Hispanic families live at low-income levels and 30% at poverty levels (Staveteig &Wigton, 2000). Social and economic oppression and discrimination can be a regular feature of life for Hispanic families (Garcia-Preto, 2005). The literature describes the racism targeted at Hispanics as embedded in the social institutions that were designed to provide help: "They tend to reinforce the feelings of shame and failure that Latinos feel when their dreams about improving their lives are truncated" (Garcia-Preto, 2005, p. 157). They must fall back on their extended families, but shortcomings there can lead to resentments and conflicts within families (Garcia-Preto, 2005).

Asian American Families

There are almost 14 million Asian Americans and Pacific Islanders living in the U.S. This represents approximately 8% of the national population. The terms

"Asian American" describe a number of ethnic subgroups including Chinese, Filipino, Asian Indian, Japanese, and Korean which are the most numerous groups.

Economic data for Asian families show them to be relatively stronger when compared to other ethnic minority groups. Only 29% of Asian families are categorized as low-income and only 14% as poor (Staveteig &Winston, 2000). For this and a variety of other reasons, including the stereotypical image of a relative docile group, Asians are held up to be a "model minority" (Lee & Mock, 2005).

Lee and Mock (2005) described a number of experiences that Asian Americans have in common. Family unity is of central importance to Asian traditions in contrast to the traditional Western perspective which values individual autonomy and self-sufficiency. Immigration history is also important as each Asian ethnic minority has a unique and complex story of the circumstances of their arrival to the U.S., which often includes exposure to war and political violence. Despite their contribution to American society, Asian Americans may be victims of racism, discrimination, and hate crimes in the U.S.

The importance of the family unit to Asian traditions is well documented. Asian families have the highest percentage of two-parent families, with 77% of Asian families categorized as two-parent households (Staveteig & Winston, 2000). Lee and Mock described how "the individual is seen as the sum of all the generations of his or her family" (Lee & Mock, 2005, p. 274). As a result of this, actions of individuals reflect not only on them but on their family and ancestors (Hong & Ham, 2001; Wong & Mock, 1997). Loyalty to the family as a whole and obligation to particular kin are highly valued in Asian American families. In the interest of smooth family functioning, individual expression of feeling and sentiments is normally not encouraged and is reinforced by guilt and shame (Lee & Mock, 2005). In traditional families, women are identified by their relationship to men throughout their lives, and women are valued primarily for their ability to give birth to a son. In Asian Indian and Pakistani families, while families are still strongly patriarchal, mothers-in-law have a significant amount of power over their daughters-in-law.

Within the traditional Asian family system, experts have identified and described three different subsystems: the marital subsystem, the parent-child subsystem, and the sibling subsystem. The marital subsystem refers to the relationship between husband and wife. This is usually not the primary relationship and is usually arranged by parents or grandparents. The husband will be the leader of the family and the provider and protector, the women assumes the role of homemaker, mother, and nurturer. Divorce is uncommon and disagreements between the husband and wife are addressed by a mediator or other family member. Women are dominated by their husband, father, in-laws, and sometimes eldest son (Lee & Mock, 2005).

The parent-child subsystem is the primary relationship and strongest bond in an Asian family. Women's strongest attachment is usually to their children, especially their sons. While the woman nurtures and supports, the father is responsible for the maintenance of discipline. Similar to other ethnic groups, children can be cared for by a wide variety of family members from their extended family even though they are most often raised by their parents. These members can be uncles, aunts, cousins, grandparents, and close non-blood relatives. In turn, elder members are highly respected and cared for in their old age.

The sibling subsystem refers to the child-caring role that the eldest sibling can often play. It is common for Asian families to have a large number of children. Often, the eldest daughter has the greatest responsibility to her siblings. Cooperation and sharing between siblings is very important and enforced in families (Lee & Mock, 2005).

Asian families may be in various stages of cultural transition. Traditional families are composed of members born and raised in Asian countries and who are unacculturated and have very limited exposure to Western culture. They usually choose to live in ethnic Asian communities. "Families in culture conflict" have children who were born in the U.S. or came to the country when they were very young. These families are characterized by a great deal of conflict between the acculturated children and the unacculturated parents. Conflict can also occur between one spouse who is more acculturated than the other. Bicultural families are characterized by well-acculturated parents who were exposed to Western culture and values before moving to the U.S. Additionally, these families tend to be more professional and egalitarian in terms of the marital relationship. Highly acculturated families or "Americanized" families are Asian families that have for the large part adopted mainstream American culture. They communicate largely in English. New millennium families are alternatively titled "interracial families." These families are characterized by their ability to integrate multiple cultures successfully and harmoniously. "New millennium families are at the cutting edge of what it means to be an Asian American family, yet at the same time keep their cultural backgrounds in some perspective" (Lee & Mock, 2005, p. 277).

Muslim American Families

Muslims are one of the fastest growing population groups in the United States. There are between 4 and 11 million in the U.S., of which 80% are Sunnis and 20% are Shiites (Hodge, 2005). Media attention on Muslims has intensified considerably since September 11, 2001. This has allowed awareness of Islam and Muslims to grow, but it has also spread misinformation and stereotypes.

While this section will be addressing Muslims as a single group, Muslims in the U.S. come from many different racial, ethnic, and cultural groups. More than 30% of U.S. Muslims are African Americans and most of them are Sunnis. Most of the remaining Muslims are foreign-born hailing from diverse regions around the world. As Daneshpour notes, "local ethnic, social, and historical factors affect the ways in which the Islamic faith is interpreted and applied" (Daneshpour, 1998, p. 355). Regardless, Daneshpour adds, Islamic ideology still is a fundamental link between cultures and has been used to guide family life. The emerging literature on Muslim families finds that, "Islam is not so much a belief system as a way of life that unifies metaphysical and materialistic dimensions" (Hodge, 2005, p. 162). The principles of Islam enter into and inform every aspect of life including family life. Islam regards the family as the basic social unit. Obligation to their family is an important duty of all Muslims.

Research shows that among certain ethnic Muslims, such as Indian Muslims and Pakistani Muslims, marriage is considered one of the most important events in one's life. Almeida (2005) describes how the family begins planning for the event even while the children are young. A marriage is seen not only as a union of two people but a joining of two families. As such, the family is often very involved in the process. Nath (2005) points out in her description of Pakistani Muslims that a Muslim marriage is a civil contract. In the United States, intermarriage may be more prevalent, but it is still discouraged and frowned upon and "viewed as a threat to the integrity of the family, culture, and faith" (Almeida, 2005).

Like most other minority immigrant families, Muslim family systems often include the extended family and may follow a hierarchical, patriarchal construct. Almeida (2005) has noted that an extended family system can include up to three to four generations in which elders are hugely respected and valued and obedience is demanded. Elders are expected to be cared for in their old age. The family system is also described as one that encourages harmony and interdependence and discourages women and younger members from changing the family order (Almeida, 2005).

Almeida identified marriage and adolescence as among the major sources of conflicts that bring Muslim families to seek mental health care. She explains that leaving home and family during adolescence or even marriage is not a part of the family life cycle of Muslim families. Thus, leaving home for these or other reasons can cause conflicts to emerge amongst immigrant families. Marriages between Muslims from the United States and Muslims from home countries can be troubled due to a lack of congruence between American and homeland values. As a result, couples may find it difficult to reach a level of intimacy with their partner. Almeida explained that each may view the other as a "stranger," one of them with "values of friendship from the homeland and the other with friendship values of this country" (Almeida, 2005, p. 383). In such cases, men can resort to violence and abuse to gain the position of power and authority that they hold in traditional families (Almeida, 2005).

It has been reported that the most common reason for suicide among Muslim populations is problems arising from spousal relations and the family (Khan & Reza, 2000). Very often, it is the extended family that mediates and addresses domestic problems and also takes care of and supports members with mental illness. However, as research has noted, immigrant families in the United States are most probably separated from their extended network and, as a result, find it difficult to adequately deal with family problems and mental illness (Nath, 2005).

Contrary to popular belief, Arabs as a group comprise a small proportion of total Muslims. The U.S. Census Bureau defines Arabs as individuals with ancestry originating from Arabic-speaking countries or parts of the world (U.S. Census Bureau, 2003); over 85% of the world's Muslims are not Arabic in this sense (Almeida, 2005). While Arab Muslim families are similar to other Muslim families described, there are some differences. One feature of Arab families that Nuha Abudabbeh singles out as characteristic is the style of communication. It is described as, "hierarchical, creating vertical as opposed to horizontal communication between those in authority and those subservient to that authority" (Abudabbeh, 2005, p. 427). The literature suggests that such a style of communication may lead to parents resorting to anger and punishment toward their children and children responding by crying, self-censorship, covering up, or deception. Furthermore, Abudabbeh adds that preferential treatment toward boys over girls in a family is not uncommon.

Among Arabs with a social history embedded in tribal society, the practice of endogamy has been found to be much more common. Endogamy, or marriage within the same lineage to a cousin, reflects a valuation of the family and the tribe over the individual (Abudabbeh, 2005). Islam allows women the power of choice in deciding among their suitors. However, this is often not practiced in Arab traditions and the father or the family may determine who the woman is to marry.

Evidence-Based Family Determinants of Minority Mental Health and Wellness

In this section, we consider some of the existing research evidence regarding family determinants of minority mental health and wellness. We do not claim this to be a systematic review of all existing research evidence, which would be beyond the scope of this chapter. In conducting this selective review we faced several difficulties. First, the existing studies are found in different disciplinary domains of the literature, which may not recognize analogous research of other disciplines. Second, the studies range greatly in their size, scope, and methodological rigor. Third, the studies are often not expressly identified as studies of family determinants. Fourth, some determinants have been the focus of much research, whereas others have had hardly any scientific attention. Acknowledging these four limitations, we set out to review some of the existing literature and to consider the implications for clinical and research work.

Given that much of this research has focused on specific types of mental illnesses, where possible we have organized this section in terms of categories of mental illnesses. In a subsequent section, we will summarize family determinants as either risk or protective factors.

Mental Health and Illness

We found several studies that found a relationship between family roles and global mental health. A national study of adults found that occupying familial roles are associated with improved mental health in Blacks, Mexicans, and Puerto Ricans (Jackson, 1997). Data from a family research project with low income women (White, Black, Puerto Rican, and other Hispanic) were analyzed to find that conflict with family predicted adverse mental health outcomes. Conflict with siblings was a stronger predictor than parental conflict (Bassuk, Mickelson, Bissel, & Perloff, 2002). In African American youth, family support helped to protect against the mental health consequences of poverty (Li, Nussbaum, & Richards, 2007). Separation and divorce were found to have differing mental health consequences in Blacks and Whites (e.g. separation was more stressful for Whites, whereas divorce was more stressful for Blacks) (Barrett, 2003).

Psychiatric disorders were less prevalent in Mexican immigrants than in persons of Mexican descent born in the U.S. (Burnam et al., 1987). Several studies pointed to a negative effect of acculturation upon the mental health of Mexican immigrants (Escobar & Randolph, 1982). This was thought to be due to diminishing traditional cultural values and practices amongst immigrant families.

Depression

In another study of risk and protective factors for urban African American youth, an increased level of family support was related to lower levels of depressive symptoms (Li et al., 2007). The study concluded that family support can have a mitigating effect when present with other risk factors. For example, in the presence of hassles (e.g. teasing, ostracism by peers, and racism), higher levels of family support were related to lower levels of symptoms. Amongst women, depression symptoms worsened with decreased income and poverty status in the three years post-childbirth (Dearing, Taylong, & McCartney, 2004). Amongst Asian immigrant elders, 40% were depressed, and depression was associated with a perceived acculturation gap between themselves and their better acculturated adult children (Mui & Kang, 2006). Amongst Chinese immigrants, those who experienced domestic violence were more likely to be depressed (Yick, Shibusawa, & Agbayani-Siewert, 2003). Amongst low income African Americans, those with positive beliefs regarding the benefits of children were significantly less depressed (Roxburgh, Stephens, Toltzis, & Adkins, 2001). In U.S. Latino families support mediated the relationship between acculturation and depression. More highly acculturated Latinos had less family support and greater depression (Rivera, 2007).

Trauma and PTSD

Ethnic minorities have a greater lifetime exposure to victimization (e.g. sexual assault, witnessing family violence), as well as to other forms of adversity (parental alcoholism, family problems) (Graham-Bermann, DeVoe, Mattis, Lynch, & Thomas, 2006). For children who were exposed to intimate partner violence, maternal mental health problems were a risk factor for traumatic stress symptoms, whereas social support to the mother was a protective factor (Graham-Bermann et al., 2006). Immigrant youth had high rates of victimization within past years and a higher prevalence of PTSD and Depression (Stein et al., 2000). A study of women survivors of childhood sexual abuse found that Hispanic women reported less intrusive traumatic stress symptoms than non-Hispanic Whites (Andres-Hyman, Cott, & Gold, 2004).

Expressed Emotion and Relapse of Schizophrenia

Early research studies on schizophrenia amongst Whites in Great Britain investigating the relationship between family factors and relapse found that high expressed emotion (as measured by the Campbell Family Interview) in family members predicted relapse (Bebbington & Kuipers, 1994; Kavanaugh, 1992; Leff & Vaughn, 1985). Cross-cultural investigations of this finding have yielded variable results. Several studies of Mexican American samples found that (1) expressed emotion was lower in Mexican American families in comparison with non-Hispanic Whites (Karno et al., 1987); (2) Mexican Americans tend to think of schizophrenia as an illness for which the individual is not responsible (Jenkins, 1988); and (3) high expressed emotion still predicted relapse (Kopelowicz et al., 2002). Another study found that in Mexican American families, distance or lack of warmth in the family predicted relapse (Lopez & Guarnaccia, 1998).

Living with Severe Mental Illness

Research comparing African American and White families found that for African American families, high levels of critical and intrusive behaviors by family members predicted better outcomes (Rosenbarb, Bellack, & Aziz, 2006). This finding was interpreted to mean that cultural beliefs in African American families hold that confrontation is an expression of concern. In Latino families, severely mentally ill persons were more likely to be living with relatives and to have family contact than average (Garcia, Chang, Young, Lopez, & Jenkins, 2006). African Americans with a first episode schizophrenia spectrum diagnosis, and a history of child abuse had higher rates of cannabis dependence (Comptom, Furman, & Kaslow, 2004).

Suicide

Suicide rates amongst American Indians and Alaska Natives between ages 15 and 24 were 3.3 times higher than the U.S. average (Barlas, 2005). Asian American women between ages 15 and 24 had the second highest suicide rate amongst all ethnic and racial groups (Mental Health Weekly, 2003). Negative life events associated with family (e.g. separation, divorce, death, abuse, and interpersonal violence) have been believed to increase the rate of suicide. A study of 200 African American men and women found that the rate of suicide was increased with lower levels of family adaptability and family cohesion (Compton, Thompson, & Kaslow, 2005; Harris & Molock, 2000).

Child Mental Disorders

A study of Hawaiian multiethnic adolescents found that Hawaiian adolescents experienced more family adversity (e.g. criminality) and that this was significantly related to their psychiatric symptomatology (Goebert et al., 2000). A community-based sample of youths and caregivers found that ethnic minority adolescent and parent dyads were less likely to be concordant in their views of mental health problems. Ethnic minority parents had a higher threshold for recognizing problems (Roberts, Alegria, Roberts, & Chen, 2005). One study of families of children with autism found evidence for resilience processes, such as "becoming united and closer as a family" (Bayat, 2007).

HIV Risk Behaviors

Family-oriented mental health professionals have focused on the risks of racial and ethnic minority youth for acquiring HIV/AIDS. This has led them to study the roles of family processes in preventive behaviors and to develop family-focused preventive interventions and to study their effectiveness. For example, CHAMP (Collaborative HIV Prevention and Adolescent Mental Health Project) found that parent-youth communication about difficult-to-talk-about topics, and parental monitoring and supervision of youth, were associated with lower HIV risk behaviors (McKay et al., 2004).

Family Caregiving

Analysis of a large sample of persons receiving public mental health services found that Latino and Asian American consumers, in comparison with non-Hispanic White consumers, were more likely to report living with family members and receiving family support (Snowden, 2007). African Americans have been found to be more likely to fear mental health treatment and to keep mentally ill persons within the community (Sussman, Robins, & Earls, 1987). African Americans also reported lower caregiver strain (or family burden of care) than other racial groups (Guarnaccia & Parra, 1996; Stueve, Vine, & Struening, 1997). In their study of family support and medication usage among Mexican American individuals with schizophrenia, Garcia et al. (2006) reported that a higher level of family support was associated with a greater likelihood of medication usage. Furthermore, they discovered that family support was a more significant factor in predicting medication usage than the psychiatric status of the patient and the family-expressed emotion. They also reported that instrumental family support was associated with a greater probability of regular medication usage (Ramirez, Chang, Young, López, & Jenkins, 2006).

Family Risk and Protective Factors in Ethnic Minorities

This selective review of research evidence indicates that multiple family determinants are playing a role in ethnic minority mental health and wellness. These may be roughly classified as risk factors and protective factors.

The *risk factors* with some basis in research evidence include the following :

- Victimization in the family
- Adverse family events (e.g. conflict, separation)
- Conflict within families (especially siblings)
- Maternal mental health problems (for youth exposed to intimate partner violence)
- Parents with higher threshold for problem recognition (for migrant youth)
- Lower parent-youth concordance regarding views of mental health problems.
- Lower family adaptability and cohesion (for suicide)
- Lack of warmth in families (for severely mentally ill)
- Perceived cultural gap with their adult children (for elderly immigrants)
- More highly acculturated families (for migrants)
- Lower family income (for depression)

The *protective factors* with some basis in research evidence include the following:

- Living with relatives
- Family contact
- Family support (both instrumental and emotional)
- Occupying family roles
- Traditional cultural values and practices
- Social support to the mother (for youth exposed to intimate partner violence)

- Parent-youth communication about difficult to talk about topics (for HIV prevention)
- Parental monitoring and supervision of youth (for HIV prevention)
- High levels of confrontational behavior by family members (for severely mentally ill)
- Parents' perceived benefits of having children

By no means is this a definitive list of family determinants for mental health and wellness. It certainly reflects a bias toward focusing on mental illness in the professional and scientific literatures. Nor is this list meant to imply either that these family determinants of either risk or protection are either universal or particular to a given culture. Some were investigated in only one minority group, and some were investigated in several groups. Far more research would need to be done among more ethnic minorities, especially newer immigrant and refugee groups, to better understand both the potential generalizability and particularity of any of these determinants.

Presently, insufficient research has been conducted to speak to these important concerns. Furthermore, the existing research on family determinants has not consistently utilized the strongest methodologies. Future investigations should utilize the best possible methods for research design, sampling, measures, and analysis.

This list of research-based family determinants, in comparison with the family determinants that we discussed based on the family therapy literature, has a large degree of overlap. That is to say, the majority of the determinants that were mentioned in family therapy have been investigated in research studies on the family determinants of minority mental health and wellness. However, this comparison also reveals that the psychiatric research, with its emphasis upon standardization of terms, constructs, and measures, often has a difficult time approaching the variability of family situations that are described in the family therapy literature. In addition, this comparison also brings out the following deficiencies in the research-based literature. These include our understanding and construction of culture, the characterization of family determinants, and consideration of biological and other factors.

To better understand the role of culture in relation to family determinants, culture has to be regarded as much more than simply membership in a particular ethnic group. Components of culture deserving of inquiry include (1) the linguistic dimensions of family determinants (e.g. the precise meaning of family terms); (2) the cultural history of family determinants (e.g. how they have evolved over historical time); (3) the particular subjective meanings of determinants for family members; and (4) the processes by which determinants work in the day-to-day lives of ethnic minority families (e.g. families undergoing cultural transition). Each of these requires different types of conceptualizations and research methodologies than prior studies have used. Overall, they would require a multidisciplinary approach that draws upon both the clinical sciences and the social sciences, including anthropology, linguistics, and sociology.

As great as the need is to focus on the role of culture, it is no less important to attend to the roles of other dimensions, including those in the economic, social, and biological realms. Yet what are we to make of the fact that largely these factors do not appear on the list of research-based family determinants? They were mentioned in the family therapy literature's consideration of family determinants and of the families from particular ethnic groups. We may not consider a variable such as "poverty" a "family determinant" proper, but if we do not take that into account, we are losing valuable information about families. For example, we need to be able to say that, under the condition of poverty, a particular family determinant functions as a risk or protective factor, rather than emphasizing a family determinant under nonspecific conditions. This calls for a way of conceptualizing family determinants in social and economic context, which relates broad socioeconomic conditions to proximal family-level factors that then drive individual behavior. One such model for this approach to research is provided by Felner's ecological-mediation format (Felner, Brand, DuBois, Adan, Mulhall, & Evans, 1995).

Simply characterizing family determinants as either risk or protective factors can be misleading. This is because family determinants may function as either risk or protective factors exclusively in different phases or dimensions in relation to mental illness or wellness. For example, there may be risk/protection for acquiring the diagnosis, risk/protection for higher levels of symptoms and dysfunction, risk/protection for lower levels of treatment, and risk/protection for shorter versus longer term outcomes.

We have another concern regarding an underlying premise of many of these studies: the belief that family determinants must be bound with ethnicity. Might there be instances when this belief, which is a basic tenet of multiculturalism, is drawing too much emphasis? Instead of laboring to build or sustain ethnic stereotypes, which can be false and hurtful, perhaps we should be working our hardest to investigate the multidimensional factors that appear to determine mental health and wellness. The leading candidates would have to include cultural, socioeconomic, familial, and biological factors. But culture as a dynamic force, not a frozen stereotype, as will be discussed further in the subsequent section related to services.

Consideration of the roles of medical conditions and biological factors is largely absent from the research that we reviewed. This is a significant deficiency. We recognize that there is a vast body of literature that focuses on the genetics of schizophrenia, bipolar disorder and major depression, and substance use and dependence; another chapter in this book focuses on these issues in the context of minority populations. For purposes of this discussion, we note that a consideration of family determinants should also take into account the biological vulnerability or invulnerability that some ethnic groups or subgroups may possess with respect to mental health problems, although we caution that we do not expect a focus on genetics to be any kind of substitute for the careful conceptualization and study of the cultural and socioeconomic dimensions that we are also calling for.

Understanding the Role of Families in the Treatment of Mental Illness in Minorities

The landmark 2001 *Mental health: A report of the Surgeon General* which included a supplementary section on cultural diversity and mental health services, is useful because it extends our discussion of family determinants into the topic of mental health service utilization for ethnic minorities. (Health systems and access to care for mental health are discussed in detail by Koroukian in Chapter 7 of this volume.)

The Report's supplementary section argued that racial and ethnic minority groups face multiple barriers to mental health care and have been underserved by mental health systems of care. For example, less mental health care is provided to African American and Hispanics than to Whites (Cook, McGuire, & Miranda, 2007); Latino children have high rates of unmet mental health needs (Kataoka, Zhang, & Wells, 2002); African American parents have received less information about attention deficit-hyperactivity disorder (ADHD) than White parents (Bussing, Schoenberg, & Perwien, 1998).

The Surgeon General's *Report* questioned why many members of racial and ethnic minorities appear to be less inclined than Whites to seek mental health treatment. It noted that, in addition to the constellation of barriers deterring Whites, such as cost, fragmentation of services, and the societal stigma on mental illness, racial and ethnic minorities are also hindered in seeking care due to mistrust and limited English proficiency (DHHS, 1999). The *Report* also found that racial and ethnic minorities may have specific cultural attitudes toward mental illness which carry a strong sense of stigma and shame and a distrust of mental health professionals. Low levels of acculturation are associated with less mental health service utilization (Wells, Golding, Hogh, Burnam, & Karno, 1989).

The *Report* called for greater linguistic and cultural competency of mental health services. However, as this chapter's discussion of family determinants suggests, the issue is not only helping minorities to overcome barriers in accessing mainstream mental health treatment but understanding whether or not the forms of promotion and treatment are congruent with the culture and practices of families and whether or not these forms are responsive to family determinants that are functioning as either risk or protective factors. In trying to achieve a better understanding of these issues, the question not so often asked is "what are those families doing that is genuinely helpful and how can services better learn from and promote those behaviors?"

This takes us back to the observation that racial and ethnic minorities often have especially strong family ties and that these ties may serve as a resource and strength for individuals who either are at risk for or have been diagnosed with mental health problems. As we have already discussed, many families from ethnic minorities would much prefer to try to take care of mental health problems within the family. Some families are able to offer much needed support for their members with mental illness. Others may offer them less than acceptable care. Snowden (2007) found that living with a family reduced disparities to a level of statistical insignificance. The Surgeon General's *Report* also found that instead of seeking care from mental health professionals, culturally diverse families were more likely to ask for help from primary care providers, clergy, traditional healers, and family and friends (Neighbors & Jackson, 1984; Peifer, Hu, & Vega, 2000).

The Surgeon General's *Report* (1994, Chapter 2) also called for "strategies to strengthen families to function at their fullest potential and to mitigate the stressful effects of caring for a relative with mental illness or serious emotional disturbance." Our review of family determinants indicated that there are inherent properties of ethnic minority families that are associated with greater protection from disorder and promotion of wellness. Accordingly, systems of care should design programs and policies that are effective in enhancing protective factors that prevent and/or ameliorate the consequences of mental disorders, or promote mental health and wellness. Do the evidence-based culturally diverse family-focused programs and policies yet exist? As far as we know, although there are some programs that have been found to be helpful with ethnic minority groups, little research has been done with culturally diverse family-focused programs.

Some of the best examples of family-focused services with ethnic minorities come not in the treatment and care of mental illness but from mental health efforts focusing on HIV prevention. One prime example is CHAMP (Collaborative HIV Prevention and Adolescent Mental Health Project), a family-based HIV prevention program that targets youth and their families and has been implemented in Chicago, New York, South Africa, and Trinidad/Tobago. Research on the CHAMPS' program has demonstrated that a multiple-family group intervention model changes family processes that mediate important health and mental health outcome variables (e.g. lowers HIV risk, enhances HIV preventive skills in families facing a range of health and mental health adversities). McKay and colleagues are working on extending the evidence-based interventions with HIV to address child mental health outcomes, especially in conditions of extreme poverty (McKay, 2007).

More research is called for regarding mental health service-related behaviors in ethnic and racial minorities. The focus on psychopathology and treatment is important, but it is not necessarily going to help to develop effective mental health service programs and policies. Interventions must be adapted to specific groups; it is necessary to adapt the intervention to fit with varying social and cultural contexts that may reflect variation in how familiar family determinants (e.g. family support) operate. There are likely to be considerable differences not only between ethnic minority groups, but also within groups as well, due to differing phases of cultural transition, educational level, economic status, and other factors. Given the complexities of adapting interventions for new cultures and contexts, investigators have explored alternatives to the randomized control trial, which is perceived as being too rigid to facilitate intervention adaptation. One such alternative, the comprehensive dynamic trial, is characterized by multiple sources of information and recurring mechanisms for feedback and response and is particularly suited to community prevention research (Rapkin & Trickett, 2005).

Family interventions require a conceptualization that is not only based upon family illness or pathology but upon family strengths and resources. For example, to build preventive interventions for refugee youth, we have developed a family resilience perspective upon refugee youth and their families (Walsh, 1998). A family resilience perspective understands that refugee youth live in families, where there is the possibility that multiple traumas and losses interact with social and economic difficulties, cultural transitions, and parental mental illness (Weine, 2007). However, their families may also contain resources that may be protective against negative outcomes for youth. To deploy them effectively in their new circumstances, families may need additional knowledge, skills, relationships, or practice. Because families do not function in isolation, a family resilience conceptualization also encompasses ecological protective resources such as those involving the school and community. This view of family resilience is linked with family eco-developmental theory, which envisions youth in the context of a family system that interacts with larger social systems (Szapocznik & Coatsworth, 1999). Overall, family services for mental health promotion and treatment need to find ways to acknowledge and draw upon the family resiliency that lies in family protective factors such as family support; however they are expressed in particular ethnic groups.

It is also important to clarify the conceptualization of multiculturalism that underlies many mental health approaches. Cultural diversity is more than simply an issue of difference where one ethnic group is different from the other. Cultural diversity must incorporate the notion of interaction where cultural and families in relation to culture are engaged in ongoing processes of change. For many immigrants and refugees, it is these processes of change (e.g. being in cultural transition) and not the absolute difference between themselves and the dominant group that account both for their day-to-day difficulties and achievements. This calls both for a closer study of the cultural theory of cultural change (Weine, Ware, & Lezic, 2004).

Qualitative and ethnographic methods and mixed methods have been underutilized in the research on family determinants and could play a very helpful role in explaining or interpreting the findings from the quantitative studies and in identifying emergent themes or generating hypotheses concerning behaviors, attitudes, or contexts. For example, ethnographic research, which has been very helpful in providing an insiders' perspective on mental health services, is especially well suited to investigating the dynamic interactions involving cultural, socioeconomic, familial, and biological factors which are at play with family determinants of minority mental health and wellness.

Conclusion

It is straightforward to conclude that not enough is known about the family determinants of minority mental health and wellness. It is somewhat less clear to suggest what concerns should guide research and services. This focused review and discussion has described family determinants based upon the family therapy and psychiatric research literatures. Further conceptual and research work on family determinants and minority mental health and wellness is needed. It should attend to the multidimensional complexities of determinants and be aimed at developing new family focused services for mental health treatment and promotion for ethnic minority families.

References

Abudabbeh, N. (2005). Arab families. In M. McGoldrick, J. Giordano, & N. Garcia-Preto (Ed.), *Ethnicity & family therapy* (3rd ed., pp. 423–436). New York: Guilford Press.

Almeida, R. (2005). Asian Indian families. In M. McGoldrick, J. Giordano, & N. Garcia-Preto (Ed.), *Ethnicity & family therapy* (3rd ed. pp. 377–394). New York: Guilford Press.

Andres-Hyman, R. C., Cott, M. A., & Gold, S. N. (2004). Ethnicity and sexual orientation as PTSD mitigators in child sexual abuse survivors. *Journal of Family Violence, 19*(5), 319–325.

Bae, S., & Kung, W. W.-M., (2000). Family intervention for Asian Americans with a schizophrenic patient in the family. *American Journal of Orthopsychiatry, 70*(4), 532–541.

Barlas, S. (2005. September 1). Concerns raised about high suicide rates in Native Americans. *Psychiatric Times,* 83, 44–45.

Barrett, A. E. (2003). Race differences in the mental health effects of divorce a reexamination incorporating temporal dimensions of the dissolution process. *Journal of Family Issues, 24*(8), 995–1019.

Bassuk, E. L., Mickelson, K. D., Bissel, H. D., & Perloff, J. N. (2002). Role of kin and nonkin support in the mental health of low-income women. *American Journal of Orthopsychiatry, 72*(1), 39–49.

Bayat, M. (2007). Evidence of resilience in families of children with autism. *Journal of Intellectual Disability Research, 51*(9), 702–714.

Bebbington, P., & Kuipers, L. (1994). The predictive utility of expressed emotion in schizophrenia: an aggregate analysis. *Psychological Medicine, 24*(3), 707–718.

Bell, J. M., Watson, W. L., & Wright, L. M. (1996). *Beliefs: The heart of healing in families and illness.* New York: Basic Books.

Billingsley, A. (1968). *Black families in White America.* Englewood Cliffs, NJ: Prentice-Hall.

Boss, P. (2000). *Ambiguous loss: learning to live with unresolved grief.* Cambridge, MA: Harvard University Press.

Boss, P., Doherty, W., LaRossa, R., Schumm, W., & Steinmetz, S. (1993). *Sourcebook of family theories and methods: A contextual approach.* New York: Plenum Press.

Boyd-Franklin, N. (2003). *Black families in therapy: Understanding the African American experience* (2nd ed.). New York: Guilford Press.

Bronfenbenner, U. (1986). Ecological of the family as a context for human development: Research perspectives. *Developmental Psychology, 22,* 723–742.

Burnham, M. A., Hough, R. L., Karno, M., Escobar, J. I., & Telles, C. A. (1987). Acculturation and lifetime prevalence of psychiatric disorders among Mexican Americans in Los Angeles. *Journal of Health and Social Behavior, 28,* 89–102.

Bussing, R., Schoenberg N. E., & Perwien A. R. (1998). Knowledge and information about ADHD. *Social Science & Medicine, 46*(7), 919–928.

Compton, M. T., Furman, A. C., & Kaslow, N. J. (2004). Preliminary evidence of an association between childhood abuse and cannabis dependence among African American first-episode schizophrenia-spectrum disorder patients. *Drug and Alcohol Dependence, 76,* 311–316.

Compton, M., Thompson, N., & Kaslow, N. (2005). Social environment factors associated with suicide attempt among low-income African Americans: The protective role of family relationships and social support. *Social Psychiatry & Psychiatric Epidemiology, 40*, 175–185.

Cook, B., McGuire, T., & Miranda, J. (2007). Measuring trends in mental health care disparities, 2000–2004. *Psychiatric Services, 58*(12), 1533–1540.

Daneshpour, M. (1998). Muslim families and family therapy. *Journal of Marital and Family Therapy, 24*(3), 355–368.

Dearing, E., Taylor, B., & McCartney, K. (2004). Implication of family income dynamics for women's depressive symptoms during the first 3 years after childbirth. *American Journal of Public Health, 94*(8), 1372–1377.

Escobar, J. I. (1998). Why are immigrants better off? *Archives of General Psychiatry, 55*, 781–782.

Falicov, C. R.(2004). Ambiguous loss: Risk and resilience in Latino immigrant families. In M. Suarez-Orozco, C. Suarez-Orozco, & D. B. Qin (Eds.), *The new immigration: An interdisciplinary reader* (pp. 274–288). New York: Routledge.

Felner, R., Brand, S., DuBois, D., Adan, A., Mulhall, P., & Evans, E. (1995). Socioeconomic disadvantage, proximal environmental experiences, and socioemotional and academic adjustment in early adolescence: Investigation of a mediated effects model. *Child Development, 66*, 774–792.

Fink, A. (2003). A school-based mental health program for traumatized Latino immigrant children school children. *Journal of the American Academy of Child & Adolescent Psychiatry, 42*(3), 311–318.

Friedman, M. J., & Jaranson, J. (1994). The applicability of the post-traumatic stress disorder concept to refugees. In A. M. Marsella, T. Bornemann, S. Ekblad, & J. Orley (Eds.), *Amidst peril and pain* (pp. 207–227). Washington, DC: American Psychological Association.

Frisbie, W. P. & Bean, F. D. (1995). The Latino family in comparative perspective: Trends and current conditions. In C. K. Jacobson (Ed)., *American families: Issues in race & ethnicity* (pp. 29–71). New York: Garland Press.

Garcia, J. I. R., Chang, C. L., Young, J. S., Lopez, S. R., & Jenkins, J. H. (2006) Family support predicts psychiatric medication usage among Mexican American individuals with schizophrenia. *Social Psychiatry & Psychiatric Epidemiology, 41*, 624–631.

Garcia-Preto, N. (2005). Latino families: An overview. In M. McGoldrick, J. Giordano, & N. Garcia-Preto (Ed.), *Ethnicity & family therapy* (3rd ed., pp. 153–165). New York: Guilford Press.

Goebert, D., Nahulu, L., Hishinuma, E., Bell, C., Yuen, N., Carlton, B., et al. (2000). Cumulative effect of family environment on psychiatric symptomatology among multi-ethnic adolescents. *Journal of Adolescent Health, 27*, 34–42.

Graham-Bermann, S., DeVoe, E., Mattis, J., Lynch, S., & Thomas, S. (2006). Ecological predictors of traumatic stress symptoms in Caucasian and ethnic minority children exposed to intimate partner violence. *Violence against Women, 12*(7), 663–692.

Greenstein, T. (2006). *Methods of family research*. Thousand Oaks, California: Sage Publications.

Harris, T. L. & Molock, S. D. (2000). Cultural orientation, family cohesion, and family support in suicide ideation and depression among African American college students. *Suicide and Life-Threatening Behavior, 30*(4), 341–353.

Hill, R. (1999). *The strengths of African American families: Twenty-five years later*. Lanham, MD: University Press of America.

Hill, R. (1993). Dispelling myths and building on strengths: Supporting African American families. *The Roundtable – Journal of the National Resource Center for Special Needs Adoption, 7*(2), 1–6.

Hines, P. M., & Boyd-Franklin, N. (2005). African American families. In M. McGoldrick, J. Giordano, & N. Garcia-Preto (Ed.), *Ethnicity & family therapy* (3rd ed., pp. 87–100) New York: Guilford Press.

Hodge, D. R. (2005). Social work and the house of Islam: Orienting practitioners to the belief and values of Muslims in the United States. *Social Work, 50*(2), 162–173.

Hong, G., & Ham, M. (2001). *Psychotherapy and counseling with Asian American clients.* Thousand Oaks, CA: Sage Publishing.

In case you haven't heard. (2003). *Mental Health Weekly, 13*(25), 8, 1.

Jackson, P. B. (1997). Role occupancy and minority mental health. *Journal of Health & Social Behavior, 38*, 237–255.

Kamya, H. (2005). African Immigrant families. In M. McGoldrick, J. Giordano, & N. Garcia-Preto (Ed.), *Ethnicity & family therapy* (3rd ed., pp. 101–116). New York: Guilford Press.

Karno, M., Jenkins, J. H., de la Selva, A., Santana, F., Telles, C., Lopez, S., & Mintz, J. (1987). Expressed Emotion and schizophrenic outcome among Mexican American families. *Journal of Nervous Mental Disease, 175*, 143–151.

Kataoka, S., Zhang, L., & Wells, K. (2002). Unmet need for mental health care among u.s. children: variation by ethnicity and insurance status. *American Journal of Psychiatry, 159*(9), 1548–1555.

Khan, M. M., & Reza, H. (2000). The pattern of suicide in Pakistan. *Journal of Crisis Intervention and Suicide Prevention, 21*(1), 31–35.

Kopelowicz, A., Zarate, R., Gonzalez, V., Lopez, S. R., Ortega, P., Obregon, N., & Mintz, J. (2002). Evaluation of expressed emotion in schizophrenia: a comparison of Caucasians and Mexican Americans. *Schizophrenia Research, 55*, 179–186.

Kottak, C., & Kozaitis, K. (2007). *On being different: Diversity and multiculturalism in North America.* New York: McGraw Hill

Lee, E., & Mock, M. (2005). Chinese families. In M. McGoldrick, J. Giordano, & N. Garcia-Preto (Ed.), *Ethnicity & family therapy* (3rd ed., pp. 302–318). New York: Guilford Press.

Leff, J. P., & Vaughn, C. (1985). *Expressed emotion in families.* New York: Guildford Press.

Lewis, O. (1964). *A death in the Sanchez family.* New York: Random House.

Li, S. T., Nussbaum, K. M., & Richards M. H. (2007) Risk and protective factors for urban African-American youth. *American Journal of Community Psychology, 39*, 21–35.

Lopez, S., R. & Guarnaccia, P. J. (1998). The mental health and adjustment of immigrant and refugee children. *Child and Adolescent Psychiatry Clinics of North America, 7*(3), 537–553.

McGoldrick, M. (1998a). Introduction: revisioning family therapy through a cultural lens. In M. McGoldrick (Ed.), *Re-visioning family therapy* (pp. 3–10). New York: Guilford Press.

McGoldrick, M. (1998b). Belonging and liberation: finding a place called home. In M. McGoldrick (Ed.), *Re-visioning family therapy* (pp. 215–228). New York: Guilford Press.

McGoldrick, M., Giordano, J., & Garcia-Preto, N. (2005). *Ethnicity & family therapy* (3rd ed.). New York: Guilford Press.

McKay, M. (2007). Inner-city adversity: Child mental health & service use. K01 Proposal to the National Institute of Mental Health.

McKay, M., Paikoff, R., Baptiste, D., Bell, C., Coleman, D., Madison, S., et al. (2004). Family-level impact of the CHAMP Family Program: A community collaborative effort to support urban families and reduce youth HIV risk exposure. *Family Process, 43*(1), 77–91.

McKinnon, J. (2003). The Black Population in the United States: March 2002. *Current population reports*, Series P20-541. Washington, DC: U.S. Bureau of the Census.

Minuchin, S., Montalvo, B., Guerney, B., Rosman, B., & Schumer, F. (1967). *Families of the slums.* New York: Basic Books.

Mui, A. C., & Kang, S. K. (2006). Acculturation stress and depression among Asian immigrant elders. *Social Work, 51*(3), 243–255

Nath, S. (2005). Pakistani families. In M. McGoldrick, J. Giordano, & N. Garcia-Preto (Ed.), *Ethnicity & family therapy* (3rd ed., pp. 407–420). New York: Guilford Press.

Neighbors, H. W., & Jackson, J. S. (1984). The use of informal and formal help: Four patterns of illness behavior in the black community. *American Journal of Community Psychology, 12*(6), 629–644.

Newbigging, K., & McKeown, M. (2007). Mental health advocacy with black and minority ethnic communities: conceptual and ethical implications. *Current Opinions in Psychiatry*, *20*(6), 588–93.

Nobles, W. (2004). African philosophy: Foundations for Black psychology. In R. Jones (Ed.), *Black psychology* (4th ed.). New York: Harper & Row.

Peifer, K. L., Hu, T. W., & Vega, W. (2000). Help seeking by persons of Mexican origin with functional impairments. *Psychiatric Services*, *51*, 1293–1298.

Pollard, K. M., & O'Hare, W. P. (1999). America's racial and ethnic minorities. *Population Bulletin*, *54*(3), 48.

Ramrez-Garca, J. I., Chang, C. L., Young, J. S., López, S. R., & Jenkins, J. H. (2006). Family support predicts psychiatric medication usage among Mexican American individuals with schizophrenia. *Social Psychiatry Epidemiology*, *41*, 624–631.

Rapkin, B., & Tricket, E. J. (2005). Comprehensive dynamic trial designs for behavioral prevention research with communities: Overcoming inadequacies of the randomized controlled trial paradigm. In E. J. Trickett & W. Pequegnat (Eds.), *Community intervention and AIDS* (pp. 249–277). New York: Oxford University Press.

Rivera, F. (2007). Contextualizing the experience of young Latino adults: Acculturation, social support and depression. *Journal of Immigrant & Minority Health*, *9*, 237–244.

Roberts, R. E., Alegria, M., Roberts, C. R., & Chen, I. G. (2005). Concordance of reports of mental health functioning by adolescents and their caregivers. *Journal of Nervous and Mental Disease*, *192*(8), 528–534.

Rosenfarb, I. S., Bellack, A. S, & Aziz, N. (2006). Family interactions and the course of schizophrenia in African American and White patients. *Journal of Abnormal Psychology*, *115*(1), 112–120.

Roxburgh, S., Stephens, R. C., Toltzis, P., & Adkins, I. (2001). The value of children, parenting strains, and depression among urban African American mothers. *Sociological Forum*, *16*(1), 55–72.

Sabogal, F., Marín, G., Otero-Sabogal, R., Marín, B. V., & Perez-Stable, E. (1987). Hispanic familism and acculturation: What changes and what doesn't? *Hispanic Journal of Behavioral Sciences*, *9*(4), 397–412.

Snowden, L. R. (2007). Explaining mental health treatment disparities. *Culture of Medical Psychiatry*, *31*, 389–402.

Stein, M., McQuaid, J., Pedrelli, P., Lenox, R., & McCahill, M. (2000). Posttraumatic stress disorder in the primary care medical setting. *Gen Hosp Psychiatry*, *22*, 261–9.

Stueve, A., Vine, P., & Struening, E. L. (1997). Perceived burden among caregivers of adults with serious mental illness: comparison of Black, Hispanic, and White families. *American Journal of Orthopsychiatry*, *67*, 199–209.

Sussman, L. N., Robins, L. N., & Earls, F. (1987). Treatment seeking for depression by black and white Americans. *Social Science & Medicine*, *24*, 187–96.

Sutton, C. T. & Broken Nose, M. A. (2005). American Indian families: An Overview. In M. McGoldrick, J. Giordano, & N. Garcia-Preto (Eds.), *Ethnicity & family therapy*. (pp. 43–54). New York: Guilford Press.

Szapocznik, J., & Coatsworth, J. D. (1999). An ecodevelopmental framework for organizing risk and protection for drug abuse: A developmental model of risk and protection. In M. Glantz & C. R. Hartel (Eds.), *Drug abuse: Origins and interventions* (pp. 331–366). Washington, DC: American Psychological Association.

Tafoya, T. (1989). Coyote's eyes: Native cognition styles. *Journal of American Indian Education* [special issue], 29–40.

United Nations High Commission on refugees. (2002). Special Feature on the 50th Anniversary of the Convention (available at www.unhcr.org/ 1951convention/index.html)

U.S. Census Bureau. (2006). *2006 American community survey*. Last accessed January 18, 2008; Available at factfinder.census.gov/servlet/ADPTable?_bm = y&-geo_id = 01000US&-qr_name = ACS_2006_EST_G00_DP5&-ds_name = &-_lang = en&-redoLog = false

U.S. Census Bureau. (2003). *The Arab population: 2000 – Census 2000 Brief.* Last accessed January 20, 2008; Available at www.census.gov/prod/2003pubs/c2kbr-23.pdf.

U.S. Department of Health and Human Services. (1999). *Mental health: A report of the Surgeon General.* Rockville, MD: U.S. Department of Health and Human Services, Substance Abuse and Mental Health Services Administration, Center for Mental Health Services, National Institutes of Health, National Institute of Mental Health.

U.S. Department of Health and Human Services. (2001). *Mental health: Culture, race, and ethnicity—a supplement to mental health: A report of the Surgeon General.* Rockville, MD: U.S. Department of Health and Human Services, Substance Abuse and Mental Health Services Administration, Center for Mental Health Services.

Vega, W. A., Kolody, B., Aguilar-Gaxiola, S., Alderete, E., Catalano, R. Caraveo-Anduaga, J. (1998). Lifetime prevalence of *DSM-III-R* psychiatric disorders among urban and rural Mexican Americans in California. *Archives of General Psychiatry, 55*, 771–778.

Walsh, F. (1998). *Strengthening family resilience.* New York: Guilford Press.

Weine, S. M. (2008). Family roles in refugee youth resettlement from a prevention perspective. *Child and Adolescent Psychiatric Clinics of North America, 17*(3), 515–532.

Weine, S. M. (2006). A Services Approach to Preventive Mental Health for Adolescent Refugees. (1 R01 MH076118-01A2).

Weine, S. M. (1999). *When history is a nightmare: Lives and memories of ethnic cleansing in Bosnia-Herzegovina.* New Brunswick, New Jersey: Rutgers University Press.

Weine, S. M., Ware, N., & Lezic, A. (2004). An ethnographic study of converting cultural capital in teen refugees and their families from Bosnia-Herzegovina. *Psychiatric Services, 55*, 923–927.

Wells, K. D., Golding, J. M., Hogh, R. L., Burnam, M. A., & Karno, M. (1989). Factors affecting the probability of use of general and medical health and social/community services for Mexican-Americans and Non-Hispanic Whites. *Medical Care, 26*, 441–452.

Weissbourd, B., & Kagan, S. L. (1989). Family support programs: catalysts for change. *American Journal of Orthopsychiatry, 59*(1), 20–31.

Williams, D., Haile, R., González, H., Neighbors, H., Baser, R., & Jackson, J. (2007). The mental health of Black Caribbean immigrants: Results from the National Survey of American Life. *American Journal of Public Health, 97*(1), 52–59.

Williams, K., & Dunne-Bryant, A. (2006). Divorce and adult psychological well-being: clarifying the role of gender and child age. *Journal of Marriage and Family, 68*, 1178–1196.

Williams, B., Sawyer, S. C., & Wahlstrom, C. M. (2005). *Marriages, families & intimate relationships.* Boston, MA: Pearson.

Wong, L., & Mock, M. R. (1997). Asian American young adults. In E. Lee (Ed.), *Working with Asian Americans: A guide for clinicians.* New York: Guilford Press.

Yeung, A., & Kung, W. W. (2004). How culture impacts on the treatment of mental illnesses among Asian-Americans. *Psychiatric News, 21*, 34–36.

Yick, A. G., Shibusawa, T., & Agbayani-Siewert, P. (2003). Partner violence, depression, and practice implications with families of Chinese descent. *Journal of Cultural Diversity, 10*(3), 96–104.

Zambrana, R. E. (Ed.). (1995). *Understanding Latino families: Scholarship, policy, and practice.* Thousand Oaks, CA: Sage

Zayas, L. H., & Palleja, J. (1988). Puerto Rican familism: Considerations for family therapy *Family Relations, 37*(3), 260–264.

Zemore, S. E. (2007). Acculturation and alcohol among Latino adults in the United States: a comprehensive review. *Alcoholism: Clinical and Experimental Research, 31*(12), 1968–1990.

Chapter 12
Family-Focused Psychoeducational Programs for Minorities with Serious Mental Illness

Amy Weisman de Mamani, Radha Dunham, Stephanie Aldebot, Naomi Tuchman and Stephanie Wasserman

Overview

This chapter will provide an overview of family-focused psychoeducational programs for minorities with serious mental illness. Psychoeducation refers to treatments that impart information about mental and physical health by way of didactic and structured methods (Rummel-Kluge & Kissling, 2008). Psychoeducation for serious mental disorders typically involves providing specific information on the symptoms of the illness, the biological and psychosocial processes contributing to the development of an illness, factors impacting the course of the illness, coping, and problem-solving strategies, as well as information on available treatments and resources for ongoing care for patients and family members coping with the disorder (Goldstein & Miklowitz, 1995). Family-focused psychoeducational approaches are useful in a variety of settings and with a variety of clients, but they appear to be particularly well-suited for minorities, as researchers consistently recommend including the family in mental health treatments for minorities (Flaskerud, 1986; Szapocznik, 1994; McGoldrick, Giordano, & Garcia-Preto, 2005).

This chapter will address how psychoeducational interventions can be tailored to better serve minorities. By way of example, we will describe a family-focused, culturally informed therapy for schizophrenia, that was developed by the first author and which is currently being pilot tested at the University of Miami.

Background

Why is family psychoeducation important in mental illness? Over the last several decades, managed care restrictions have increased, leaving families with a greater responsibility for the care of their ill relatives (Goldstein &

A. Weisman de Mamani (✉)
Department of Psychology, University of Miami, Coral Gables, FL
e-mail: aweisman@psy.miami.edu

S. Loue, M. Sajatovic (eds.), *Determinants of Minority Mental Health and Wellness*, DOI 10.1007/978-0-387-75659-2_12,
© Springer Science+Business Media, LLC 2009

Miklowitz, 1995; Mueser & Glynn, 1999). This responsibility is especially pronounced for many minorities in the U.S., who are even more likely to take on the care of an ill relative, often with fewer economic resources and social service options and more limited housing alternatives (Guarnaccia & Parra, 1996; Snowden, 2007). In addition, minorities are often socially isolated.

Psychoeducation for mental illness appears to work best when offered as a family affair (Magliano et al., 2005). In this format, families are educated on how best to assist the patient while also attending to their own needs in order to prevent burnout and counteract common strains. The stress and burden of caregiving should not be underestimated as the impact on the family is often far-reaching, with caregivers reporting high rates of depression, anxiety, and stress (Magliano, Fiorillo, Malangome, De Rosa, & Maj, 2006). Some common challenges include limited access and time for social activities, feelings of loss and isolation, and drainage of emotional and financial support (McFarlane, Dixon, Lukens, & Lucksted, 2003). Minorities often face additional burdens including racial discrimination, challenges of acculturation and assimilation, as well as language barriers. Psychotic spectrum mental illnesses (such as schizophrenia) present further challenges in that family members frequently become the focus of a patient's symptoms (particularly paranoid delusions). As a result, individuals with severe mental illness may refuse to participate in family-based treatments and may express strong convictions that their family members be kept out of their psychiatric care. Minorities may be particularly distressed by this because family trust is often paramount in many traditional ethnic cultures (Triandis, McCusker, & Hui, 1990). Thus, minorities may be even more vulnerable to feelings of hurt and despair if feared or shunned by a mentally ill relative.

While biological/genetic factors are clearly involved in the development and course of schizophrenia and other severe disorders such as bipolar illness (e.g., Torrey, Bowler, Taylor, & Gottesman, 1994), the patient's family and psychosocial environment also largely impacts the course of the illness (Mueser, Torrey, Lynde, Singer, & Drae, 2003; Dixon et al., 2001; Pitschel-Walz, Leucht, Bauml, Kissling, & Engel, 2001). For example, when individuals with schizophrenia are in close contact with family members who express critical, hostile, or emotionally overinvolved attitudes (defined as high expressed emotion, or high EE) about them, they have a substantially greater risk for psychiatric relapse than do patients whose relatives are designated as low EE. This finding is based on 40 years of research in multiple countries and cultures (Hooley & Hiller, 2000) and will be addressed further below.

On the positive side, research has indicated that the effects of mental illness sometimes pose beneficial effects on patients, individual family members, and the entire family system. For example, helping a loved one can result in greater self-esteem and self-worth and successfully coping with mental illness can result in a feeling of enhanced personal resilience and a reassessment of life's priorities (Chen & Greenberg, 2004; Marsh & Lefley, 1996). Families often rally together, and this frequently has the effect of increasing perceived family unity. This may be particularly important for minorities. Weisman, Rosales, Kymalainen, and Armesto (2005) found that for Black and Latino/Hispanic families with schizophrenia, increased perceived family cohesion was associated with lower levels of depression, anxiety, and stress for both patients and family members and fewer psychiatric symptoms for patients.

Family-focused, psychoeducational treatments can be an excellent resource for increasing the likelihood of these positive consequences, as well as decreasing the negative sequalae often associated with mental illness in the family. The importance of including family members in the treatment of mental illness has been well documented, with reviews demonstrating that family treatments can reduce relapse rates for schizophrenia by 20–50% (Pitschel-Walz et al., 2001; McFarlane et al., 2003). Meta-analyses and reviews of the literature on family psychoeducation have shown the following benefits: reductions in family member perceived burden, greater family member well-being, increased employment and participation in vocational rehabilitation for patients, change in EE behaviors, increased knowledge of illness, better treatment and medication adherence, better social functioning and adjustment for patients, increased quality of life, reduced medical costs, reduced psychiatric relapse, and less severe psychiatric symptoms (Pitschel-Walz et al., 2001; McFarlane et al., 2003). As the domains for improvement are so varied, it is important to think of psychoeducation as more than just a means to reduce hospitalization rates. Furthermore, treatment gains from family psychoeducation have been shown in diverse cultures, including the U.S. (Goldstein & Miklowitz, 1995), China (Ling et al., 1999), Spain (Muela Martinez & Godoy Garcia, 2001), Scandinavia (Rund et al., 1994), and Britain (Barrowclough et al., 2001).

Unfortunately, very few families of any ethnicity who are coping with severe mental illness receive family psychoeducation or therapy, with estimates ranging from .7% to 8% receiving formal help depending on the sample and method of data collection (Dixon et al., 1999). Furthermore, in general, there are disparities for ethnic minorities. First, minorities tend to utilize services less frequently. (For an in-depth discussion of utilization, see the chapter by Koroukian in this volume.) Second, when they do utilize services, they appear to receive poorer quality care (National Institute of Mental Health, 1999). For example, a large-scale study with 4,249 patients with schizophrenia found only a 17% utilization rate of case management services among Blacks and a 19% utilization rate for Latinos/Hispanics. Utilization rates for Whites were at 30% (Barrio et al., 2003). Efforts to close the gap in health care disparities are sorely needed.

Including family members in treatment may help in this aim. Members of ethnic minorities tend to have a more interdependent and interconnected view of family (Weisman de Mamani, Kymalainen, Rosales, & Armesto, 2007; Oyserman, Coon, & Kemmelmeier, 2002). Additionally, research shows that Blacks and Latinos/Hispanics with serious mental illness turn to other family members for advice more so than do non-Hispanic Whites. Whites are more likely to seek help from mental health professionals (Guarnaccia & Parra, 1996). Thus, family treatments may be more culturally syntonic for these ethnic groups. This may make minorities more willing to enroll and attend family therapy than they might for more individually oriented treatment approaches.

Structured family treatments can provide specific skills and information that are critical in managing a severe mental illness. The following three sets of skills have been found to be invaluable for both patients and families dealing with mental illness: education about illness, communication training, and problem solving (for schizophrenia: Falloon, Boyd, & McGill, 1984; for bipolar disorder: Goldstein & Miklowitz, 1995; Miklowitz et al., 2000). These components are also well suited to minorities, particularly low socioeconomic status (SES) families, as problem-focused and didactic styles of therapy appear to be more culturally sanctioned and less threatening (Organista & Muñoz, 1996).

In addition to education and skills training, therapists should also include information about supplementary resources available to families (in clients' preferred languages, if possible). These include support groups, consumer-run meetings, or membership in national organizations. In our experience, the National Alliance on Mental Illness (NAMI) has been a particularly helpful resource for many of our clients coping with severe mental illness. In many cities, groups are available in Spanish and other languages. Additional information about this organization can be found at www.nami.org/multicultural.

Culturally Relevant Domains of Psychoeducational Intervention

Successful family-focused programs for mental illness tend to focus on educating the family about the illness, improving communication and expressing negative feelings more effectively, teaching problem-solving skills and active listening, and helping family members develop more realistic expectations for the patient (Goldstein & Miklowitz, 1995). Below we use a multicultural perspective to discuss significant factors that impact the course of mental illness.

Expressed Emotion (EE)

EE is both a universal and a culturally bound construct. The majority of cross-cultural studies have supported the predictive validity of EE (Hashemi & Cochrane, 1999). A relative is rated as high EE if he/she expresses high degrees of criticism, hostility, or emotional overinvolvement (e.g., overly self-sacrificing behavior) toward a relative with a mental illness. However, the different components of EE predict outcome differentially across cultures and are moderated by culture (López et al., 2004). For example, criticism is significantly less prominent in collective cultures. Also, it is important to note that what is considered critical, hostile, or emotionally overinvolved varies across cultures (Jenkins & Karno, 1992). White family members tend to criticize undesirable, individual personality traits that violate norms of autonomy. Latino/Hispanic relatives and Black relatives, on the other hand, appear more likely to condemn behaviors that disrespect and shame other family members and defy collectivism and interdependence (Jenkins, Karno, de la Selva, & Santana, 1986; Kymalainen, Weisman, Rosales, & Armesto, 2006).

In general, Latinos/Hispanics and other minorities appear to have significantly lower rates of high EE and better course of illness when compared to their White counterparts (Weisman de Mamani et al., 2007; Karno et al., 1987). Less blameworthy attributions, greater reliance on adaptive religiosity/spirituality, high degrees of family cohesion, and the suppression of negative affect may begin to explain lower rates of high EE among Latin Americans (Jenkins, 1991; Weisman & López, 1996; Weisman, Gomes, & Lopez, 2003; Weisman, Duarte, Koneru, & Wasserman, 2006). Family member warmth has also been found to predict relapse for Latinos/Hispanics and may be an even better predictor than high EE in this ethnic group (López, Nelson, Snyder, & Mintz, 1999; Kopelowicz et al., 2002; López et al., 2004). This is not surprising given that family affection and harmony are highly prized among Latinos/Hispanics (Marín & Marín, 1991). Thus, high degrees of warmth from a loved one may be especially soothing to Latino/Hispanic patients with a mental illness.

The study of EE has also been exported to several Asian countries, and in most studies appears to be associated with poor course of illness. For example, studies in China and Japan indicate that patients from high EE homes relapse sooner and more frequently than those from low EE homes (Mino et al., 1995; Ng, Mui, Cheung, & Leung, 2001). However, base rates of high EE may be lower in Asian countries. In India (Leff et al., 1987) and in China (Ran, Leff, Hous, Xiang, & Chan, 2003) only about a quarter of relatives were rated as high EE, compared to approximately 67% of non-Hispanic Whites in the U.S. (Vaughn, Snyder, Jones, Freeman, & Falloon, 1984). The comparatively low base rates of high EE may be due to the centrality of collectivism, conformity, modesty, and suppression of negative emotions among traditional cultures (Ran et al., 2003). Low occurrence of high EE and these protective values may explain why patients with schizophrenia living in developing countries have a better prognosis than do patients living in more developed countries (Saravanan et al., 2007; Murphy & Raman, 1971; Wing, 1978).

Blacks are one of the only cultural groups for which high EE has not been found to predict poorer prognosis for schizophrenia. (Moline, Singh, Morris, & Meltzer, 1985; Tompson et al., 1995). In fact, criticism may serve as a protective factor against relapse in this ethnic group. Rosenfarb, Bellack, and Aziz (2004) found that the more critical Black relatives were, the less likely their ill relative was to relapse. Weisman, Rosales, Kymalainen and Armesto's (2006) found no association between the number of relatives' criticisms toward patients rated from the Camberwell Family Interview (to assess EE) and Black patients' own perception of their relatives' criticism. This may explain why high EE does not predict relapse among Blacks. It may be that conversations perceived as angry and aggressive by Whites are experienced as culturally syntonic by Blacks (Tompson et al., 1995), whose communication patterns are often characterized as effusive and emotionally and physically expressive (Millhouse, Asante, & Nwosu, 2001). Moreover, Blacks may feel that their relatives' critical statements are reflective of engagement, affection, caring, and support (Rosenfarb et al., 2004). Although criticisms as traditionally measured by EE instruments do not predict relapse among Blacks, Black patients' perceptions of relatives as critical may be predictive (Tompson et al., 1995). Because criticisms may actually serve as a buffer against relapse (they are thought to be perceived as statements of care and concern), interventions that attempt to reduce relatives' criticisms may inadvertently increase the risk of relapse in Black patients with schizophrenia. Instead, patients' perceptions of criticism may be particularly important to address in psychotherapy with Black families. Psychosocial programs aimed at lowering EE in most ethnic groups, and perceived criticism in Blacks are important.

Attributions

Attributions address causal worldviews and are inherently cultural. Some evidence exists for cross-cultural differences in attributions and affect toward relatives with schizophrenia that may account for some of the cultural differences observed in base rates of high EE and in illness prognosis. In line with this, Weisman and Lopez (1997) found that Mexicans were more likely to perceive the negative behavioral symptoms of schizophrenia as less controllable than were Whites. In turn, Whites expressed much more intense unfavorable emotion (anger, frustration) toward a person described to meet the criteria for schizophrenia.

This research suggests that a less blaming view of schizophrenia and the associated symptoms may lead to lower levels of negative emotion and high EE (Weisman & Lopez, 1997). There is a fair amount of evidence to support this view in Whites and minorities alike. For example, in a Mexican American sample (Weisman, Lopez, Karno, & Jenkins, 1993) and again in a non-Hispanic White sample (Weisman, Nuechterlein, Goldstein, & Snyder, 1998), Weisman and colleagues found that relatives designated as high EE were more likely to perceive the patient's illness and the associated symptoms as within the patient's personal control. In other words, they were less likely to buy into the notion that the patient was genuinely ill and that the symptoms were an unintended side effect. Others (e.g., Brewin, Maccarthy, Duda, & Vaughn, 1991, Hooley and Campbell, 2002) have found similar results. When family members attribute patients' symptoms to external (e.g., a biochemical/organic disease), rather than to internal controllable factors (e.g., laziness), they are less likely to blame them for their symptoms. Thus, increasing knowledge about the causes of serious mental illness, as well as fostering a more realistic understanding regarding the extent of a patient's ability to control his or her symptoms, should be a major aim of psychoeducational programs.

Stigma

Stigma is an another important construct to explore in family-focused treatment for severe mental illness because it sometimes prevents patients and their relatives from fully accepting the illness and taking steps to treat it (Kravetz, Faust, & David, 2000). It is interesting and important to note that persons from minority ethnic groups with severe mental illness may experience a double stigma. Primarily, these individuals face stigma as a result of belonging to a cultural minority group and may further face discrimination due to the fact that they have a serious mental illness. Terms such as *nervios* and *fallo mental* among Latinos/Hispanics and neurasthenia among Asians are frequently supplemented to decrease perceived stigma (Guarnaccia, Parra, Deschamps, Milstein, & Arqiles, 1992). These terms have been used to describe a variety of common and not so common experiences and symptoms such as heart palpitations, anxiety, depression, panic attacks, and schizophrenia (Guarnaccia et al., 1992). These terms can be useful in diminishing feelings of embarrassment and disgrace, but they can also have the effect of decreasing the likelihood that patients and families will seek and/or remain in treatment. Thus, it may be particularly important to target feelings of stigma when conducting psychoeducational interventions with minority groups.

Family Collectivism

While strong family ties are likely beneficial to everyone, as discussed above, perceived family collectivism appears to be especially important to the emotional well-being and symptom severity of minorities with schizophrenia (Weisman et al., 2005). While there is substantial heterogeneity between and within minority groups in the United States, one factor that stands out to differentiate certain minority cultures from the mainstream is the emphasis on interdependence over individualism. In a meta-analysis of cross-national studies and studies within the U.S., Oyserman et al. (2002) found that European Americans are both more individualistic and less collectivist than others. In many ways, mainstream American culture is founded on the ideals of individualism; these ideals include a focus on self-expression, direct communication, and the promotion of one's own goals (Singelis, 1994). Collectivists, by contrast, share a number of opposing defining attributes, which include the belief in a common fate, emotional dependence, and the desire to maintain harmony within groups (Triandis et al., 1990; Brewer & Chen, 2007). It is, therefore, essential for therapists to be aware that many minorities living in the U.S. may come from cultures that ascribe to a more collectivist orientation with an emphasis on family values and interdependence.

This may pose unique challenges to the therapeutic alliance. One contentious issue that is likely to arise at the beginning of treatment with minorities, for example, is the intense focus on individual thoughts and feelings in mainstream U.S. therapy. This can be highly uncomfortable for families from collectivist cultures (Aponte & Johnson, 2000). A culturally conscious therapist should ease this discomfort by understanding and applying the concept of contextualism. In their work on family therapy with minority clients, Szapocznik and Kurtines (1993) define contextualism as a system for understanding an individual as embedded within the context of the family, which is itself embedded within the context of the culture. In this way, the therapist begins to understand the contextual factors working on family and individual issues. Educating the family about ways to capitalize on their collectivist orientation is a main goal of psychoeducation in family therapy.

Spirituality

Spirituality/religion is another critical component to consider when helping families to conceptualize and cope with mental illness (Weisman et al., 2006). The issue of whether or not to address spirituality and religiosity in the treatment of individuals with serious mental illness has been hotly debated among mental health professionals. On one hand, it has been argued that addressing these issues might lead to increased religious delusions in patients with schizophrenia, which are already highly common and distressful (Getz, Fleck, & Strakowski, 2001; Torrey, 1995). Others, however, have argued that ignoring spiritual issues in treatment provides a disservice to those patients who are religiously oriented (Fallot, 1998; Pargament, 1997).

Whether or not a therapist decides to address spiritual or religious issues in treatment often depends on the patient's particular personality and symptom profile. For example, a religious intervention would likely be contraindicated for a patient who is highly opposed to one or for a patient with frequent religious delusions. In general, however, there is a growing body of evidence highlighting the benefits of religion. For example, a meta-analysis conducted by McCullough, Hoyt, Larson, Koenig, and Thoresen (2000) found a strong association between religious involvement and lower mortality rates. Furthermore, a review article by Koenig, Larson, and Weaver (1998) summarizes the breadth of data showing that religious individuals have lower rates of depression, less alcohol and drug abuse, and lower rates of anxiety disorders.

Another benefit of religion that is more specific to minorities is the accessibility and centrality of the religious community. In many minority cultures, churches and religious communities play a central role in the lives and coping processes of their members. In Latino/Hispanic cultures, for example, strong religious beliefs inform the conceptualization of both physical and mental illness (Musgrave, Allen, & Allen, 2002). Furthermore, where access to mental health care is limited, as it is for many minorities of lower SES, individuals often turn to religious coping for strength and support (Pargament, 1997; Lincoln & Mamiya, 1990). This is because adaptive uses of religion may share many of the same functions as psychotherapy. Some of these overlapping functions include providing meaning to life, utilizing social support networks, and facilitating positive change (Stander, Piercy, Mackinnon, & Helmeke, 1994). Educating clients about the overlap between religion and psychotherapy and providing information regarding how to use faith to access positive therapeutic processes can be very effective in religious patients. It is important to note that spirituality education is indicated for nonreligious clients as well, as the main focus is on the development of empathy, forgiveness, and appreciation, all of which are essential therapeutic processes (Sperry, 2001).

Language

While there are many issues to take into consideration when working with ethnic minority clients, one of the most obvious barriers to treatment is language use. Of course, it is ideal if mental health practitioners are able to provide services in the client's preferred language. If both the therapist and clients are bilingual, some researchers suggest using the language preferred by older family members (Santisteban & Szapocznik, 1994) so as to respect the common age hierarchy in many minority families (Szapocznik, Rio, Perez-Vida, & Kurtines, 1986). If translators are needed, it is critical to select a person with training in mental health interpretation, rather than drafting a family member or friend into this role (Leung & Boehnlein, 2005, p. 370). This can be problematic because informal translators may provide incorrect or insufficient information important for diagnosis and treatment, increase mistranslations or omissions of the therapists' questions, and supply shortened or misconstrued representations of the clients' responses (Monroe & Shiranzian, 2004).

In our work with families with schizophrenia at the University of Miami, we have found that flexibility is more important than following a specific formula dictating which language to use. The first author of this chapter has described this with a case example in Weisman et al. (2006, p. 182):

In one of our cases, the family included a mother who understood English extremely well but reported feeling comfortable speaking only Spanish, and her two children who were young adults raised primarily in the United States. The children understood Spanish very well but reported being uncomfortable speaking it. In this case, the family actually recommended to the therapist that she direct the mother in Spanish and the children in English, and that family members would each respond in their dominant language. As this was a pilot case, we agreed to try the approach requested by the family and found that it worked extremely well. Everyone was able to speak in the language that they were most at-home in and comfortable speaking. In fact, this approach appeared to strengthen the bond between the therapist and the family.

As Weisman and colleagues (2006) describe, strict adherence to their original treatment manual would have prescribed speaking in Spanish with the family. In hindsight, however, we believe that following strict guidelines to use the mother's dominant language would have proven less effective with this particular family. Thus we believe this demonstrates the importance of flexibility with respect to language and accommodating to a particular family's style and wishes.

Culturally Informed Therapy for Schizophrenia (CIT-S)

We will now describe an example of one treatment that has been informed by the literature and developed specifically so as to be relevant for minority families coping with schizophrenia. Culturally Informed Therapy for Schizophrenia (CIT-S) is a 15-session family therapy currently being pilot tested at the University of Miami. Specifically, the treatment is broken into five 3-session modules on the following topics: Family Collectivism, Education, Spiritual/Religious Coping, Communication Training, and Problem Solving. The Education, Communication Training, and Problem-Solving modules are based on the work of Falloon et al. (1984) and Miklowitz and Goldstein (1997). Although we believe CIT-S will be effective for many minority and majority groups, it has been especially designed to be relevant for people of Latino/Hispanic decent. All assessment and therapy tools and procedures have been developed in both English and Spanish. Handouts are used to guide each session. For more information or copies of handouts, please email the first author (Dr. Amy Weisman de Mamani, aweisman@miami.edu). The treatment is also described in more detail in Weisman, Duarte, Koneru, and Wasserman (2006).

Family Collectivism

The first module of CIT-S is family collectivism. The overarching objective of this segment is to foster or enhance family unity and help family members to see one another as team members working toward shared goals. Furthermore, blame for the patient's illness is deflected off of any one individual. Initially, family members are praised for attending treatment; the therapist frames their attendance as indicative of a commitment to the patient and to the family unit. To further highlight family cohesion, the therapist asks participants about their expectations for treatment and points out commonalities among the family members. Specific topics covered during this segment, with the aid of handouts, include what the concept of family means to each member, each family member's perception of his or her role in the family, each family member's perception of other family members' roles in the family, how family members view generational and gender roles, whether family members see a clear hierarchy within the family, and whether family members see any significant conflicts or alliances between members.

An example from one of our CIT-S cases illustrates how the collectivism segment can be used to examine and improve individual family member's roles and contributions to the family unit and dissipate conflicts. The family members were recent Cuban immigrants and consisted of the mother of the patient and the adolescent brother of the patient. Upon discussing each member's role, it became clear that the mother held all the responsibility for the family's well-being and felt very overburdened. Her son, and the patient's brother, had largely withdrawn from the family unit and from assisting his mother because of the resentment he harbored toward his sibling, the identified patient. This was evidenced by his silence and animosity during the initial session. During the collectivism sessions, we reframed the brother's potential contribution as assisting the mother and the family as a whole and discussed ways in which each family member might contribute more equally. As treatment progressed, the mother and brother of the patient became a more cohesive unit. The brother of the patient became highly involved during the sessions. He regularly contributed ideas as to how he might help his mother in caring for the patient and often aided his mother in obtaining services for the patient.

Education

In this segment of CIT-S, therapists present information on the symptoms of schizophrenia, the factors contributing to the development of the illness, exacerbating factors, warning signs of a relapse, and ways to create an environment that is protective against relapse. The role of high-EE attitudes and attributions and its relationship to psychiatric relapse is emphasized. This didactic approach is especially well suited to Hispanic and other minorities who may expect therapy to provide more immediate information, advice, and problem-solving techniques. Additionally, minority families may associate a large amount of stigma regarding therapy, and a more information-oriented approach may help make therapy more concrete and less daunting (Organista & Muñoz, 1996).

One particular challenge during the education module is if the patient becomes defensive about symptoms of the illness. For example, we worked with one family in which the patient had difficulty accepting his diagnosis of schizophrenia. He was upset by the focus of the sessions on his symptoms and as a reaction would minimize his experiences or provide alternative explanations for his symptoms involving esoteric religious beliefs he formed after developing the illness. To diffuse this defensiveness, the therapist asked other family members to discuss their experiences with some of the symptoms within their own lives (e.g., periods of poor hygiene, lack of motivation, distrusting others, etc.). Once the focus was less directly on the patient's own symptoms, he seemed to feel more comfortable discussing his symptoms without relying on the religious explanations as a defense.

Spiritual/Religious Coping

The spirituality module begins with a discussion of the family's spiritual and religious history. Family members are encouraged to discuss beliefs about God, morality, and the meaning of life, as well as more behavioral components of religion, such as attendance of religious services or private prayer. In therapy, the clinician helps family members cultivate important spiritual practices, including emotional wisdom through forgiveness and empathy. Outside therapy, families are encouraged to utilize the available social support inherent in most religious congregations to help cope with the illness and to continue their spiritual growth. Therapists also suggest that patients and family members read spiritual/religious texts and find passages that may provide inspiration for more active ways to manage or come to terms with the illness, such as "God helps those who help themselves."

It is important to note that within families, individuals often present with very different spiritual beliefs and practices. This can be viewed as a point of contention or, preferably, as a jumping-off point for a rich and meaningful conversation about beliefs and purpose. In one of our cases, we saw a Cuban American patient and his mother. The patient had been diagnosed with schizophrenia but also exhibited a number of obsessive-compulsive symptoms, including a fear of being in a car and driving to new locations. During the spirituality module, it was established that going to church was a culturally sanctioned behavior that the highly religious mother desired to share with her son. The patient felt positively about attending church but had been limited because of his symptomology. Over the course of these three sessions, the patient and mother agreed to try driving to church with the ultimate goal of attending services. The religious underpinning of this behavioral intervention proved useful in that it provided a meaningful goal for the family to meet together. By the end of treatment, the patient had driven to church with his mother and was optimistic about attending services in the future.

Communication Training

The communication training segment of treatment aims to enhance the quality and effectiveness of the family's verbal interactions. Communication training involves teaching the families four basic skills: expressing positive feelings, active listening, making positive requests for change, and expressing negative feelings about specific behaviors. Role playing is the primary technique used to teach these skills. These skills are drawn largely from the work of Falloon, Boyd, and McGill (1984) and from Miklowitz and Goldstein (1997). Using this method, family members practice new ways of communicating in a setting that is safe and nonjudgmental.

In one of our CIT-S cases, we had a family from Panama, including the son (identified patient), his mother and his father. During the communication training module, we noticed a pattern whereby the mother frequently served as the primary spokesperson for the entire family. She would often talk over other family members and they would often collude by yielding the floor to her. Furthermore, when the son did speak he would often look to his mother for confirmation that what he was saying was acceptable. Through the use of role playing, the mother became a much more conscientious communicator. She was better able to refrain from interrupting when others spoke, maintain eye contact, and demonstrate that she understood what her relatives were saying by paraphrasing the information back in her own words. This change appeared to have many benefits. For example, the mother reported enjoying learning more about her son's and husband's perspective on things. Moreover, the son appeared to gain confidence in expressing himself more clearly and directly. This is a skill that will serve him well when interacting with doctors and mental health counselors in managing his illness and eventually in other areas of his personal and professional life.

Problem Solving

This module teaches family members more concrete ways of discussing problems, brainstorming strategies to address problems, discussing the pros and cons of each idea, agreeing on a solution, and implementing the plan. Family members work through several examples with the therapist and use homework to practice the techniques between sessions. As this is the final module in CIT-S, families practice a "relapse drill," where they use problem-solving strategies to develop a detailed course of action in the event of a psychiatric relapse.

Culture can play a huge role in relapse-prevention strategies, particularly when family members have different levels of acculturation. For example, one Hispanic family we worked with consisted of a couple and their adult son, who was the patient. The patient, who was more acculturated to U.S. culture than his parents, was returning to college and desired more independence. The mother, however, wanted to call and visit the patient frequently in order to monitor his symptoms and be more involved in his life. These behaviors made the patient feel like his parents did not trust him to manage his own illness and expected him to relapse. The problem-solving module provided an opportunity to come to a solution that was decided on by all family members in which the patient agreed to take more initiative to call his parents and keep them informed of his symptoms so they felt connected to his life, but he felt more in control.

While data collection for the CIT-S project is still underway, preliminary analyses using a 7-point scale (1 = "Very Dissatisfied"; 7 = "Very Satisfied") have indicated a very high degree of consumer satisfaction with the treatment for both family members ($M = 6.26$, $SD = .88$) and for patients ($M = 5.75$, $SD = 1.27$). Furthermore, in a recent study we have found that greater therapist competence/adherence to the various modules of CIT-S is strongly associated with greater treatment retention and greater consumer satisfaction for family members (Dunham & Weisman de Mamani 2007).

Conclusions

In conclusion, the use of psychoeducational programs in the treatment of schizophrenia and other serious mental illness is essential for reducing relapse and improving quality of life for minority and nonminority patients and their family members. Including techniques that emphasize family collectivism, adaptive spiritual/religious coping techniques, as well as tailoring discussions of constructs such as EE, attributions, and stigma may increase the effectiveness of psychoeducational approaches when working with ethnic minorities. Of course, more work needs to be done to eliminate the language and other cultural barriers to treatment that minorities often face.

References

Aponte, J. F., & Johnson, L. R. (2000). The impact of culture on the intervention and treatment of ethnic populations. In J. F. Aponte & J. Wohl (Eds.), *Psychological intervention and cultural diversity* (pp. 18–39). Boston, MA: Allyn and Bacon.

Barrio, C., Yamada, A. M., Hough, R. L., Hawthorne, W., Garcia, P., & Jeste, D. V. (2003). Ethnic disparities in use of public mental health case management services among patients with schizophrenia. *Psychiatric Services, 54*, 1264–1270.

Barrowclough, C., Haddock, G., Tarrier, N., Lewis, S. W., Moring, J., O'Brien, R., et al. (2001). Randomized controlled trial of motivational interviewing, cognitive behavior therapy, and family intervention for patients with comorbid schizophrenia and substance use disorders. *American Journal of Psychiatry, 158*, 1706–1713.

Brewer, M. B. & Chen, Y. (2007) Where (who) are collectives in collectivism? Toward conceptual clarification of individualism and collectivism. *Psychological Review, 114*, 133–151.

Brewin, C. R., Maccarthy, B., Duda, K., & Vaughn, C. E. (1991). Attribution and expressed emotion in the relatives of patients with schizophrenia. *Journal of Abnormal Psychology, 100*, 546–554

Chen, F., & Greenberg, J. S. (2004). A positive aspect of caregiving: The influence of social support on caregiving gains for family members of relatives with schizophrenia. *Community Mental Health Journal, 40*, 423–435.

Dixon, L., Lyles, A., Scott, J., Lehman, A., Postrado, L., Goldman, H., & McGlynn, E. (1999). Services to families of adults with schizophrenia: From treatment recommendations to dissemination. *Psychiatric Services, 50,* 233–238.

Dixon, L., McFarlane, W., Lefley, H., Luckstead, A., Cohen, C., & Falloon, I. (2001). Evidence-based practices for services to family members of people with psychiatric difficulties. *Psychiatric Services, 52,* 903–910.

Dunham, R., & Weisman de Mamani, A. (2007). Therapist competence and adherence as a predictor of treatment efficacy in families enrolled in Culturally Informed Therapy for Schizophrenia. Poster presented at the annual meeting of the Society for Research in Psychopathology, Iowa City, IA.

Falloon, I. R. H., Boyd, J. L., & McGill, C. W. (1984). *Family care of schizophrenia: A problem-solving approach to the treatment of mental illness.* New York: Guilford Press.

Fallot, R. D. (1998). The place of spirituality and religion in mental health services. *New Directions for Mental Health Services, 80,* 3–12.

Flaskerud, J. H. (1986). The effects of culture-compatible intervention on the utilization of mental health services by minority clients. *Community Mental Health Journal, 22,* 127–141.

Getz, G. E., Fleck, D. E., & Strakowski, S. M. (2001). Frequency and severity of religious delusions in Christian patients with psychosis. *Psychiatry Research, 103,* 87–91.

Goldstein, M. J., & Miklowitz, D. J. (1995). The effectiveness of psychoeducational family therapy in the treatment of schizophrenic disorders. *Journal of Marital and Family Therapy, 21,* 361–376.

Guarnaccia, P. J., & Parra, P. (1996). Ethnicity, social status, and families' experiences of caring for a mentally ill family member. *Community Mental Health Journal, 32,* 243–260.

Guarnaccia P. J., Parra, P., Deschamps, A., Milstein, G., & Arqiles, N. (1992). Si Dios quiere: Hispanic families' experiences of caring for a seriously mentally ill family member. *Culture, Medicine and Psychiatry, 16,* 187–215.

Hashemi, A., & Cochrane, R. (1999). Expressed emotion and schizophrenia: A review of studies across cultures. *International Review of Psychiatry, 11,* 219–224.

Hooley, J. M., & Campbell, C. (2002). Control and controllability: beliefs and behaviour in high and low expressed emotion relatives. *Psychological Medicine, 32,* 1091–1099

Hooley, J. M., & Hiller, J. B. (2000). Personality and expressed emotion. *Journal of Abnormal Psychology, 109,* 40–44.

Jenkins, J., Karno, M., De La Selva, A., & Santana, F. (1986). Expressed emotion in cross-cultural context: Familial responses to schizophrenic illness among Mexican-Americans. In M. Goldstein, I. Hand, & K. Hahlweg (Eds.), *Treatment of schizophrenia: Family assessment and intervention* (pp. 35–49). New York, NY: Springer-Verlag.

Karno, M., Jenkins, J., De La Selva, A., Santana, F., Telles, C., Lopez, S., et al. (1987). Expressed emotion and schizophrenic outcome among Mexican-American families. *Journal of Nervous and Mental Disease, 175,* 143–151.

Koening, H. G., Larson, D. B., & Weaver, A. J. (1998). Research on religion and serious mental illness. *New Directions for Mental Health Services, 80,* 81–95.

Kopelowicz, A., Zarate, R., Gonzalez, V., Lopez, S., Ortega, P., Obregón, N., et al. (2002). Evaluation of expressed emotion in schizophrenia: A comparison of Caucasians and Mexican-Americans. *Schizophrenia Research, 55,* 179–186.

Kravetz, S., Faust, M., & David, M. (2000). Accepting the mental illness label, perceived control over the illness, and quality of life. *Psychiatric Rehabilitation, 23,* 323–332.

Kymalainen, J. Weisman, A., Rosales, G., & Armesto, J. (2006). Ethnicity, expressed emotion, and communication deviance in family members of patients with schizophrenia. *The Journal of Nervous and Mental Disease, 194,* 1–6.

Leff, J., Wig, N., Ghosh, A., Bedi, H., Menon, D., Kuipers, L., et al. (1987). Influence of relatives' EE on the course of schizophrenia in Chandigarh. *British Journal of Psychiatry, 151,* 166–173.

Lueng, P. K., & Boehnlein, J. K. (2005). Vietnamese families. In M. McGoldrick, J. Giordano, & N. Garcia-Preto (Eds.), *Ethnicity and family therapy* (pp. 363–373). New York: Guilford Press.

Lincoln, C. E., & Mamiya, L. H. (1990). *The Black church in the African American experience*. New York: Duke University Press.

Ling, S., Zhao, C., Yang, W., Wang, R., Jin, Z., Ma, T., et al. (1999). Efficacy of family intervention on schizophrenics in remission in community: Result of one year follow-up study. *Chinese Mental Health Journal, 13*, 325–327.

López, S., Hipke, K., Polo, A., Jenkins, J., Karno, M., Vaughn, C., et al. (2004). Ethnicity, expressed emotion, attributions, and course of schizophrenia: Family warmth matters. *Journal of Abnormal Psychology, 113*, 428–439.

Mak, W. W., & Wu, C. F. (2006). Cognitive insight and causal attribution in the development of self-stigma among individuals with schizophrenia. *Psychiatric Services, 57*, 1800–1802.

Magliano, L., Fiorillo, A., Fadden, F., Gair, F., Economou, M., Kallert, T., et al. (2005). Effectiveness of a psychoeducational intervention for families of patients with schizophrenia: Preliminary results of a study funded by the European Commission. *World Psychiatry, 4*, 45–49.

Magliano, L., Fiorillo, A., Malangome, C., De Rosa, C., & Maj, M. (2006). Patient functioning and family burden in a controlled, real-world trial of family psychoeducation for schizophrenia. *Psychiatric Services, 57*, 1784–1791.

Marín, G., & Marín, B. V. (1991). Research with Hispanic populations. *Applied social research method series*, 23. Newbery Park, CA: Sage Publications.

Marsh, D. T., & Lefley, H. P. (1996). The family experience of mental illness: Evidence for resilience. *Psychiatric Rehabilitation Journal, 20*, 3–12.

McCullough, M. E., Hoyt, W. T., Larson, D. B., Koenig, H. G., & Thoresen, C. (2000). Religious involvement and mortality: A meta-analytic review. *Health Psychology, 19*, 211–222.

McFarlane, W. R., Dixon, L., Lukens, E., & Lucksted, A. (2003). Family psychoeducation and schizophrenia: a review of the literature. *Journal of Marital and Family Therapy, 69*, 3–12.

McGoldrick, M., Giordano, J., & Garcia-Preto, N (Eds.). (2005). *Ethnicity and family therapy*. New York: Guilford Press.

Miklowitz, D. J., & Goldstein, M. J. (1997). *Bipolar disorder. A family focused treatment approach*. New York: Guilford Press.

Miklowitz, D. J., Simoneua, T. L., George, E. L., Richards, J. A., Kalbarg, A., Sachs-Ericcson, et al. (2000). Family focused treatment of bipolar disorder: 1-year effects of a psychoeducational program in conjunction with pharmacotherapy, *Biological Psychiatry, 48*, 582–592.

Millhouse, V. H., Asante, M. K. & Nwosu, P. O. (2001). *Transcultural realities: Interdisciplinary perspectives on cross-cultural relations*. Thousand Oaks, CA: Sage.

Mino, Y., Tanaka, S., Inoue, S., Tsuda, T., Babazono, A., & Aoyama, H. (1995). Expressed emotion components in families of schizophrenic patients in Japan. *International Journal of Mental Health, 24*, 38–49.

Moline, R., Singh, S., Morris, A., & Meltzer, H. (1985). Family EE and relapse in schizophrenia in 24 urban American patients. *American Journal of Psychiatry, 142*, 1169–1177.

Monroe, A. D., & Shiranzian, T. (2004). Challenging linguistic barriers to health care: Students as medical interpreters. *Academic Medicine, 79*, 118–122.

Muela Martinez, J. A., & Godoy Garcia, J. F. (2001). Family intervention program for schizophrenia: Two-year follow-up of the Andalusia Study. *Apuntes de Psicología, 19*, 421–430.

Mueser, K. T., & Glynn, S. M. (1999). *Behavioral family therapy for psychiatric disorders* (2nd ed.). Oakland, CA: New Harbinger.

Mueser, K. T., Torrey, W. C., Lynde, D., Singer, P., & Drae, R. (2003). Implementing evidence based practices for people with severe mental illness. *Behavior Modification, 27*, 387–411.

Murphy, H. B.M. & Raman, A. C. (1971). The chronicity of schizophrenia in indigenous tropical peoples: Results of a 12-year follow-up on Muritius. *British Journal of Psychiatry, 118*, 489–497.

Musgrave, C. F., Allen, C. E., & Allen, G. J. (2002). Spirituality and health for women of color. *American Journal of Public Health, 92*, 557–560.

National Institute of Mental Health. (1999). *Strategic plan on reducing health disparities.* Rockville, MD: Author.

Ng, R., Mui, J., Cheung, H., & Leung, S. (2001). Expressed emotion and relapse of schizophrenia in Hong Kong. *Hong Kong Journal of Psychiatry, 11*, 4–11.

Organista, K. C., & Munoz, R. F. (1996). Cognitive behavioral therapy with Latinos. *Cognitive and Behavioral Practice, 3*, 255–270.

Oyserman, D., Coon, H. M., & Kemmelmeier, M. (2002). Rethinking individualism and collectivism: Evaluation of theoretical assumptions and meta-analyses. *Psychological Bulletin, 128*, 3–72.

Pargament, K. I. (1997). *The psychology of religion and coping: Theory, research, and practice.* New York: Guilford Press.

Pitschel-Walz, G., Leucht, S., Bauml, J., Kissling, W., & Engel, R. (2001). The effect of family interventions on relapse and rehospitalization in schizophrenia: A meta-analysis. *Schizophrenia Bulletin, 27*, 73–92.

Ran, M., Leff, J., Hou, Z., Xiang, M., & Chan, C. (2003). The characteristics of expressed emotion among relatives of patients with schizophrenia in Chengdu, China. *Culture, Medicine and Psychiatry, 27*, 95–106.

Rosenfarb, I., Bellack, A., & Aziz, N. (2004). Race, family interventions and patient stabilization in schizophrenia. *Journal of Abnormal Psychology, 113*, 109–115.

Rummel-Kluge, C., & Kissling, W. (2008). Psychoeducation in schizophrenia: new developments and approaches in the field. *Current Opinions in Psychiatry, 21*, 168–172.

Rund, B. R., Moe, L., Sollien, T., Fjell, A., Borchgrevink, T., Hallert, M., et al. (1994). The Psychosis Project: Outcome and cost-effectiveness of a psychoeducational treatment programme for schizophrenic adolescents. *Acta Psychiatrica Scandinavica, 89*, 211–218.

Santisteban, D. A., & Szapocznik, J. (1994). Bridging theory, research and practice to more successfully engage substance abusing youth and their families into therapy. *Journal of Child and Adolescent Substance Abuse, 3*, 9–24.

Saravanan, B., Jacob, K. S, Johnson, S., Prince, M., Bhugra, D., & David, A. S. (2007). Assessing insight in schizophrenia: East meets West. *British Journal of Psychiatry, 190*, 243–247.

Singelis, T. M. (1994). The measurement of independent and interdependent self-construals. *Personality and Social Psychology Bulletin, 20*, 580–591.

Snowden, L. R. (2007). Explaining mental health treatment disparities: Ethnic and cultural differences in family involvement. *Culture, Medicine and Psychiatry, 31*, 389–402.

Sperry, L. (2001). *Spirituality in clinical practice: Incorporating the spiritual dimension in psychotherapy and counseling.* Ann Arbor, MI: Sheridan Books.

Stander, V., Piercy, F. P., Mackinnon, D., & Helmeke, K. (1994). Spirituality, religion and family therapy: competing or complementary worlds? *The American Journal of Family Therapy, 22*, 27–41.

Szapocznik, J. (Ed.). (1994). *A Hispanic/Latino family approach to substance abuse prevention.* Rockville, MD: Center for Substance Abuse Prevention.

Szapocznik, J., & Kurtines, W. M. (1993). Family psychology and cultural diversity: opportunities for theory, research, and application. *American Psychologist, 48*, 400–407.

Szapocznik, J., Rio, A., Perez-Vida, A., & Kurtines, W. (1986). Bicultural effectiveness training: An experimental test of an intervention modality for families experiencing intergeneration/intercultural conflict. *Hispanic Journal of Behavioral Sciences, 8*, 303–330.

Tompson, M., Goldstein, M., Lebell, M., Mintz, L., Marder, S., & Mintz, J. (1995). Schizo-phrenic patients' perceptions of their relatives' attitudes. *Psychiatry Research, 57*, 155–167.

Torrey, E. F. (1995). *Surviving schizophrenia: A manual for families, consumers, and providers* (3rd ed.). New York: Harper Perennial.

Torrey, E. F., Bowler, A. E., Taylor, E. H., & Gottesman, I. I. (1994). *Schizophrenia and manic-depressive disorder*. New York: BasicBooks.

Triandis, H. C., McCusker, C., & Hui, C. H. (1990). Multimethod probes of individualism and collectivism. *Journal of Personality and Social Psychology, 59*, 1006–1020.

Vaughn, C. E., Snyder, K. S., Jones, S., Freeman, W. B., & Falloon, I. R. (1984). Family factors in schizophrenic relapse: Replication in California of British research on expressed emotion. *Archives of General Psychiatry, 41*, 1169–1177.

Weisman, A. G., Duarte, E., Koneru, V., & Wasserman, S. (2006). The development of a culturally informed, family focused treatment for schizophrenia. *Family Process, 45*, 171–186.

Weisman, A. G., Gomes, L. G., & Lopez, S. R. (2003). Shifting blame away from ill relatives: Latino families' reactions to schizophrenia. *Journal of Nervous and Mental Disorders, 191*, 574–581.

Weisman de Mamani, A. G., Kymalainen, J., Rosales, G., & Armesto, J. (2007). Expressed emotion and interdependence in White and Latino/Hispanic family members of patients with schizophrenia. *Psychiatry Research, 151*, 107–113

Weisman, A. G., & Lopez, S. R. (1997). An attributional analysis of emotional reactions to schizophrenia in Mexican and Anglo American cultures. *Journal of Applied Social Psychology, 27*, 223–244.

Weisman, A. G., Lopez, S. R., Karno, M., & Jenkins, J. (1993). An attributional analysis of expressed emotion in Mexican-American families with schizophrenia. *Journal of Abnormal Psychology, 102*, 601–606.

Weisman, A. G., Nuechterlein, K. H., Goldstein, M. J., & Snyder, K. S. (1998). Expressed emotion, attributions, and schizophrenia symptom dimensions. *Journal of Abnormal Psychology, 107*, 355–359.

Weisman, A., Rosales, G., Kymalainen, J., & Armesto, J. (2005). Ethnicity, family cohesion, religiosity and general emotional distress in patients with schizophrenia and their relatives. *Journal of Nervous & Mental Disease, 193*, 359–368

Weisman, A. G., Rosales, G. A., Kymalainen, J. A., & Armesto, J. C. (2006), Ethnicity, expressed emotion, and schizophrenia patients' perceptions of their family members' criticism. *The Journal of Nervous and Mental Disease, 194*, 644–649.

Wing, J. K. (1978). Social influences on the course of schizophrenia. In L. C. Winny, R. L. Cromwell, & S. Matthysse (Eds.), *The nature of schizophrenia* (pp. 599–616). New York: Wiley.

Chapter 13
Socioeconomic Status: Risks and Resilience

Lara M. Stepleman, Dustin E. Wright, and Kathryn A. Bottonari

Introduction

In the discussion of race, ethnicity, sexual orientation, and mental illness, it is essential to consider the impact of socioeconomic status (SES) as one of the most influential variables in health morbidity and mortality research (Angell, 1993). SES has been conceptualized as "a broad concept that refers to the placement of persons, families, households, and census tracts or other aggregates with respect to the capacity to consume goods that are valued in society" (Miech & Hauser, 2001). Given that the risk for psychiatric disorders is about two-fold for individuals in the lowest SES groups compared to those in higher SES groups (Holzer et al., 1986), it is acutely troublesome that Hispanics and African Americans experience poverty at rates two to three times that of White, non-Hispanics (DeNavas-Walt, Proctor, & Lee, 2006). Research indicates that the inverse linear relationship between SES and mental health spans the entire economic spectrum (Adler & Snibbe, 2003; Gallo, Bogart, Vranceanu, & Matthews, 2005). Furthermore, SES appears to have both causative and consequential relationships to psychiatric variation and severity (Huurre, Rahkonen, Komulainen, & Aro, 2005) such that both social selection and social causation explanations have been proposed (Stansfeld, Bosma, Hemingway, & Marmot, 1998).

Although the relationship between SES and mental health is inversely linear, the interactive effects of race, sexual orientation, and low SES appear to more adversely affect minorities than when examining either variable alone. Some researchers propose that with regards to low-SES, minority status adds a unique set of disadvantages, such as experiences of discrimination, segregation, and racism/homophobia that further explain differences in health access and outcomes (Adler & Snibbe, 2003). Additionally, even when racial minorities raise their level of SES, they do not experience the same rate of return regarding

L.M. Stepleman (✉)
Medical College of Georgia, Augusta, GA
e-mail: lsteplem@mail.mcg.edu

S. Loue, M. Sajatovic (eds.), *Determinants of Minority Mental Health and Wellness*, DOI 10.1007/978-0-387-75659-2_13,
© Springer Science+Business Media, LLC 2009

improvement in health outcomes as non-Hispanic Whites, (i.e., "diminishing returns hypothesis"; Farmer & Ferraro, 2005).

In order to examine more carefully the impact of SES on minority mental health, concurrence regarding the construct of SES, its measurement, and its relationship to related variables is necessary. SES is typically an indication of social position (Adler & Snibbe, 2003) measured through proxies such as income, education, and occupation, with income having the strongest tie to health outcomes in the literature (Stronks, van de Mheen, van den Bos, & Mackenbach, 1997). With reference to the measurement of SES, both objective (i.e., Hollingshead's four factor index social status; Hollingshead, 1975) and subjective measures (i.e., MacArthur Scale of Subjective Social Status; Adler, Epel, Castellazzo, & Ickovics, 2000) have been used. Additionally, SES can be assessed using single, multiple, or composite measures (Shavers, 2007) across individuals, families, and neighborhoods (Chen & Paterson, 2006). Most frequently, SES is measured cross-sectionally, which presents limitations regarding interpretation and extrapolation of the impact of SES status at one life point on SES, mental health, and other variables of interest across the life span (Shavers, 2007; Whitfield, Weidner, Clark, & Anderson, 2002). For example, Adler and Snibbe (2003) state that SES appears to have the strongest relationship to health at birth and in mid-to-late adulthood but that additional research findings have suggested actual duration of time spent in low-SES environments during childhood may also be predictive of adult health.

Cross-sectional designs are not the only challenge to SES research. Shavers (2007) adds that there is a lack of precision and reliability in SES measurement and that sampling irregularities impact the generalizability of findings. Furthermore, as SES is frequently linked with the male working head of household, data for women, children, retired individuals, and the unemployed may be misclassified or not included at all. Moreover, Siefert, Finlayson, Williams, Delva, and Ismail (2007) point out that the traditional means of measuring SES may not allow for adequate discrimination of mental health risk factors because of their universality within low-SES groups.

One solution has been to examine variables specific to poverty and mental health, particularly those more proximal and amenable to direct intervention (e.g., homelessness, hunger; Siefert et al., 2007; Whitfield et al., 2002). Although there is an established link between poverty, mental health, and well-being, there is still a need to better delineate the influence of chronic versus time-restricted poverty (Seifert et al., 2007). Moreover, though poverty-related "access to care" difficulties have been suggested as a likely contributor to health disparities, similar differential outcomes are found even when universal access is offered (Adler & Snibbe, 2003). Due to the inherent problems with SES and poverty as variables in mental health research, it is essential for investigators and consumers to be aware of measurement issues, methodological limitations, and their influence on interpretation of findings.

Social Causation and Selection in Mental Health

There are two primary models (with multiple iterations there of) used to conceptualize the relationship between mental health and SES. The first is the Social Causation model, which postulates that increased stress associated with low-SES environments contributes to higher rates of psychiatric disorders (Hollingshead, Ellis, & Kirby, 1954). For example, Gallo and Matthews (2003) propose that people in low-SES environments have greater exposure to stress and an imbalance of negative life experiences over positive ones, necessitating increased usage of psychological resources with less opportunity to replenish them. Similarly, Adler and Ostrove (1999) discuss allostatic load, referring to the cumulative wear and tear on the body from the stress of low-SES environments that contributes to worsening emotional and physical health. Stress in these models can come from a variety of sources including environmental, emotional, social, economic, and physical. There has been some evidence supporting Social Causation, such as research examining the connection between high levels of stress and increased rates of PTSD, depression, and anxiety (Wadsworth & Achenbach, 2005).

In contrast, the Social Selection model proposes that genetic and environmental factors predispose individuals to psychiatric disorders, which subsequently results in an inability to perform expected social roles, such as remaining employed, having effective social relationships, and eventual SES decline (Wadsworth & Achenbach, 2005; Wender, Rosenthal, Kety, Schlusinger, & Welner, 1973). This phenomenon has also been referred to as "downward drift" and suggests that individuals with good mental and physical health move up the social hierarchy whereas those with poor mental and physical health move down (Huurre et al., 2005). Although Social Causation and Selection are often presented as mutually exclusive theories, empirical evidence suggests that both contribute to the relationship between SES and mental illness (Johnson, Cohen, Dohrenwend, Link, & Brook, 1999). It is also likely that racism and discrimination provide unique contributions to models of mental illness among minorities. Therefore, the remainder of this chapter is devoted to examining the research on SES and mental health for minority populations, in either direction, with a focus on the risk factors, potential for resiliency, and future directions for this area of research.

Risk Factors

There is a substantial body of research examining the SES risk factors associated with poor mental health and well-being. Impoverished individuals and/or those from low-SES families do not live as long as individuals in higher income groups (National Center for Health Statistics, 1998 as cited in Williams,

1999), have a higher mortality rate from chronic illnesses (Carnon et al., 1994; Dayal, Power, & Chiu, 1982), and are at increased risk of mental health problems (Bratter & Eschbach, 2005; Lorant et al., 2003; Williams & Collins, 1995). This pattern is especially true among minorities, who are disproportionately represented in low-income groups. However, the relationship between SES and mental health is incredibly complex, and the most direct measures of SES (e.g., income, education, etc.) explain only a portion of the differences in mental and physical health outcomes in minorities. An ever-increasing body of research has focused on the specific mediating risk factors (e.g., parental education, exposure to discrimination and racism, segregated housing, etc.) that more fully explain the relationship between SES and mental health/well-being. Developing a better understanding of these mediating factors and processes holds promise for intervention and policy changes aimed to improve the health and quality of life of minorities. In this section, we will review the community/system, family/social, and individual/intrapsychic risk factors that mediate the relationship between SES and mental health problems in minorities.

Community/System Factors

Access to care. Low-SES minorities tend to have limited access to resources (e.g., money, insurance coverage), quality care, and follow-up, despite being more frequently exposed to adverse physical and psychological events. Many of the poor are unemployed or underemployed and have limited access to insurance coverage. Minority women, in particular, have higher rates of unemployment and lower paying jobs, while relying more on public health insurance than their White counterparts. Minorities are also more likely to receive less comprehensive and lower quality care than Whites. Studies comparing health service usage patterns have found that Black patients are more likely to live in areas where the rates of specialized medical procedures and quality of care are low, and to receive medical care in a hospital clinic or emergency room, with different providers at each visit, and thus receive less continuous care (Baicker, Chandra, Skinner, & Wennberg, 2004; Blendon, Aiken, Freeman, & Corey, 1989).

Individuals from low-SES backgrounds are also less likely to use mental health services (Barker & Adelman, 1994) for a number of reasons. Physical proximity is an obviously vital component to treatment seeking, and individuals living in isolated, rural communities (e.g., American Indian/Alaska Natives) are limited in their mental health treatment options. Stigma and acceptability of services are two other significant barriers. As noted by Gary (2005): "Stigmatization of mental illness is one of the major reasons why persons who need treatment do not readily seek assistance, decide to delay treatment and support until a crisis develops, or the disorder becomes overpowering and debilitating." Moreover, the stigma of mental illness is compounded by being poor and a member of a minority group. Individuals who are uneducated, unemployed, poor, and from chaotic families are more likely to report barriers to mental health care unrelated to cost or availability (Steele, Dewa, & Lee, 2007). Finally, at least one study has reported that low-SES individuals are less likely to receive antidepressants and psychotherapy, and have less favorable mental health outcomes (Lorant et al., 2003).

Minorities' attitudes and experiences with the health care system are additional factors influencing their access to care. A long history of discrimination and exploitation of minorities in medical care and research have led to increased distrust of the health care system and health care providers and decreased their usage of health and mental health care. One recent study found that negative stereotypes and beliefs about the health and mental health care systems remain common among low-income Blacks and continue to negatively influence their likelihood of seeking care, adhering to treatment recommendations, and overall satisfaction with their care (Bogart, Bird, Walt, Delahanty, & Figler, 2004). In addition, one analysis of data from the National Comorbidity Study found an interaction between race and attitudes about mental health care, with African Americans having more positive attitudes than Whites toward *seeking* services, but being less likely to use them and having *less* positive attitudes after using mental health services than Whites (Diala et al., 2000). Similarly, gay/lesbian/bisexual/transgendered (GLBT) patients with negative attitudes toward the health care system or who perceive that their physicians have "gay-negative" attitudes are less likely to seek care (Heck, Sell, & Gorin, 2006; Owens, Riggle, & Rotosky, 2007; Steele, Tinmouth, & Luc, 2006). Finally, many Hispanic individuals face major language barriers in health care, resulting in difficulty communicating in ways to obtain proper treatment. Clearly, interventions seeking to increase access to health care services for minorities must be multifaceted in their approach by eliminating cost and convenience barriers, considering the ethnic/cultural match between provider and patient, educating providers on minorities' attitudes toward the health care system, and reducing the impact of stigma on help-seeking.

Neighborhood/Environmental Issues. Minorities are more likely to live in neighborhoods that are crowded, polluted, high in crime and discrimination, and have poor educational facilities and work environments (Baum, Garofalo, & Yali, 1999; Evans & Kantrowitz, 2002; Logan & Stults, 1999). Further, many of these low-income neighborhoods have become racially segregated, which impacts residents' access to education and employment opportunities, reduces access to social services, and accounts for the vast majority of Black-White differences in earnings, high school graduation rates, employment, and single-motherhood (Alba & Logan, 1993; Williams & Harris-Reid, 1999; Williams & Jackson, 2005). Individuals living in poor neighborhoods perceive their lives as more stressful, report more stressful life events, and experience increased social strain (Cohen, Kaplan, & Salone, 1999; Gallo et al., 2005). This chronic stress results in increased physical risk factors, subsequently increasing an individual's "allostatic load" and reducing their physical and mental health (Karlamangla, Singer, McEwen, Rowe, & Seeman, 2002; McEwen, 1998). Neighborhood quality and SES are associated with negative psychosocial experiences and mental health problems (Chen & Paterson, 2006). Two reports of large inner city samples found that the incidence of major depression increased in areas with a greater proportion of residents living below the poverty line, deteriorated housing, insufficient household food, and more prevalent social disorder, regardless of individual factors (Cutrona et al., 2005; Siefert et al., 2007). Individuals in low-SES neighborhoods are also more likely to have low life satisfaction and to become depressed when exposed to negative life events than individuals from higher SES areas (Cutrona et al., 2005; Schulz et al., 2000). Finally, drugs and alcohol are more prevalent, available, and marketed in low-income neighborhoods (Hacker, Collins, & Jacobson, 1987; MacIntyre, Maciver, & Sooman, 1993; Maxwell & Jacobson, 1989) resulting in as much as a two-fold increase in usage among residents of those communities (Lillie-Blanton, Anthony, & Schuster, 1993).

Experiences of racism/discrimination. Ethnic and sexual minorities of varied socioeconomic backgrounds are frequently exposed to racism and discrimination. A lifetime of adverse experiences and other forms of chronic psychological and physical stress arising from general social disadvantage (e.g., poverty, unemployment, limited resources, etc.) result in an additive negative affect on physical and mental well-being among low-SES ethnic minorities (Taylor & Turner, 2002). Among ethnic minorities, perceived discrimination is associated with reduced happiness and life satisfaction, lowered self-esteem, more negative health behaviors (e.g., smoking, alcohol use), and a reduced sense of mastery/control, purpose in life, autonomy, and potential for personal growth (Landrine & Klonoff, 2000; Ryff, Keyes, & Hughes, 2003; Schulz et al., 2000; Taylor & Turner, 2002; Williams & Jackson, 2005; Williams, Neighbors, & Jackson, 2003; Yen, Ragland, Greiner, & Fisher, 1999a,b). Men, African Americans, and those of low social status are especially vulnerable to the negative physical and psychological effects of discrimination and racism (Karlsen & Nazroo, 2002a,b; Krieger & Sidney, 1996), although one study found decreased life satisfaction and psychological distress among professional Hispanic women experiencing employment discrimination (Amaro, Russo, & Johnson, 1987). The effects of discrimination across the life span are cumulative in nature. One study of Black and Latino patients found that individuals with more lifetime exposure to discrimination were more likely to perceive new negative events as threatening and to cope with the experiences using anger (Brondolo et al., 2005). Also, risk for specific psychiatric diagnoses including major depression, generalized anxiety disorder, psychosis, anger problems, and substance use are elevated among individuals experiencing discrimination (Karlsen, Nazroo, McKenzie, Bhui, & Weich, 2005; Williams & Jackson, 2005; Williams et al., 2003). Perceptions of discrimination are also predictive of reduced quality of life and increased psychiatric disorder among GLBT individuals (Cochran, Mays, Alegria, Ortega, & Takeuchi, 2007; Diaz, Ayala, Bein, Henne, & Marin, 2001; Mays & Cochran, 2001). The physical and mental health problems arising from perceived discrimination are exacerbated if one responds and engages in passive or avoidant coping in response to the experiences, as opposed to taking a stand against discriminatory treatment (Krieger & Sidney, 1996). These findings indicate that experiences of discrimination play a primary role in health disparities, and that providers should seek to understand how these experiences influence individuals' response to treatment.

Acculturation. Among U.S. ethnic minorities, Hispanics and Asians are much more likely to have immigrated than to have been born in the U.S. These two groups, in general, face a number of significant stressors associated with acculturation, including separation from family, a lack of community, language barriers, and experiences of discrimination/racism (Caplan, 2007; Finch, Kolody, & Vega, 2000). However, the relationship between level of acculturation and mental health outcomes is very complex and has conflicting evidence. Some studies have found an inverse relationship between morbidity and acculturation (Cheung, 1995; Takeuchi et al., 1998), while others have found that increased acculturation is associated with an increased risk of psychiatric disorder (Guglani, Coleman, & Sonuga-Barke, 2000). One reason for the differences in these findings is that acculturation is associated both with increased SES and increased stress, which are mediated by factors such as social support, increased optimism, and perceptions of health (Shen & Takeuchi, 2001). These varied findings also reflect differences in the economic and political circumstances under which different groups arrive in the United States. For example, Uehara, Takeuchi, and Smukler (1994) found differences in the psychological functioning between Asian ethnic groups (e.g., Vietnamese, Japanese, Cambodian), much of which was explained by participants' refugee status, suggesting that contextual factors likely mediate the relationship between ethnic background and psychological functioning.

Family and Social Factors

Growing up in an unstable, low-SES household with uneducated parents, and/ or with a single-parent has been shown to have both short and long-term effects on physical and mental health. First, at least two published reports of a longitudinal study of over 700 families across an 18-year period found increased rates of adult anxiety, depression, conduct, and personality disorders among children from low-SES families, even after controlling for offspring demographic characteristics and parental depression (Johnson et al., 1999; Ritsher, Warner, Johnson, & Dohrenwend, 2001). Similar results have been reported in retrospective surveys of adults (Gilman, Kawachi, Fitzmaurice, & Buka, 2003). An increased risk for depression has also been observed among children from disrupted, low-income families, and families who move frequently (Lynch & Kaplan, 1997). In addition to income, parental education is associated with health outcomes and children's perception of the world. An examination of low-SES teenagers found that teens living in homes with uneducated parents perceive their lives as more stressful and are less optimistic about the future (Finkelstein, Kubzansky, Capitman, & Goodman, 2007). Chen, Martin, and

Matthews (2006) found that poor health among children was associated with fewer years of parent education among White and Black children, while psychological/behavioral problems in children appear to be more strongly linked to the cumulative effects of stressful experiences, parental distress, and adverse events than parental education, housing status, or family income (Masten, Miliotis, Graham-Bermann, Ramirez, & Neemann, 1993). However, these relationships were virtually nonexistent among Hispanic and Asian children, suggesting that the negative effects of limited parental education may be mediated by differences in health behaviors and other lifestyle characteristics of low-SES Hispanic and Asian children.

Family structure plays a role in the well-being and health of minority children and their parents. Single parent households are strongly linked to poverty and minority status, placing children in these homes at increased risk of having limited resources, food, etc. Children in single-parent households are also at higher risk for emotional, behavioral, and educational problems (Fendrich, Warner, & Weissman, 1990; McLeod & Shanahan, 1993). In addition, single mothers report higher levels of psychological distress and psychiatric morbidity than mothers in two-parent families. This difference appears to be more strongly linked to their increased exposure to perpetual financial and caregiving strain than other mothers, as opposed to deficits in social competence or coping skills (Avison, 2002). Finally, several studies have reported no difference in access to health care between children from single-parent homes and those from two-parent homes, primarily due to the availability of public health insurance (Chen & Escarce, 2006; Heck & Parker, 2002).

Individual Factors

Race. Research investigating the relationship between race and mental health has been mixed. Some studies have found that African Americans report fewer lifetime psychiatric disorders (Breslau et al., 2006) and lower levels of distress (Bratter & Eschbach, 2005) compared to Whites and other minorities. However, others have reported greater levels of psychological distress (Williams & Harris-Reid, 1999) and higher rates of dementia and psychotic disorders (Husaini et al., 2002) in African Americans than in their White counterparts. American Indian/Alaska Natives (AIAN) have particularly high rates of mental health problems, with the lifetime prevalence of psychiatric disorders in this population being reported as high as 21% (Harris, Edlund, & Larson, 2005) and rates of suicide and drug/alcohol use disorders that are significantly higher than those of both Whites and other minority groups (Duran et al., 2004; Fingerhut & MaKuc, 1992). Differences in mental health outcomes between ethnic groups tend to disappear or even reverse after accounting for psychosocial variables such as neighborhood income, experiences of discrimination, and individual experiences (Schulz et al., 2000). For example, among Asian Americans, occupational and educational indicators of SES are more strongly linked to self-esteem than income (Twenge & Campbell, 2002). These studies indicate that race likely affects mental health through multiple pathways, with some groups being especially susceptible to the effects of the chronic stressors (e.g., poverty, chronic illness, nonmarriage) that are common in low-SES populations.

Sexual orientation. Several investigations have demonstrated that sexual minorities tend to be at higher risk for psychiatric disorders than their heterosexual counterparts (Cochran et al., 2007; Mays & Cochran, 2001). GLBT populations are at higher risk for suicidal behavior (Cochran & Mays, 2000; Garofalo, Wolf, Wissow, Woods, & Goodman, 1999; Remafedi, French, Story, Resnick, & Blum, 1998). Rather than attributing these higher rates of psychopathology to the impact of sexual orientation, researchers tend to attribute these higher incidences to the impact of stigma and discrimination against sexual minorities (e.g., emotional, financial/occupational, and interpersonal impact; Mays & Cochran, 2001; Mays, Cochran, & Roeder, 2004; Meyer, 2003). These individuals are also less likely to receive treatment for their psychiatric disorders, in part due to actual and perceived discrimination by treatment providers (e.g., Cochran & Mays, 1988; Owens et al., 2007; Willging, Salvador, & Kano, 2006).

Gender. Several studies have reported a relationship between gender and health outcomes in low-SES populations. Women are at increased risk of poverty as a result of wage disparities compared to men, gender discrimination, and the disproportionate need to be a single parent, which also limits their access to health insurance. Low-SES women more frequently report health problems, drug use, and poor mental health (Gold et al., 2006; Nyamathi, Berg, Jones, & Leake, 2005), and are a greater mortality risk than similar samples of men (Backlund, Sorlie, & Johnson, 1996). Furthermore, in the extreme poor, female mortality is more strongly connected to income than that of males (Backlund et al., 1996), as is females' self-esteem (Twenge & Campbell, 2002). Men, on the other hand, account for a greater proportion of total health care costs than women, primarily due to their more frequent use of emergency/inpatient services and less frequent use of outpatient services compared to women (Husaini et al., 2002). Finally, analyses from the Epidemiological Catchment Area (ECA) study found an interaction between gender and race with low-SES White males having higher rates of psychiatric disorders than Black males and low-SES Black females having higher rate of substance abuse disorders than White females (Williams, Takeuchi, & Adair, 1992).

Age. Older minorities are at somewhat increased risk for health and mental health problems compared to younger minorities and Whites, at least part of which is explained by cumulative life experiences of racism, discrimination, and decreasing socioeconomic status (Peters, 2004; Tiffin, Pearce, & Parker, 2005). Older African Americans are more likely to be distressed by experiences of racism, but are more likely to internalize their anger, increasing their risk for stress-related health problems (e.g., hypertension). Old age also attenuates the impact of SES on psychological variables, such as self-esteem (Twenge & Campbell, 2002), and on overall mortality rates (Backlund et al., 1996).

Psychological Factors. SES is associated with a number of psychological factors that play a role in the mental health and well-being of minorities. First, lower family and neighborhood SES is associated with increased levels of anger and hostility in both adults and adolescents (Cohen et al., 1999; Gallo & Matthews, 2003). One investigation of the perceptions of a diverse sample of inner city residents reported that lower SES subjects described their social worlds as more hostile and less friendly and perceived more exposure to dominant/controlling behavior by others compared to higher SES subjects (Gallo, Smith, & Cox, 2006). In turn, higher levels of anger and chronic hostility increase the risk of cardiovascular disease and poor health in general (Helmers, Posluszny, & Krantz, 1994). Second, SES is strongly linked to self-esteem, particularly status- or aptitude-related indicators of SES such as occupation and education (Turner, Lloyd, & Roszell, 1999; Twenge & Campbell, 2002). Adler and colleagues (2000) found that subjective social standing was more predictive of depression, self-rated health, and obesity than objective measures of SES. Third, having an external locus of control negatively impacts physical and mental health. One notable study by Gallo and colleagues (2005) found lower levels of perceived control and higher levels of social strain among women of a lower SES. This reduced sense of control and increased strain from the social environment contributed to higher rates of negative affect as did having more instrumental and psychological resources. Next, the way in which individuals interpret negative events and their ability to cope effectively can influence their overall physical and mental health. An investigation by Chen, Langer, Raphaelson, and Matthews (2004) found that low-SES children were more likely to interpret ambiguous events as a threat, and that a lack of positive experiences in life was a stronger predictor of this relationship than specific negative experiences (e.g., trauma, exposure to violence). Finally, employing passive coping responses appears to increase the risk of stress-related health problems. One study found that low-SES African American men who employed a passive coping style were three times more likely to be hypertensive than African American men of higher SES who used a more active coping style (James, 1994).

Resiliency Factors

Overview

Despite the strong positive correlation between SES and health outcomes (e.g., Adler & Snibbe, 2003; Gallo et al., 2005), positive mental health outcomes do occur in low-SES minority populations. Recently, the National Comorbidity Survey Replication (NCS-R; Breslau et al., 2006) examined rates of mental illness among Hispanic, Black, and White groups and found lower lifetime risk for common internalizing disorders (i.e., depressive and anxiety disorders) among both minority groups. Moreover, the NCS-R found that lower risk among minorities was more pronounced at lower levels of education, suggesting the presence of protective factors among low-SES minorities. Likewise, Keyes (2007) has argued that African Americans have better mental health outcomes than Caucasians and suggests that differences between these two groups could be even more pronounced in the absence of discrimination. Thus, despite the large number of risk factors that are associated with being a member of a minority group (e.g., racism & discrimination), the presence of any number of resiliency factors provide the opportunity for improved mental health. Resiliency has been defined as "adaptation despite risk" (Arrington & Wilson, 2000). More specifically, resilience factors are mechanisms that allow an individual to flourish taking into account the impact of person-level, family-level, and community-level risk factors that may put them at risk of negative outcome (e.g., Murry, Bynum, Brody, Willert, & Stephens, 2001; Rutter, 1987). Given that low-SES minority individuals face numerous barriers to optimal physical and mental health, it is particularly important to isolate mechanisms that help people to combat negative outcomes.

Improving resiliency among low-SES minorities cannot be achieved simply by adding an influx of resources and money. Results from the National Survey of Black Americans, a nationally representative sample of the adult Black population, demonstrated that the negative relationship between SES and distress was not eliminated for those receiving financial assistance (Neighbors & Laveist, 1989). Rather, there is a complex interaction between personal goals, resources (e.g., social role, external possessions including finances, or personal characteristics), and well-being, such that psychological well-being is influenced by concordance between personal resources and goals (Diener & Fujita, 1995). Therefore, it is imperative to identify factors which improve both access to resources and encourage identification of personally meaningfully goals to improve psychological well-being among low-SES minorities. In this section, we will highlight community-level, family-level, and person-level variables that have been empirically identified as resiliency factors.

Community Level

Cultural identification. Both the Social Causation model (Hollingshead et al., 1954) and the Social Selection model (Wender et al., 1973) suggest a complex interaction between environmental factors and health/well-being. Although environmental factors are typically examined as risk factors, there is evidence to suggest that several community-level variables may influence mental health resilience among low-SES minorities. Several empirical investigations have demonstrated that more positive identification with one's cultural background influences the strength of the relationship between stress and health outcomes among low-SES minorities. Walters, Simoni, and Evans-Campbell (2002) have theorized that Native American cultural practice influence the relationship between sociocultural stressors and health outcomes. Walters and colleagues' indigenist "stress-coping" model identified the following cultural factors as resiliency factors, which aid in coping following traumas or other life stressors:

family and community social support, enculturation, identity attitudes, spiritual coping, and participation in traditional ceremonies and health practices (Walters, 1995, 1999; Walters, Simoni, & Evans-Campbell, 2002). Mossakowski (2003) also found that higher levels of ethnic pride among Filipino Americans were predictive of fewer depressive symptoms. Likewise, Farver, Bhadha, and Narang (2002) demonstrated that newly immigrated Asian Indian adolescents who had more integrative acculturation (e.g., identification with both Indian and American cultures) had better psychological functioning in contrast to those who either identified primarily with one culture and/or felt disconnected from both cultures. Relatedly, Crawford, Allison, and Zamboni (2002) reported similar results with gay and bisexual African American men, such that men with more integrated positive beliefs about their race and sexual orientation reported better mental health (e.g., self-esteem) than those with less integrated beliefs. Collectively, these empirical findings suggest that feeling connected to one's culture of origin and to the culture of one's community may function as resiliency factors to improve psychological well-being among low-SES minorities.

Access to health care. When minority individuals have better access to care, they experience improved mental health well-being (e.g., Miranda & Cooper, 2004). However, acceptance of cultural values and beliefs about health care may also influence psychological well-being via help-seeking behavior among low-SES minorities. For example, although the traditional "American" health care system relies on the expertise of physicians and traditional Western medicine, Pumariega, Rogers, & Rothe (2005) have theorized that cultural beliefs/ attitudes about health care may influence whether minority individuals choose to seek assistance from neighborhood wise ladies (i.e., "co-madres") and traditional healers or from physicians and mental health professionals. Racial and ethnic concordance, i.e., members of same racial/ethnic group, between patient and provider has also been identified as a factor that improves health outcome and patient experience among minorities (Cooper et al., 2003). Alternatively, when formal health care facilities are not available, capitalizing on community resources often leads to improved resiliency. For example, Rasheed and Rasheed (2003) found that rural older African Americans generally have limited access to formal health care services compared to urban elders. As such, rural minority elders tend to make use of church-based and community-based services to improve their physical and mental health well-being in spite of limited resources. Taken together, these findings suggest that incorporation of cultural attitudes and beliefs about health care into mental health care treatment facilities may improve both access to treatment and the impact of the treatments provided in these centers for low-SES minorities.

Family Level

Social support. Families are embedded within communities, and there are a number of family-level variables that promote mental health among low-SES minority families. Social support has been identified as a robust indicator of health and well-being (Cohen et al., 1999; Cohen & Syme, 1985). However, familial and social support may be particularly important in the context of other risk factors such as poverty. First, we see lower rates of psychological disorders and suicide attempts (Barrett & Turner, 2005; Compton, Thompson, & Kaslow, 2005; deGroot, Auslander, Williams, Sherraden, & Haire- Joshu, 2003) and higher rates of usage of mental health resources (Barker & Adelman, 1994) when individuals have supportive networks. It may be that with additional emotional (e.g., listening) and instrumental support (e.g., offer of tangible goods), resource-poor individuals are better able to cope with their circumstances. Several investigations have examined coping and mental health outcome among low-SES minority women. Belle has argued that poor women are able to persevere because they care for and sustain each other in times of stress (Belle, 1990; Belle & Doucet, 2003). Support from family and friends has been associated with more effective coping and reduced psychological distress in several studies of low-income African American women (Durden, Hill, & Angel, 2007; Ennis, Hobfoll, & Schroder, 2000; Jackson, Gyamfi, Brooks-Gunn, & Blake, 1998; Schulz et al., 2006). McKelvey and McKenry (2002) have also reported associations between well-being and use of formal support (e.g., religious leader or therapist) among Black women following divorce. Moreover, it is noteworthy that having support from nonresident family members is associated with positive outcomes. Jackson (1999) found that single minority mothers reported that nonresident fathers' involvement in the lives of their children is associated with lower levels of depression. Further, in the absence of support from biological families, sexual minorities often create informal families to provide support (Oswald, 2002). Finally, social support may be needed to improve mental health outcomes when formal resources are lacking for low-SES minorities. For example, Willging and colleagues (2006) reported that low-income, rural lesbian, gay, bisexual, and transgendered individuals tended to utilize social support to improve their mental health as they found available formal programs to be unsupportive of their particular needs. Thus, future interventions may need to examine the idiographic impact of social support on the mental health of low-SES minorities, rather than examining social support as a broad factor.

Parenting Style and Childcare. There is a complex, multidirectional relationship between SES, parenting style, and mental health status of low-SES minority families. First, access to childcare is vital for parental mental and physical well-being. Research has determined that minority women are more likely to utilize both friends and family for childcare than nonminority women. Furthermore, African American women are more likely than White women to share housing with adult kin (Hogan, Hao, & Parish, 1990). Reliance on a kinship network allows low-SES minority women greater access to resources (e.g., childcare and support) than financial resources would provide otherwise. Relatedly, several investigations have demonstrated that both resident and nonresident fathers' participation in childcare had salutary effects on child and maternal well-being (Black, Dubowitz, & Starr, 1999; Jackson, 1999).

Furthermore, Taylor and Roberts (1995) have also demonstrated that mothers with adequate support engage in more supportive parenting practices. Finally, parenting style has salutary effects on childhood wellbeing. Sullivan and Farrell (1999) demonstrated that frequent parent–child communication, positive parental role modeling, negative parental attitudes toward deviance, parents' insistence upon school attendance, and parents' efforts to maintain healthy relationships with their children are all parenting variables that are associated with less substance use. Furthermore, Formoso, Gonzales, & Aiken (2000) found that parenting style has differential effects on girls versus boys. Whereas parental attachment and monitoring were protective for low-SES girls, these variables served as risk factors for boys. Third, supportive parent-child relationships are protective with respect to child mental health (e.g., Gorman-Smith, Tolan, Henry, & Florsheim, 2000; Klein & Forehand, 2000; Murry & Brody, 1999; Ruiz, Roosa, & Gonzales, 2002). Finally, parental encouragement, involvement, and motivation have all been shown to improve adolescent adjustment and psychological well-being (e.g., greater self-reliance, greater school engagement, less problem behavior, and less psychological distress; Smokowski, Reynolds, & Bezruczko, 1999; Taylor, 1996). Given the bidirectional effects between childhood and adult SES and mental well-being, interventions to improve childhood mental and physical health will likely lead to exponential gains in adulthood (Adler & Snibbe, 2003).

Availability of Resources. By definition, low-SES individuals have limited financial and educational resources. Improving this deficit may occur either by improving the acquisition of new resources or by slowing the loss of existing resources. Hobfoll and Johnson (2003) have demonstrated that loss of resources has relatively more damaging effects on mental health than an influx of resources can have to improve mental health among poor women. These findings suggest that interventions should work to reduce resource loss, rather than encouraging resource gain. Among the existing resilience factors that aid low-SES minority families in maintaining psychological well-being are the availability of instrumental support, a loan during a time of crisis, childcare, transportation, and home ownership (deGroot et al., 2003; Israel, Farquhar, Schulz, James, & Parker, 2002; McLoyd, Jayaratne, Ceballo, & Borquez, 1994; Siefert et al., 2007).

Person Level

Gender. The psychological literature had demonstrated gender differences in the prevalence of psychological disorders with higher rates of depression among women (Nolen-Hoeksema, 2002) and higher rates of substance use disorders (Office of Applied Studies, 2004) among men. Therefore, gender may function as both a risk and resiliency factor for low-SES minorities. First, it appears that female adolescents may have lower rates of alcohol and drug use than males (Barker & Adelman, 1994). Second, decision-making ability is predictive of improved psychological wellness for males but not females (Epstein, Griffin, &

Botvin, 2002). Third, although perceived discrimination is consistently a negative predictor of psychological well-being, Ryff and colleagues (2003) only found adverse effects of high levels of perceived discrimination among women for measures of well-being including self-acceptance, environmental mastery, positive relations with others, personal growth, and autonomy. These results suggest that being female may be protective against substance abuse, whereas being male may be protective with regards to psychological well-being in the face of perceived discrimination.

Marital/Relationship Status. The literature has demonstrated the positive effect of marriage on mental health (e.g., Simon, 2002; Marcussen, 2005). However, marriage does not have a beneficial impact for all; rather, the literature demonstrates that mental health benefits are contingent upon marital satisfaction (Barrett, 2000; Bradbury, Fincham, & Beach, 2000) and the absence of negative influences such as partner violence (e.g., Leone, Johnson, Cohan, & Lloyd, 2004). Several empirical investigations demonstrate the health benefits of marriage among low-SES minorities, such that married individuals experience less distress and discrimination than single individuals (Durden, Hill, & Angel, 2007; Gary, 1995). Stimpson, Peek, & Markides (2006) demonstrated a contagion effect within older Mexican American couples such that wives' mental health was influenced by husbands' well-being. However, husbands' mental health was not influenced by wives' functioning (see also Peek, Stimpson, & Townsend, 2006). Thus, given that marital satisfaction appears to be a resiliency factor, interventions should encourage and foster healthy marriages among heterosexual couples. Research has also identified that committed relationships among sexual minorities improve their mental health outcomes, particularly with respect to coping in response to stress and availability of economic and emotional resources (Kirkpatrick, 1987; Peplau & Fingerhut, 2007; Rostosky, Riggle, Gray, & Hatton, 2007). As similar relational processes predict relationship satisfaction among heterosexual and homosexual couples (Gottman et al., 2003), healthy relationships likely improve mental health outcomes among low-SES minorities regardless of marital status. Policy researchers may want to examine how legal recognition of committed relationships among low-SES minority couples will influence mental and physical health (e.g., health insurance coverage; King & Barlett, 2006).

Psychological Factors. Numerous psychological variables have been shown to influence overall psychological well-being among low-SES minorities. First, higher levels of perceived control/mastery are associated with better health, greater life satisfaction, less anger, and lower depressive symptoms (Ennis et al., 2000; Hobfoll, Jackson, Hobfoll, Pierce, & Young, 2002; Hobfoll & Jackson, 2003; Hobfoll, Schroeder, Wells, & Malek, 2002; Lachman & Weaver, 1998). Furthermore, Lachman and Weaver's (1998) investigation demonstrated that a high sense of control among the lowest income individuals results in similar mental health outcomes compared to individuals with much higher income and resources. Second, feelings of competence appear to predict overall well-being, as well as lower substance use. Several studies by Epstein and colleagues

(2000a,b; 2002) found that higher levels of competence among high-school students (as measured by decision making and self-efficacy) are associated with higher levels of positive mental health (as measured by psychological wellness) and reduced use of use of alcohol and cigarettes. Finally, personality characteristics may influence psychological well-being among low-SES minorities. Results from a culturally sensitive intervention with minority youth found that prevention efforts lowered risk-taking behavior and decreased substance use (Botvin, Schinke, Epstein, Diaz, & Botvin, 1995). Finally, self-esteem has been shown to be a protective factor against poor mental health outcomes for African Americans, with strongest effects at lowest level of SES (deGroot et al., 2003; Gray-Little & Hafdahl, 2000; Murry et al., 2001).

Religion/Spirituality. Participation in organized religion and level of spirituality are prevalent among low-SES minority individuals and are associated with positive mental health outcomes (Franzini et al., 2005; Schieman, Pudrovska, Pearlin, & Ellison, 2006). In particular, many low-SES minority individuals may rely on religion to improve health and well-being due to the high cost of "Westernized" mental health care (Constantine, Myers, Kindaichi, & Moore, 2004). Furthermore, higher levels of religiosity, attendance at church, and/or belief in divine influence is associated with improved mental health, reduced level of distress, decreased use of alcohol and drugs among low-SES minority adolescents (see Rotosky, Danner, & Riggle, 2007 for disconfirming results), lowered self-reported hostility, and improved parenting practices and parent-child relationships (Brody & Flor, 1998; Schieman, Pudrovska, & Milkie, 2005; Schieman et al., 2006; Strayhorn, Weidman, & Larson, 1990; Sullivan & Farrell, 1999). Of particular interest is Schieman and colleagues' (2006) finding that a sense of divine control is highest among African Americans and individuals of low SES. Furthermore, the sense of divine control was negatively associated with distress among low-SES African Americans but was found to be positively associated with distress among low-SES White elders, suggesting that a sense of divine control is protective for minority but not majority individuals.

Education/Work. The empirical literature is somewhat mixed regarding the impact of education and work status on the psychological well-being of low-SES minorities. Some studies have demonstrated that education level and employment are protective against depression and other measures of poor psychological well-being (deGroot et al., 2003; Jackson et al., 1998; Smokowski, Mann, & Reynolds, 2004). However other studies have identified complex relationships between education, employment status, and psychological health. For example, Brody and Flor's (1997) investigation of economically stressed, single, African American mothers living in rural communities found that women with higher levels of education also perceived their financial status to be more adequate, which in turn, led to lower levels of depression and higher self-esteem. Ryff and colleagues (2003) also found that poorly educated African Americans had higher levels of self-acceptance than Whites and, conversely, that more highly educated African Americans reported an increased sense of purpose relative to Whites.

Finally, the NCS-R results also indicated a lower risk of psychological disorders among individuals at lower levels of education (Breslau et al., 2006). Collectively, these findings suggest that the relationship between education and psychological well-being is not necessarily linear in nature.

Future Directions

Given that the relationship between mental health and SES in minorities is multifactorial, it is crucial that intervention efforts reflect this and are culturally relevant to affected populations, address risk factors at individual, family, and community levels, and capitalize on the expanding base of knowledge on resiliency. As such, innovations are needed within mental health delivery, policy, and research that are synergistic and steered by community leaders and experts from a variety of disciplines (e.g., mental health, social work, legal, environmental). The remainder of this chapter is devoted to intervention, policy, and research pathways that seek to reduce mental health risks and increase resiliency in low-SES populations.

Mental Health Care Delivery

To improve mental health service delivery to low-SES minorities, a variety of systemic, cultural, and individual factors must be considered. Steele and colleagues (2007) provide a useful conceptual framework for examining barriers to mental health care in low-SES populations. They offer that barriers can be categorized into three primary groups: *accessibility* (e.g., cost, transportation, child care), *acceptability* (e.g., stigma, help-seeking beliefs, and cultural attitudes), and *availability* of convenient and culturally competent providers. Accessibility barriers are often those first addressed by clinics attempting to increase service utilization, such as expanding hours of operation or assisting with applications for social service benefits. However, many clinics have insufficient resources and/or conflicting priorities that prevent true accessibility. For example, GLBT individuals must be able to find clinics that are both financially and logistically accessible and staffed by clinicians who are sensitive to the unique needs of GLBT consumers (Owens et al., 2007). Camacho and colleagues (2002) offer that specialized health programs tailored to the complex needs of indigent populations are scarce and need to be more widely available in low-income communities. Further, when difficulties like transportation, childcare, and housing are reconceptualized as *health issues* impacting health and quality of life outcomes, they can be woven into our health care practices instead of treating them as ancillary.

Although accessibility difficulties are commonly thought to be primary deterrents to care, acceptability of mental health services may actually be more predictive of service utilization (Owens et al., 2007; Sareen et al, 2007; Steele et al., 2007). Low levels of acceptability for mental health care can stem from stigma, cultural beliefs systems that are not consistent with the use of formal mental health services, and individuals' perceptions and knowledge about mental issues (e.g., Pumariega et al., 2005). For example, many GLBT individuals may be reluctant to seek mental and physical health treatment for fear of the reaction and response of their treatment providers to their sexuality and lifestyle (Cochran & Mays, 1988; Owens et al., 2007; Willging et al., 2006). Thus, altering service delivery to better fit with patients' health beliefs and value systems may encourage increased use. For example, Yeung and colleagues (2006) demonstrated increased acceptability of and engagement in psychiatric services by Chinese Americans when those services were integrated into primary care services. Provider education is also important with respect to improving acceptability of services. Culturally sensitive screening and motivational interventions performed within the context of environments accessed by low-SES minority groups can create a bridge into mental health care by identifying patient needs, debunking myths and stereotypes about mental health treatment, and problem-solving treatment obstacles (Stepleman, Hann, Santos, & House, 2006).

While availability barriers vary by geography and population, shortages of mental health providers for rural dwellers (Hinton, Dembling, & Stern, 2003), children (Kim, 2003; Pumariega et al., 2005), GLBT populations (Willging et al., 2006), and non-English speaking minorities (Musser-Granski & Carillo, 1997) are well documented. The use of bicultural, bilingual outreach workers in local community environments (Musser-Granski & Carillo, 1997), telepsychiatry services (Rohland, Saleh, Rohere, & Romitti, 2000), and loan repayment as incentives for new providers to work in low-SES, minority communities (Gamm, 2004) are promising. However, these interventions also have drawbacks, such as providers leaving these communities as soon as contractual obligations are met or patient apprehension about using technology to facilitate care. Capitalizing on natural leaders within communities as partners in mental health prevention and intervention is another possible alternative (Blank, Mahmood, Fox, & Guterbock, 2002) but necessitates ongoing commitment to training, relationship building, and resources for success. Furthermore, community-based education on coping and stress management techniques (Adler & Snibbe, 2003) and neighborhood improvement programs that foster community pride, interpersonal connectivity and social control (Wen, Hawkley, & Cacioppo, 2006) are other nontraditional means for buffering individuals and families from stress and improving well-being that may circumvent availability issues.

Mental Health Policy

Health care reform is a crucial component of reducing the mental health risks and treatment disparities that exist in this country. One issue plaguing the

United States has been the lack of mental health parity, such that lifetime benefits of mental health services are not equivalent to those of medical and surgical benefits. As low-SES minorities are frequently unable to pay out of pocket for uncovered services, they are severely affected by this lack of parity by being limited to high premium, high deductible, low coverage insurance plans. The initial Mental Health Parity Act (MHPA) was passed by Congress in 1996 but had many loopholes and resulted in some companies actually decreasing benefits (Ault, 2007). MHPA was set to expire in 2001 but has been extended since and is up again for renewal in 2007. Although most states now have mental health parity laws, the benefits and exclusions vary widely. In many cases, continued revision of the laws to create actual parity is needed.

According to Alegria, Perez, and Williams (2003), mental health disparities will not be ameliorated through mental health care reform alone. Rather, alteration of the social conditions that increase risks for mental illness must also change. Given the disparities in housing, education, and poverty between minorities and Whites, and their association with stress and poorer mental health, they argue that corresponding public policy can affect mental health through improvement of these conditions (Alegria et al., 2003). For example, the Earned Income Tax Credit (EITC) has resulted in decreased poverty rates and increased entrance into the labor force, with African Americans and Latinos appearing to benefit the most (Porter, Primus, Rawlings, & Rosenbaum, 1998). Sexual minorities also struggle for partner-based health insurance as many health insurance plans extend coverage only to marital partners, excluding same-sex partners and nonmarried heterosexual life partners from needed health benefits. Extension of benefits coverage would likely lead to improved health outcomes among low-SES racial and sexual minorities (King & Barlett, 2006). Similarly, additional funding to combat hunger and nutritional deficits (Siefert et al., 2007) and incorporation of behavioral health education into welfare-related employment programs (Jayakody, Danziger, & Pollack, 2000) have been suggested. However, as mentioned earlier in the resiliency section of the chapter, there must also be a stronger focus on policies that assist low-SES families in not only acquiring new resources, but on preventing the loss of currently held resources, such as safe housing and employment.

Mental Health Research

Future directions for research need to support intervention and policy efforts while also filling in the gaps in our understanding about mental health and low-SES minorities. In particular, more longitudinal studies are necessary to better discern the causal relationships between SES and mental health across the life span for different minorities groups (Adler & Snibbe, 2003). Studies that examine the independent and interactive contributions of race, sexual orientation, and SES for mental health outcomes are also a priority, as are intervention studies that examine the influence of transportation, support systems, attitudes and other potentially amenable variables in order to enhance interventions (Shavers, 2007). Moreover, it is important to determine the influence of neighborhood level interventions (Chen & Paterson, 2006) and social policy changes on reducing mental health disparities, such as the Individuals with Disabilities Education Act (IDEA) or the EITC, as they have the ability to reach a large numbers of individuals.

Summary

Although there appear to be significant mental health risks for low-SES minorities, there is also compelling evidence of resiliency within individuals, families, and communities. We are optimistic that the growing efforts to reduce health care disparities through the cultivation of novel mental health interventions, social reform, and applied research targeting low-SES minorities will result in genuine and durable change.

References

Adler, N. E., Epel, E. S., Castellazzo, G., & Ickovics, J. R. (2000). Relationship of subjective and objective social status with psychological and physical health: Preliminary data in healthy white women. *Health Psychology, 19*(6), 585–591.

Adler, N.E., & Ostrove, J. M. (1999). Socioeconomic status and health: What we know and what we don't. *Annals of the New York Academy of Sciences, 896*, 3–15.

Adler, N. E., & Snibbe, A. C. (2003). The role of psychosocial processes in explaining the gradient between socioeconomic status and health. *Directions in Psychological Science, 12*(4), 119–123.

Alba, R. D., & Logan, J. R. (1993). Minority proximity to whites in suburbs: An individual-level analysis of segregation. *The American Journal of Sociology, 98*(6), 1388–1427.

Alegria, M., Perez, D. J., & Williams, S. (2003). The role of public policies in reducing mental health disparities for people of color. *Health Affairs, 22*(5), 51–64.

Amaro, H., Russo, N. F., & Johnson, J. (1987). Family and work predictors of psychological well-being among Hispanic women professionals. *Psychology of Women Quarterly, 11*(4), 505–521.

Angell, M. (1993). Privilege and health–What is the connection? *The New England Journal of Medicine, 329*(2), 126–127.

Arrington, E.G., & Wilson, M.N. (2000). A re-examination of risk and resilience during adolescence: Incorporating culture and diversity. *Journal of Child and Family Studies, 9*(2), 221–230.

Ault, A. (2007, November 6). Equal coverage for mental health? The Washington Post. Retrieved November 29, 2007, from the World Wide Web: www.washingtonpost.com/wp-dyn/content/article/2007/11/02/AR2007110201764.html

Avison, W. R. (2002). Family structure and mental health. In A. Maney & J. Ramos (Eds.), *Socioeconomic conditions, stress and mental disorders: Toward a new synthesis of research and public policy*. Bethesda, MD: NIH Office of Behavioral and Social Research.

Backlund, E., Sorlie, P.D., & Johnson, N.J. (1996). The shape of the relationship between income and mortality in the United States: Evidence from the national longitudinal mortality study. *Annals of Epidemiology, 6*(1), 12–23.

Baicker, K., Chandra, A., Skinner, J. S., & Wennberg, J. E. (2004). Who you are and where you live: How race and geography affect the treatment of Medicare beneficiaries. Health Affairs, Web Exclusive.

Barker, L. A., & Adelman, H. S. (1994). Mental health and help-seeking among ethnic minority adolescents. *Journal of Adolescence, 17*(3), 251–263.

Barrett, A. E. (2000). Marital trajectories and mental health. *Journal of Health and Social Behavior, 41*(4), 451–464.

Barrett, A. E., & Turner, R. J. (2005). Family structure and mental health: The mediating effects of socioeconomic status, family process, and social stress. *Journal of Health and Social Behavior, 46*(2), 156–169.

Baum, A., Garofalo, J. P., & Yali, A. M. (1999). Socioeconomic status and chronic stress: Does stress account for SES effects on health? *Annals of the New York Academy of Sciences, 896*, 131–144.

Belle, D. (1990). Poverty and women's mental health. *American Psychologist, 45*(3), 385–389.

Belle, D., & Doucet, J. (2003). Poverty, inequality, and discrimination as sources of depression among U.S. women. *Psychology of Women Quarterly, 27*(2), 101–113.

Black, M. M., Dubowitz, H., & Starr, R. H., Jr. (1999). African American fathers in low income, urban families: Development, behavior, and home environment of their three-year-old children. *Child Development, 70*(4), 967–978.

Blank, M. B., Mahmood, M., Fox, J. C., & Guterbock, T. (2002). Alternative mental health services: The role of the Black Church in the South. *American Journal of Public Health, 92*(10), 1668–1672.

Blendon, R. J., Aiken, L. H., Freeman, H. E., & Corey, C. R. (1989). Access to medical care for black and white Americans. A matter of continuing concern. *Journal of the American Medical Association, 261*(2), 278–281.

Bogart, L. M., Bird, S. T., Walt, L. C., Delahanty, D. L., & Figler, J. L. (2004). Association of stereotypes about physicians to health care satisfaction, help-seeking behavior, and adherence to treatment. *Social Science & Medicine, 58*(6), 1049–1058.

Botvin, G. J., Schinke, S. P., Epstein, J. A., Diaz, T., & Botvin, E. M. (1995). Effectiveness of culturally focused and generic skills training approaches to alcohol and drug abuse prevention among minority adolescents: Two-year follow-up results. *Psychology of Addictive Behaviors, 9*(3), 183–194.

Bradbury, T.N., Fincham, F.D., & Beach, S.R.H. (2000). Research on the nature and determinants of marital satisfaction: A decade in review. *Journal of Marriage and the Family, 62*(4), 964–980.

Bratter, J. L., & Eschbach, K. (2005). Race/ethnic differences in nonspecific psychological distress: Evidence from the national health interview survey. *Social Science Quarterly, 86*(3), 620–644.

Breslau, J., Aguilar-Gaxiola, S., Kendler, K. S., Su, M., Williams, D. R., & Kessler, R. C. (2006). Specifying race-ethnic differences in risk for psychiatric disorder in a USA national sample. *Psychological Medicine, 36*(1), 57–68.

Brody, G. H., & Flor, D. L. (1997). Maternal psychological functioning, family processes, and child adjustment in rural, single-parent, African American families. *Developmental Psychology, 33*(6), 1000–1011.

Brondolo, E., Thompson, S., Brady, N., Appel, R., Cassells, A., Tobin, J. N., et al. (2005). The relationship of racism to appraisals and coping in a community sample. *Ethnicity & Disease, 15*(4, Suppl 5), S5–14.

Camacho F., Anderson, R. T., Bell, R. A., Goff, D. C. Jr, Duren-Winfield, V., Doss, D. D., et al. (2002). Investigating correlates of health related quality of life in a low-income sample of patients with diabetes. *Quality of Life Research: an International Journal of Quality of Life Aspects of Treatment, Care and Rehabilitation, 11*(8), 783–796.

Caplan, S. (2007). Latinos, acculturation, and acculturative stress: A dimensional concept analysis. *Policy, Politics, & Nursing Practice, 8*(2), 93–106.

Carnon, A. G., Ssemwogerere, A., Lamont, D. W., Hole, D. J., Mallon, E. A., George, W. D., et al. (1994). Relation between socioeconomic deprivation and pathological prognostic factors in women with breast cancer. *British Medical Journal, 309*(6961), 1054–1057.

Chen, A. Y., & Escarce, J. J. (2006). Effects of family structure on children's use of ambulatory visits and prescription medications. *Health Services Research, 41*(5), 1895–1914.

Chen, E., Langer, D. A., Raphaelson, Y. E., & Matthews, K. A. (2004). Socioeconomic status and health in adolescents: The role of stress interpretations. *Child Development, 75*(4), 1039–1052.

Chen, E., Martin, A. D., & Matthews, K. A. (2006). Understanding health disparities: The role of race and socioeconomic status in children's health. *American Journal of Public Health, 96*(4), 702–708.

Chen, E., & Paterson, L. Q. (2006). Neighborhood, family, and subjective socioeconomic status: How do they relate to adolescent health? *Health Psychology, 25*(6), 704–714.

Cheung, P. (1995). Acculturation and psychiatric morbidity among Cambodian refugees in New Zealand. *International Journal of Social Psychiatry, 41*(2), 109–119.

Cochran, S.D., & Mays, V. M. (1988). Disclosure of sexual preference to physicians by black lesbian and bisexual women. *The Western Journal of Medicine, 49*(5), 616–619.

Cochran, S. D., & Mays, V. M. (2000). Lifetime prevalence of suicide symptoms and affective disorders among men reporting same-sex sexual partners: Results from NHANES III. *American Journal of Public Health, 90*(4), 573–578.

Cochran, S.D., Mays, V.M., Alegria, M., Ortega, A.N., & Takeuchi, D. (2007). Mental health and substance use disorders among Latino and Asian American lesbian, gay, and bisexual adults. *Journal of Consulting and Clinical Psychology, 75*(5), 785–794.

Cohen, S., Kaplan, G. A., & Salone, J. T. (1999). The role of psychological characteristics in the relation between socioeconomic status and perceived health. *Journal of Applied Social Psychology, 29*(3), 445–468.

Cohen, S., & Syme, L. (1985). *Social support and health.* New York: Academic Press.

Compton, M. T., Thompson, N. J., & Kaslow, N. J. (2005). Social environment factors associated with suicide attempt among low-income African Americans: the protective role of family relationships and social support. *Social Psychiatry and Psychiatric Epidemiology, 40*(3), 175–85.

Constantine, M. G., Myers, L. J., Kindaichi, M., & Moore, J. L. (2004). Exploring indigenous mental health practices: The roles of healers and helpers in promoting well-being in people of color. *Counseling and Values, 48*(2), 110–125.

Cooper, L., Roter, D., Johnson, R., Ford, D., Steinwachs, D., & Powe, N. (2003). Patient-centered communication, ratings of care, and concordance of patient and physician race. *Annals of International Medicine, 139*(11), 907–916.

Crawford, I., Allison, K. W., & Zamboni, B. D. (2002). The influence of dual-identity development on the psychosocial functioning of African-American gay and bisexual men. *Journal of Sex Research, 39*(3), 179–189.

Cutrona, C. E., Russell, D. W., Brown, P. A., Clark, L. A., Hessling, R. M., & Gardner, K. A. (2005). Neighborhood context, personality, and stressful life events as predictors of depression among African American women. *Journal of Abnormal Psychology, 114*(1), 3–15.

Dayal, H. H., Power, R. N., & Chiu, C. (1982). Race and socio-economic status in survival from breast cancer. *Journal of Chronic Diseases, 35*(8), 675–683.

de Groot, M., Auslander, W., Williams, J. H., Sherraden, M., & Haire- Joshu, D. (2003). Depression and poverty among African American women at risk for Type 2 diabetes. *Annals of Behavioral Medicine, 25*(3), 172–181.

DeNavas-Walt, C., Proctor, B.D., & Lee, C. H. (2006). *Income, poverty, and health insurance coverage in the United States: 2005.* U.S. Government Printing Office, Washington, DC.

Diala, C., Muntaner, C., Walrath, C., Nickerson, K. J., LaVeist, T. A., & Leaf, P. J. (2000). Racial differences in attitudes toward professional mental health care and in the use of services. *American Journal of Orthopsychiatry, 70*(4), 455–464.

Diaz, R. M., Ayala, G., Bein, E., Henne, J., & Marin, B. V. (2001). The impact of homophobia, poverty, and racism on the mental health of gay and bisexual Latino men: Findings from 3 U.S. cities. *American Journal of Public Health, 91*(6), 927–932.

Diener, E., & Fujita, F. (1995). Resources, personal strivings, and subjective well-being: A nomothetic and idiographic approach. *Journal of Personality and Social Psychology, 68*(5), 926–935.

Duran, B., Sanders, M., Skipper, B., Waitzkin, H., Malcoe, L. H., Paine, S., et al. (2004). Prevalence and correlates of mental disorders among Native American women in primary care. *American Journal of Public Health, 94*(1), 71–77.

Durden, E. D., Hill, T. D., & Angel, R. J. (2007). Social demands, social supports, and psychological distress among low-income women. *Journal of Social and Personal Relationships, 24*(3), 343–361.

Ennis, N. E., Hobfoll, S. E., & Schroder, K. E. (2000). Money doesn't talk, it swears: How economic stress and resistance resources impact innercity women's depressive mood. *American Journal of Community Psychology, 28*(2), 149–173.

Epstein, J. A., Griffin, K.W., & Botvin, G. J. (2000a). Competence skills help deter smoking among inner-city adolescents. *Tobacco Control, 9*, 33–39.

Epstein, J. A., Griffin, K. W., & Botvin, G. J. (2000b). A model of smoking among inner-city adolescents: The role of personal competence and perceived social benefits of smoking. *Preventive Medicine, 31*(2), 107–114.

Epstein, J. A., Griffin, K. W., & Botvin, G. J. (2002). Positive impact of competence skills and psychological wellness in protecting inner-city adolescents from alcohol use. *Prevention Science, 3*(2), 95–104.

Evans, G., & Kantrowitz, E. (2002). Socio economic status and health: The potential role of environmental risk exposure. *Annual Review of Public Health, 23*, 303–331.

Farmer, M. M., & Ferraro, K. F. (2005). Are racial disparities in health conditional on socioeconomic status? *Social Science & Medicine, 60*(1), 191–204.

Farver, J. M., Bhadha, B. R., & Narang, S. K. (2002). Acculturation and psychological functioning in Asian Indian adolescents. *Social Development, 11*(1), 11–29.

Fendrich, M., Warner, V., & Weissman, M. M. (1990). Family risk factors, parental depression, and psychopathology in offspring. *Developmental Psychology, 26*, 40–50.

Finch, B. K., Kolody, B., & Vega, W. A. (2000). Perceived discrimination and depression among Mexican-origin adults in California. *Journal of Health and Social Behavior, 41*(3), 295–313.

Fingerhut, L. A., & MaKuc, D. M. (1992). Mortality among minority populations in the United States. *American Journal of Public Health, 82*(8), 1168–1170.

Finkelstein, D. M., Kubzansky, L. D., Capitman, J., & Goodman, E. (2007). Socioeconomic differences in adolescent stress: The role of psychological resources. *Journal of Adolescent Health, 40*(2), 127–134.

Formoso, D., Gonzales, N. A., & Aiken, L. S. (2000). Family conflict and children's internalizing and externalizing behavior: Protective factors. *American Journal of Community Psychology, 28*(2), 175–199.

Franzini, L., Ribble, J. C., & Wingfield, K. A. (2005). Religion, sociodemographic and personal characteristics, and self-reported health in whites, blacks, and hispanics living in low-socioeconomic status neighborhoods. *Ethnicity & Disease, 15*, 469–484.

Gallo, L. C., Bogart, L. M., Vranceanu, A.-M., & Matthews, K. A. (2005). Socioeconomic status, resources, psychological experiences, and emotional responses: A test of the reserve capacity model. *Journal of Personality and Social Psychology, 88*(2), 386–399.

Gallo, L. C., & Matthews, K. A. (2003). Understanding the association between socioeconomic status and physical health: Do negative emotions play a role? *Psychological Bulletin, 129*(1), 10–51.

Gallo, L. C., Smith, T. W., & Cox, C. M. (2006). Socioeconomic status, psychosocial processes, and perceived health: An interpersonal perspective. *Annals of Behavioral Medicine, 31*(2), 109–119.

Gamm, L. D. (2004). Mental health and substance abuse services among rural minorities. *The Journal of Rural Health, 20*(3), 206–209.

Garofalo, R., Wolf, R. C., Wissow, L. S., Woods, E. R., & Goodman, E. (1999). Sexual orientation and risk of suicide attempts among a representative sample of youth. *Archives of Pediatric and Adolescent Medicine, 153*(5), 487–493.

Gary, F. A. (2005). Stigma: Barrier to mental health care among ethnic minorities. *Issues in Mental Health Nursing, 26*(10), 979–999.

Gary, L. (1995). African American men's perceptions of racial discrimination. *Social Work Research, 19*(2), 207–217.

Gilman, S. E., Kawachi, I., Fitzmaurice, G. M., & Buka, S. L. (2003). Family disruption in childhood and risk of adult depression. *American Journal of Psychiatry, 160*(5), 939–946.

Gold, R., Michael, Y. L., Whitlock, E. P., Hubbell, F. A., Mason, E. D., Rodriguez, B. L., et al. (2006). Race/ethnicity, socioeconomic status, and lifetime morbidity burden in the women's health initiative: A cross-sectional analysis. *Journal of Women's Health, 15*(10), 1161–1173.

Gorman-Smith, D., Tolan, P. H., Henry, D. B., & Florsheim, P. (2000). Patterns of family functioning and adolescent outcomes among urban African American and Mexican American families. *Journal of Family Psychology, 14*(3), 436–457.

Gottman, J. M., Levenson, R. W., Gross, J., Fredrickson, B.L., McCoy, K., Rosenthal, L., et al. (2003). Correlates of gay and lesbian couples' relationship satisfaction and relationship dissolution. *Journal of Homosexuality, 45*(1), 23–43.

Gray-Little, B., & Hafdahl, A. R. (2000). Factors influencing racial comparisons of self-esteem: A quantitative review. *Psychological Bulletin, 126*(1), 26–54.

Guglani, S., Coleman, P. G., & Sonuga-Barke, E. J. (2000). Mental health of elderly Asians in Britain: A comparison of Hindus from nuclear and extended families of differing cultural identities. *International Journal of Geriatric Psychiatry, 15*(11), 1046–1053.

Hacker, G. A., Collins, R., & Jacobson, M. F. (1987). *Marketing booze to blacks: A report from the center for science in the public interest.* Washington, DC: Center for Science in the Public Interest.

Harris, K. M., Edlund, M. J., & Larson, S. (2005). Racial and ethnic differences in the mental health problems and use of mental health care. *Medical Care, 43*(8), 775–784.

Heck, J. E., Sell, R. L., & Sheinfeld Gorin, S. (2006). Health care access among individuals in same-sex relationships. *American Journal of Public Health, 96,* 1111–1118.

Heck, K. E., & Parker, J. D. (2002). Family structure, socioeconomic status, and access to health care for children. *Health Services Research, 37*(1), 171–184.

Helmers, K., Posluszny, D., & Krantz, D. S. (1994). Associations of hostility and coronary artery disease: A review of studies. In A. Siegman & T. Smith (Eds.), *Anger, hostility, and the heart.* Hillsdale: Erbaum.

Hinton, M. E., Dembling, B., & Stern, S. (2003). Shortages of rural mental health professionals. *Archives of Psychiatric Nursing, 17*(1), 42–51.

Hobfoll, S. E., & Johnson, R. (2003). Resource loss, resource gain, and emotional outcomes among inner city women. *Journal of Personality and Social Psychology, 84,* 632–643.

Hobfoll, S. E., Jackson, A., Hobfoll, I., Pierce, C. A., & Young, S. (2002). The impact of communal-mastery versus self-mastery on emotional outcomes during stressful conditions: A prospective study of Native American women. *American Journal of Community Psychology, 30*(6), 853–871.

Hobfoll, S. E., Schroeder, K. E., Wells, M., & Malek, M. (2002). Communal versus individualistic construction of sense of mastery in facing life challenges. *Journal of Social and Clinical Psychology, 21*(4), 362–399

Hogan, D. P., Hao, L. X., & Parish, W. L. (1990). Race, kin networks, and assistance to mother-headed families. *Social Forces, 68*(3), 797–812.

Hollingshead, A. B. (1975). *Four factor index of social status.* New Haven: Yale University, Department of Sociology.

Hollingshead, A. B., Ellis, R., & Kirby, E. (1954). Social mobility and mental illness. *American Sociological Review, 19*(5), 577–584.

Holzer III, C.E., Shea, B.M., Swanson, J.W., Leaf, P.J., Myers, J.K., George, L. et al. (1986). The increased risk for specific psychiatric disorders among persons of low socioeconomic status, evidence from the Epidemiologic Catchment Area Surveys. *American Journal of Social Psychiatry, 6,* 259–271.

Husaini, B. A., Sherkat, D. E., Levine, R., Bragg, R., Holzer, C., Anderson, K., et al. (2002). Race, gender, and health care service utilization and costs among Medicare elderly with psychiatric diagnoses. *Journal of Aging and Health, 14*(1), 79–95.

Huurre, T., Rahkonen, O., Komulainen, E., & Aro, H. (2005). Socioeconomic status as a cause and consequence of psychosomatic symptoms from adolescence to adulthood. *Social Psychiatry and Psychiatric Epidemiology, 40*(7), 580–587.

Israel, B., Farquhar, S. A., Schulz, A. J., James, S. A., & Parker, E. A. (2002). The relationship between social support, stress, and health among women on Detroit's east side. *Health Education & Behavior. Special Issue: Community-based participatory research–addressing social determinants of health: Lessons from the Urban Research Centers, 29*(3), 342–360.

Jackson, A. P. (1999).The effects of nonresident father involvement on single Black mothers and their young children. *Social Work, 44*(2), 156–166.

Jackson, A.P., Gyamfi, P., Brooks-Gunn, J., & Blake, M. (1998). Employment status, psychological well being, social support, and physical discipline practices of single Black mothers. *Journal of Marriage and the Family, 60*(4), 894–902.

James, S. A. (1994). John Henryism and the health of African-Americans. *Culture, Medicine and Psychiatry, 18*(2), 163–182.

Jayakody, R., Danziger, S., & Pollack, H. (2000). Welfare reform, substance use, and mental health. *Journal of Health Politics, Policy and Law, 25*(4), 623–652.

Johnson, J. G., Cohen, P., Dohrenwend, B. P., Link, B. G., & Brook, J. S. (1999). A longitudinal investigation of social causation and social selection processes involved in the association between socioeconomic status and psychiatric disorders. *Journal of Abnormal Psychology, 108*(3), 490–499.

Karlamangla, A. S., Singer, B. H., McEwen, B. S., Rowe, J. W., & Seeman, T. E. (2002). Allostatic load as a predictor of functional decline. Macarthur studies of successful aging. *Journal of Clinical Epidemiology, 55*(7), 696–710.

Karlsen, S., & Nazroo, J. Y. (2002a). Agency and structure: The impact of ethnic identity and racism on the health of ethnic minority people. *Sociology of Health & Illness, 24*(1), 1–20.

Karlsen, S., & Nazroo, J. Y. (2002b). Relation between racial discrimination, social class, and health among ethnic minority groups. *American Journal of Public Health, 92*(4), 624–631.

Karlsen, S., Nazroo, J. Y., McKenzie, K., Bhui, K., & Weich, S. (2005). Racism, psychosis and common mental disorder among ethnic minority groups in England. *Psychological Medicine, 35*(12), 1795–1803.

Keyes, C. L. M. (2007). Promoting and protecting mental health as flourishing: A complementary strategy for improving national mental health. *American Psychologist, 62*(2), 95–108.

Kim, W. (2003). Child and adolescent psychiatry workforce: A critical shortage and national challenge. *Academic Psychiatry, 27,* 277–282.

King, M., & Bartlett, A. (2006). What same sex civil partnerships may mean for health. *Journal of Epidemiology & Community Health, 60,* 188–191.

Kirkpatrick, M. (1987). Clinical implications of lesbian mother studies. *Journal of Homosexuality, 13,* 201–211.

Klein, K., & Forehand, R. (2000). Family processes as resources for African American children exposed to a constellation of sociodemographic risk factors. *Journal of Clinical Child Psychology*, *29*(1), 53–65.

Krieger, N., & Sidney, S. (1996). Racial discrimination and blood pressure: The CARDIA study of young black and white adults. *American Journal of Public Health*, *86*(10), 1370–1378.

Lachman, M. E., & Weaver, S. L. (1998). The sense of control as a moderator of social class differences in health and well-being. *Journal of Personality and Social Psychology*, *74*(3), 763–773.

Landrine, H., & Klonoff, E. A. (2000). Racial discrimination and cigarette smoking among blacks: Findings from two studies. *Ethnicity & Disease*, *10*(20), 195–202.

Leone, J. M., Johnson, M. P., Cohan, C. L., & Lloyd, S. E. (2004). Consequences of male partner violence for low-income minority women. *Journal of Marriage and Family*, *66*(2), 472–490.

Lillie-Blanton, M., Anthony, J. C., & Schuster, C. R. (1993). Probing the meaning of racial/ethnic group comparisons in crack cocaine smoking. *Journal of the American Medical Association*, *269*(8), 993–997.

Logan, J. R., & Stults, B. J. (1999). Racial differences in exposure to crime: The city and suburbs of Cleveland in 1990. *Criminology*, *37*(2), 251–276.

Lorant, V., Deliege, D., Eaton, W., Robert, A., Philippot, P., & Ansseau, M. (2003). Socio-economic inequalities in depression: A meta-analysis. *American Journal of Epidemiology*, *157*(2), 98–112.

Lorant, V., Kampfl, D., Seghers, A., Deliège, D., Closon, M. C., & Ansseau, M. (2003). Socio-economic differences in psychiatric in-patient care. *Acta Psychiatrica Scandinavica*, *107*(3), 170–177.

Lynch, J. W., & Kaplan, G. A. (1997). Understanding how inequality in the distribution of income affects health. *Journal of Health Psychology*, *2*(3), 297–314.

MacIntyre, S., Maciver, S., & Sooman, A. (1993). Area, class, and health: Should we be focusing on places or people? *Journal of Social Policy*, *22*(2), 213–234.

Marcussen, K. (2005). Explaining differences in mental health between married and cohabiting individuals. *Social Psychology Quarterly*, *68*(3), 239–257

Masten, A. S., Miliotis, D., Graham-Bermann, S. A., Ramirez, M., & Neemann, J. (1993). Children in homeless families: Risks to mental health and development. *Journal of Consulting and Clinical Psychology*, *61*(2), 335–343.

Maxwell, B., & Jacobson, M. F. (1989). *Marketing disease to Hispanics: The selling of alcohol, tobacco and junk foods*. Washington, DC: Center for Science in the Public Interest.

Mays, V. M., & Cochran, S. D. (2001). Mental health correlates of perceived discrimination among lesbian, gay, and bisexual adults in the United States. *American Journal of Public Health*, *91*(11), 1869–1876.

Mays, V. M., Cochran, S. D., & Roeder, M. R. (2004). Depressive distress and prevalence of common problems among homosexually active African American women in the United States. *Journal of Psychology and Human Sexuality*, *12*(2/3), 27–46.

McEwen, B. S. (1998). Protective and damaging effects of stress mediators. *New England Journal of Medicine*, *338*(3), 171–179.

McKelvey, M. W., & McKenry, P. C. (2000). The psychosocial wellbeing of Black and White mothers following marital dissolution. *Psychology of Women Quarterly*, *24*(1), 4–14.

McLeod, J. D., & Shanahan, M. J. (1993). Poverty, parenting, and children's mental health. *American Sociological Review*, *58*, 351–366.

McLoyd, V. C., Jayaratne, T. E., Ceballo, R., & Borquez, J. (1994). Unemployment and work interruption among African American single mothers: Effects on parenting and adolescent socioemotional functioning. *Child Development*, *65*(2), 562–589.

Meyer, I. H. (2003). Prejudice, social stress, and mental health in lesbian, gay, and bisexual populations: Conceptual issues and research evidence. *Psychological Bulletin*, *129*(5), 674–697.

Miech, R.A., & Hauser, R. M. (2001). Socioeconomic status and health at midlife. A comparison of educational attainment with occupation-based indicators. *Annuals of Epidemiology, 11*(2), 75–84.

Miranda, J., & Cooper, L. A. (2004). Disparities in care for depression among primary care patients. *Journal of General Internal Medicine, 19*(2), 120–126.

Mossakowski, K. N. (2003). Coping with perceived discrimination: Does ethnic identity protect mental health? *Journal of Health and Social Behavior, 44*(3), 318–331.

Murry, V. M., & Brody, G. H. (1999). Self-Regulation and self-worth of Black children reared in economically stressed, rural, single-mother-headed families: The contribution of risk and protective factors. *Journal of Family Issues, 20*(4), 458– 484.

Murry, V. M., Bynum, M. S., Brody, G. H., Willert, A., & Stephens, D. (2001). African American Single Mothers and Children in Context: A Review of Studies on Risk and Resilience. *Clinical Child and Family Psychology Review, 4*(2), 133–155.

Musser-Granski, J., & Carillo, D. F. (1997). The use of bilingual, bicultural paraprofessionals in mental health services: Issues for hiring, training, and supervision. *Community Mental Health Journal, 33*(1), 51–60

Neighbors, H. W., & Laveist, T. A. (1989). Socioeconomic status and psychological distress: The impact of financial aid on economic problem severity. *Journal of Primary Prevention, 10*(2), 149–165.

Nolen-Hoeksema, S. (2002). Gender differences in depression. In I.H. Gotlib & C.L. Hammen (Eds.), *Handbook of depression* (pp. 492–509). New York: Guilford.

Nyamathi, A., Berg, J., Jones, T., & Leake, B. (2005). Predictors of perceived health status of tuberculosis-infected homeless. *Western Journal of Nursing Research, 27*(7), 896–910.

Office of Applied Studies. (2004). *Results from the 2003 National Survey on Drug Use and Health: National findings* (DHHS Publication No. SMA 04–3964, NSDUH Series H–25). Rockville, MD: Substance Abuse and Mental Health Services Administration.

Oswald, R. F. (2002). Resilience within the family networks of lesbians and gay men: intentionality and redefinition. *Journal of Marriage and the Family, 64*, 374–383.

Owens, G. P., Riggle, E. D. B., & Rostosky, S. S. (2007). Mental health services access for sexual minority individuals. *Sexuality Research & Social Policy: A Journal of the NSRC, 4*(3), 92–99.

Peek, M. K., Stimpson, J. P., & Townsend, A. L. (2006). Well-being in older Mexican American spouses. *The Gerontologist, 46*(2), 258–265.

Peplau, L. A, & Fingerhut, A. W. (2007). The close relationships of lesbian and gay men. *Annual Review of Psychology, 58*, 405–424.

Peters, R. M. (2004). Racism and hypertension among African Americans. *Western Journal of Nursing Research, 26*(6), 612–631.

Porter, K., Primus, W., Rawlings, L., & Rosenbaum, E. (1998, March 9). *Strengths of the safety net: How the EITC, Social Security, and other government programs affect poverty*, Center on Budget and Policy Priorities.

Pumariega, A. J., Rogers, K., & Rothe, E. (2005). Culturally competent systems of care for children's mental health: Advances and challenges. *Community Mental Health Journal, 41*(5), 539–555.

Remafedi, G., French, S., Story, M., Resnick, M. D., & Blum, R. (1998).The relationship between suicide risk and sexual orientation: Results of a population-based study. *American Journal of Public Health, 88*(1), 57–60.

Rasheed, M. N., & Rasheed, J. M. (2003). Rural African American older adults and the Black helping tradition. *Journal of Gerontological Social Work, 41*(1/2), 137–150.

Ritsher, J. E. B., Warner, V., Johnson, J. G., & Dohrenwend, B. P. (2001). Inter-generational longitudinal study of social class and depression: A test of social causation and social selection models. *British Journal of Psychiatry, 178*(Suppl40), s84–s90.

Rohland, B.M., Saleh, S. S., Rohere, J. E., & Romitti, P. A. (2000). Acceptability of telepsychiatry to a rural population. *Psychiatric Services, 51*(5), 672–674.

Rostosky, S. S., Danner, F., & Riggle, E. D. B. (2007). Is religiosity a protective factor against substance use in young adulthood? Only if you're straight! *Journal of Adolescent Health, 40*(5), 440–447.

Rostosky, S. S., Riggle, E. D. B., Gray, B. E., & Hatton, R. L. (2007). Minority stress experiences in committed same-sex couple relationships. *Professional Psychology: Research and Practice, 38*(4), 392–400.

Ruiz, S.Y., Roosa, M.W., & Gonzales, N.A. (2002). Predictors of self-esteem for Mexican American and European American youth: A re-examination of the influence of parenting. *Journal of Family Psychology, 16*(1), 70–80.

Rutter, M. (1987). Psychosocial resilience and protective mechanisms. *American Journal of Orthopsychiatry, 57*(3), 316–331.

Ryff, C. D., Keyes, C. L. M., & Hughes, D. L. (2003). Status inequalities, perceived discrimination, and eudaimonic well-being: Do the challenges of minority life hone purpose and growth? *Journal of Health and Social Behavior, 44*(3), 275–291.

Sareen, J., Jagdeo, A., Cox, B. J., Clara, I., Ten Have, M., Belik, S., et al. (2007). Perceived barriers to mental health service utilization in the United States, Ontario, and the Netherlands. *Psychiatric Services, 58*(3), 357–364.

Schieman, S., Pudrovska, T., & Milkie, M. A. (2005). The sense of divine control and the self-concept: A study of race differences in late life. *Research on Aging, 27*(2), 165–196.

Schieman, S., Pudrovska, T., Pearlin, L. I., & Ellison, C. G. (2006). The sense of divine control and psychological distress: Variations across race and socioeconomic status. *Journal for the Scientific Study of Religion, 45*(4), 529–549.

Schulz, A. J., Israel, B. A., Zenk, S. N., Parker, E. A., Lichtenstein, R., Shellman-Weir, et al. (2006). Psychosocial stress and social support as mediators of relationships between income, length of residence and depressive symptoms among African American women on Detroit's eastside. *Social Science and Medicine, 62*(2), 510–522.

Schulz, A., Williams, D. R., Israel, B., Becker, A., Parker, E., James, S. A., et al. (2000). Unfair treatment, neighborhood effects, and mental health in the Detroit metropolitan area. *Journal of Health and Social Behavior, 41*(3), 314–332.

Shavers, V. L. (2007). Measurement of socioeconomic status in health disparities research. *Journal of the National Medical Association, 99*(9), 1013–23.

Shen, B. J., & Takeuchi, D. T. (2001). A structural model of acculturation and mental health status among Chinese Americans. *American Journal of Community Psychology, 29*(3), 387–418.

Siefert, K., Finlayson, T. L., Williams, D. R., Delva, J., & Ismail, A. I. (2007). Modifiable risk and protective factors for depressive symptoms in low-income African American mothers. *American Journal of Orthopsychiatry, 77*(1), 113–123.

Simon, R. W. (2002). Revisiting the relationships among gender, marital status, and mental health. *American Journal of Sociology, 107*(4), 1065–1096.

Smokowski, P. R., Mann, E. A., & Reynolds, A. J. (2004). Childhood risk and protective factors and late adolescent adjustment in inner city minority youth. *Children and Youth Services Review, 26*(1), 63–91.

Smokowski, P.R., Reynolds, A.J., & Bezruczko, N. (1999). Resilience and protective factors in adolescence: An autobiographical perspective from disadvantaged youth. *Journal of School Psychology, 37*(4), 425–448.

Stansfeld, S. A., Bosma, H., Hemingway, H., & Marmot, M. G. (1998). Psychosocial work characteristics and social support as predictors of sf-36 health functioning: The Whitehall ii study. *Psychosomatic Medicine, 60*(3), 247–255.

Steele, L., Dewa, C., & Lee, K. (2007). Socioeconomic status and self-reported barriers to mental health service use. *Canadian Journal of Psychiatry, 52*, 201–206.

Steele, L. S., Tinmouth, J. M., & Luc, A. (2006). Regular health care use by lesbians: A path analysis of predictive factors. *Family Practice, 23*(6), 631–636.

Stepleman, L. M., Hann, G., Santos, M., & House, A. S. (2006). Reaching underserved HIV-positive individuals by using patient-centered psychological consultation. *Professional Psychology: Research and Practice, 37*(1), 75–82.

Stimpson, J. P., Peek, M. K., & Markides, K. S. (2006). Depression and mental health among older Mexican American spouses. *Aging & Mental Health, 10*(4), 386–393.

Strayhorn, J. M., Weidman, C. S., & Larson, D. (1990). A measure of religiousness, and its relation to parent and child mental health variables. *Journal of Community Psychology, 18*(1), 34–43.

Stronks, K., van de Mheen, H., van den Bos, J., & Mackenbach, J.P. (1997). The interrelationship between income, health, and employment. *International Journal of Epidemiology, 26*(3), 592–600.

Sullivan, T. N., & Farrell, A. D. (1999). Identification and impact of risk and protective factors for drug use among urban African American adolescents. *Journal of Clinical Child Psychology, 28*(2), 122–136.

Takeuchi, D. T., Chung, R. C.-Y., Lin, K.-M., Shen, H., Kurasaki, K., Chun, C.-A., & Sue, S. (1998). Lifetime and twelve-month prevalence rates of major depressive episodes and dysthymia among Chinese Americans in Los Angeles. *American Journal of Psychiatry, 155*(10), 1407–1414.

Taylor, J., & Turner, R. J. (2002). Perceived discrimination, social stress and depression in the transition to adulthood: Racial contrasts. *Social Psychology Quarterly, 65*(3), 213–225.

Taylor, R. D. (1996). Adolescents' perceptions of kinship support and family management practices: Association with adolescent adjustment in African American families. *Developmental Psychology, 32*(4), 687–695.

Taylor, R., & Roberts, D. (1995). Kinship support and maternal and adolescent well-being in economically disadvantaged African American families. *Child Development, 66*(6), 1585–1597.

Tiffin, P. A., Pearce, M. S., & Parker, L. (2005). Social mobility over the lifecourse and self reported mental health at age 50: Prospective cohort study. *Journal of Epidemiology & Community Health, 59*(10), 870–872.

Turner, R. J., Lloyd, D. A., & Roszell, P. (1999). Personal resources and the social distribution of depression. *American Journal of Community Psychology, 27*(5), 643–672.

Twenge, J. M., & Campbell, W. K. (2002). Self-esteem and socioeconomic status: A meta-analytic review. *Personality and Social Psychology Review, 6*(1), 59–71.

Uehara, E. S., Takeuchi, D. T., & Smukler, M. (1994). Effects of combining disparate groups in the analysis of ethnic differences: Variations among Asian American mental health service consumers in level of community functioning. *American Journal of Community Psychology, 22*(1), 83–99.

Wadsworth, M.E., & Achenbach, T.M. (2005). Explaining the link between low socioeconomic strata and psychopathology: Testing two mechanisms of the social causation hypothesis. *Journal of Consulting and Clinical Psychology, 73*(6), 1146–1153.

Walters, K. L. (1995). *Urban American Indian identity and psychological wellness.* Unpublished doctoral dissertation. University of California, Los Angeles.

Walters, K. L. (1999). Urban American Indian identity attitudes and acculturative styles. *Human Behavior and the Social Environment, 2*(1/2), 163–178.

Walters, K. L., Simoni, J. M., & Evans-Campbell, T. (2002). Substance use among American Indians and Alaska natives: Incorporating culture in an "indigenist" stress-coping paradigm. *Public Health Report, 117*(Suppl. 1), S104–S117.

Wen, M., Hawkley, L. C., & Cacioppo, J. T. (2006). Objective and perceived neighborhood environment, individual SES and psychosocial factors, and self-rated health: An analysis of older adults in Cook County, Illinois. *Social Science & Medicine, 63*(10), 2575–2590.

Wender, P.H., Rosenthal, D., Kety, S. S., Schlusinger, F., & Welner, J. (1973). Social class and psychopathology in adoptees. *Archives of General Psychiatry, 28*(3), 318–325.

Whitfield, K.E., Weidner, G., Clark R., & Anderson, N. B. (2002). Sociodemographic diversity and behavioral medicine. *Journal of Consulting and Clinical Psychology*, *70*(3), 463–481.

Willging, C. E., Salvador, M., & Kano, M. (2006). Pragmatic help seeking: How sexual and gender minority groups access mental health care in a rural state. *Psychiatric Services*, *57*(6), 871-874.

Williams, D. R. (1999). Race, socioeconomic status, and health the added effects of racism and discrimination. *Annals of the New York Academy of Sciences*, *869*, 173–188.

Williams, D. R., & Collins, C. (1995). U.S. Socioeconomic and racial differences in health: Patterns and explanations. *Annual Review of Sociology*, *21*, 349–386.

Williams, D. R., & Harris-Reid, M. (1999). Race and mental health: Emerging patterns and promising approaches. In A. V. Horowitz & T. L. Scheid (Eds.), *A handbook for the study of mental health: Social contexts, theories, and systems* (pp. 295–314). Cambridge: Cambridge University Press.

Williams, D. R., & Jackson, P. B. (2005). Social sources of racial disparities in health. *Health Affairs*, *24*(2), 325–334.

Williams, D. R., Neighbors, H. W., & Jackson, J. S. (2003). Racial/ethnic discrimination and health: Findings from community studies. *American Journal of Public Health*, *93*(2), 200–208.

Williams, D. R., Takeuchi, D. T., & Adair, R. (1992). Socioeconomic status and psychiatric disorder among blacks and whites. *Social Forces*, *71*, 179–194.

Yen, I. H., Ragland, D. R., Greiner, B. A., & Fisher, J. M. (1999a). Racial discrimination and alcohol-related behavior in urban transit operators: Findings from the San Francisco muni health and safety study. *Public Health Reports*, *114*(5), 448–458.

Yen, I. H., Ragland, D. R., Greiner, B. A., & Fisher, J. M. (1999b). Workplace discrimination and alcohol consumption: Findings from the San Francisco muni health and safety study. *Ethnicity & Disease*, *9*(1), 70–80.

Yeung, A., Yu, S., Fung, F., Vorono, S., & Fava, M. (2006). Recognizing and engaging depressed Chinese Americans in treatment in a primary care setting. *International Journal of Geriatric Psychiatry*, *21*(9), 819–823.

Chapter 14
Psychiatric Genetics-An Update

Prashant Gajwani

Introduction

Over the last decade, there has been an exponential growth in understanding psychiatric illnesses with an expanded array of available treatments. The physical expression of characteristics coded by genes is known as a phenotype. The phenotype of psychiatric disorders is based on an intricate system of symptom classification which has evolved over the last several decades (American Psychiatric Association, 1994). With a better understanding of illness phenotype and comorbidities, researchers and clinicians have been able to refine treatment options.

Genetic factors play a fundamental role in the genesis of psychiatric disorders. In addition, genetic factors may also play a very important role in metabolism, distribution, and eventual response to psychotropic medications. The identification of underlying genetic variations associated with psychiatric illnesses could help us evaluate risk factors for developing phenotype targeted pharmacotherapy agents and medication doses on an individual level for an optimal outcome and relapse prevention. Most psychiatric disorders are complex in origin and are considered to have multifactorial inheritance wherein a combination of multiple susceptible genes interacts with the environment to produce a particular phenotype. In addition to genetic variance, cross-culture variations could complicate the study of prevalence and treatment of psychiatric disorders.

Culture is a broad term that includes social roles, values, and all forms of knowledge that make up a way of life. Culture may predict the way a person expresses distress, and hence symptoms of psychiatric illness expressed may be different in various cultures. Variations in interpreting illness symptoms across cultures can be challenging and may lead to imprecise or incorrect psychiatric diagnosis. Scientists have developed culture-specific screening questionnaires for emotional distress which incorporate common expressions of stress/distress

P. Gajwani (✉)
University Hospitals Case Medical Center, School of Medicine, Case Western Reserve University, Cleveland, OH
e-mail: prashant.gajwani@uhhospitals.org

S. Loue, M. Sajatovic (eds.), *Determinants of Minority Mental Health and Wellness*, DOI 10.1007/978-0-387-75659-2_14,
© Springer Science+Business Media, LLC 2009

as exhibited by that particular culture. Culture also encompasses ethnicity, race, and religion. Ethnicity and race may predispose individuals to a common genetic pool which produces phenotypic resemblance. Certain illnesses are more common in some ethnicity groups solely due to genetic makeup. Ethnicity and race confer common genes to populations and hence increase the outward expression of illnesses, inherited due to common genes.

Advances in brain research, particularly advances at the cellular and molecular level will permit us to understand cellular mechanisms responsible for psychiatric disorders. Recent attempts to understand neuronal communications in the brain have led to a rapidly expanding number of substrates that serve as neurotransmitters (compounds in the body which facilitate the transmission of nerve signals from one cell to another). Genes participate in the regulation of neurotransmitters, which play a critical role in affect modulation (how an individual feels and expresses emotion and mood) and reward systems (pleasure/pain in response to environmental stimuli). The availability of new methods for genetic analysis at the gene/ genome level (such as molecular cloning of neurotransmitters) has improved our understanding of information processing in the brain, which in turn has allowed us to improve our understanding of psychiatric disorders and mechanism of action for psychotropic medications.

Over the past two decades, research methods have been developed to determine the extent to which a specific psychiatric illness is genetically caused. All genetic illnesses have increased rate of illness among relatives of the first identified family member with the illness, known as *probands*. Psychiatric familial genetic studies have been conducted since early 20th century, although there have been some limitations to the familial studies as diagnostic criteria for psychiatric disorders have changed over time. Twin and adoption studies have demonstrated familial genetic causation in psychiatric disorders. To account for environmental factors influencing manifestation of psychiatric disorders, rates of illness amongst twins raised in the same home has been compared to twins raised apart. Advances in the field of human genetics, specifically the Human Genome Project and localization of loci for genes has improved our understanding of genes involved in psychiatric disorders.

Most psychiatric medications are administered orally. Pharmacokinetics involves ingestion, absorption, metabolism, and distribution of a drug. After oral ingestion, the drugs are absorbed by the stomach and small intestine and metabolized by the liver and then enter into systemic circulation, eventually cleared by either the liver or kidneys. Medical illnesses or other concomitant medications affecting the gastrointestinal tract, liver or kidneys can affect pharmacokinetics. Individual factors such as race, ethnicity can also affect the pharmacokinetics (absorption and breakdown of drugs in the body). Based on genetic variation between races, metabolism of psychotropic medications by hepatic P450 enzymes (those components of the liver that break down and eliminate medications from the body) can be variable depending on an individual's age, ethnicity, and use of concomitant medications. This can ultimately affect clinical efficacy of a particular compound. This is also important as frequently a combination of medications is used for management of psychiatric illnesses. Cultural factors such as a particular food intake can also affect metabolism of psychiatric medications, for example individuals from a culture that consumes more grapefruit juice can alter activity of certain hepatic enzymes involved in metabolism of medications. This chapter will focus on the genetics of psychiatric illnesses and briefly review genetic factors that influence metabolism of psychiatric medications.

Genetics of Schizophrenia

Schizophrenia affects 1% of the world's population (Robins & Regier, 1991). Clinical symptoms include hallucinations, delusions, disorganized thoughts and speech, and social withdrawal. Bipolar disorder, characterized by psychosis and cognitive changes, has been shown in familial studies to have phenotypic overlap with schizophrenia (Craddock, O'Donovan, & Owen 2005). The heritability of schizophrenia has been estimated to be approximately 80% (Cardno & Gottesman, 2000) with schizophrenia occurring worldwide and across ethnic subgroups.

A familial form of schizophrenia may be predicted by factors such as structural brain abnormalities, age at onset versus probands who suffered infections or obstetrical complications at birth may be at lower familial risk. (Bersani, Taddei, Venturi, Osborn, & Pancheri, 1995). Elevated risk of schizophrenia in the first-degree relative of schizophrenia probands has been demonstrated by familial studies. The highest risk is seen in children (12.8%), followed by siblings (10.1%) and parents (5.6%) compared to the general population (0.9%) (Gottesman & Shields, 1982). Twin and adoption studies can be used to separate the contribution of genetic and environmental causes. Monozygotic twins are genetically identical and dizygotic twins on an average share 50% of the alleles (gene materials). Genetic inheritability of schizophrenia is further strengthened by studies conducted in monozygotic and dizygotic twins. Monozygotic co-twins have three times elevated risk of developing schizophrenia (59.2%) compared to dizygotic co-twins (15.2%) (Kendler, 1986). Males and females with early onset may be at elevated familial risk (Pulver et al., 1990; Sham et al., 1994); however, this finding has not been replicated in all studies. Probands who develop schizophrenia and had suffered obstetrical complications at birth are at a lower familial risk compared to those without obstetrical complications (Bersani, Taddei, Venturi, Osborn, & Pancheri, 1994). Ventricular enlargement, a type of structural brain abnormality seen in schizophrenia, predicts lower familial risk in male probands compared to female probands (Goldstein, Tsuang, & Faraone, 1989). Various adoption studies have documented genetic heritability of schizophrenia by studying the prevalence of schizophrenia in offsprings of schizophrenic mothers separated at birth

(Tienari, 1991). The risk of developing bipolar disorder is also elevated in relatives of schizophrenic probands, indicating possible overlap in the phenotypic spectrum (Pope & Yurgelun-Todd, 1990, Craddock, O'Donovan, & Owen 2005). Relatives of patients with schizophrenia may be at an elevated risk for developing psychotic affective illnesses.

The chromosomal location of a DNA sequence is referred to as genetic locus. Genetic linkage studies have identified a large number of presumptive loci for schizophrenia including 1q21, 1q42, 5q, 6p, 6q, 8p, 10p, 10q, 13q, 17p, and 22q (Owen, Craddock, & O'Donovan, 2005). Some of the common loci are also identified in other severe psychiatric illnesses such as bipolar disorders. Many chromosomal aberrations are also being investigated in patients with schizophrenia, some with crucial role in dopaminergic pathways. An excess of the neurotransmitter dopamine and its blockage by antipsychotic medications is presumed to be the mechanism of action for medication treatment of hallucinations and delusions seen in schizophrenia.

Genetic factors that differ across ethnic subgroups may also be involved in development of side effects to schizophrenia medication treatments such as decrease in white blood cell count, also known as agranulocytosis. Previous studies have found genetic factors important in the development of agranulocytosis (cessation in the body's ability to produce infection-fighting white blood cells) to the novel antipsychotic medication, clozapine, in Ashkenazi Jewish patients suffering with schizophrenia (Lieberman et al., 1990). Other social factors across various ethnic groups can affect tolerability and response to the medications such as use of tobacco and caffeine. Cigarette smoking can cause alteration in blood levels of antipsychotics medications such as clozapine (Derenne & Baldessarini, 2005). Tobacco use via cigarette smoking can cause induction of cytochrome enzymes in liver (1A2) which can lower serum levels of clozapine and olanzapine (Zullino, Delessert, Eap, Preisig, & Baumann, 2002). Tobacco use is also influenced by cultural factors and is more prevalent in minorities such as African American and Hispanics. Tobacco use could potentially result in lower levels of antipsychotics as above and lack of clinical improvement. Tobacco smoking should always be taken into consideration especially when most of the hospitals do not allow smoking, and patients who had quit smoking during hospitalization are likely to resume upon discharge from the hospital.

Genetics of Mood Disorders

Mood disorder is a broad term that includes bipolar disorder and unipolar depression. Core features of bipolar disorder include mood elevation above the baseline (mania and hypomania) associated with depressive episodes. It affects 3–7% of the population (Calabrese et al., 2003). Core feature of Major Depressive Disorder (MDD) are depressed mood or loss in interest or pleasure with five other neurovegetative symptoms per DSM-IV to be present for at least 2 weeks. As with schizophrenia, bipolar disorder appears worldwide across ethnic subgroups.

Family studies of bipolar disorder predict a higher prevalence of psychiatric disorders among the first-degree relatives of bipolar disorder probands. These disorders include Bipolar I disorder, bipolar II disorder, schizoaffective disorder, and recurrent unipolar depression (Gershon et al., 1982; Weissman et al., 1984a; Winokur, Coryell, Keller, Endicott, & Leon, 1995).Early age at onset has been shown in multiple studies with depressed and bipolar probands to be associated with an increased rate of illness 2- to 3-fold among adult relatives (Weissman et al., 1984b). The magnitude of association of family history of depression varies by age of onset, with highest risk estimated for MDD prior to age 20, whereas family history is not associated with MDD for onset after age 50 (Tozzi et al., 2008) . Relatives of bipolar disorder probands associated with psychotic symptoms have a significantly higher risk of psychotic mood disorder compared with risk of relatives with nonpsychotic bipolar disorder probands. This reflects the partial overlap in risk for bipolar disorder and schizophrenia categories, associated with psychotic symptoms (Potash et al., 2003). Psychotic features may be mood-congruent such as delusions of deserved punishment during depression or mood incongruent such as feeling delusions of thought insertion during depressive episodes. A proband with mood incongruent psychotic features with bipolar disorder predicted mood-incongruence in relatives with bipolar I disorder. Mood-incongruent psychotic features show evidence of familial aggregation and suggest linkage to two chromosomal regions previously implicated in major mental illness susceptibility (Goes et al., 2007).

Familial studies also suggest that there may be a genetic basis for the trait of postpartum mood symptoms generally and postpartum depressive symptoms in some women with bipolar disorder (Payne et al., 2008).Twin studies of bipolar disorder have indicated an estimated heritability of 80% and some shared liability with recurrent unipolar depression (McGuffin et al., 2003). Common susceptible genes have also been identified between bipolar disorder and schizophrenia. The evidence is suggestive of five genomic regions which may represent shared genetic susceptibility for bipolar disorder and schizophrenia (Berrettini, 2003). Adoption studies have also provided clues to increased prevalence of bipolar disorder and unipolar depression in relatives of bipolar disorder probands.

The cytochrome P450 enzyme, located in the liver, is involved in metabolism and breakdown of ingested medications and toxins for elimination from the body. Genetic differences in the presence and/or activity of certain P450 enzymes can account for interindividual variability and effectiveness of psychiatric medications. Low metabolizers are individuals with low-to-no activity of an enzyme which could result in accumulation of high concentration of a drug leading to increase in side effects and toxicity of the drug. Recently the Food and Drug Administration has issued a warning that Asian patients with a specific human leukocyte antigen (HLA-B 1502) may be at increased risk of developing a severe, potentially life-threatening type of skin rash called Stevens

Johnson syndrome. About 10% of Asian people have this allele. Some anti-convulsant medications often used to treat bipolar illness (for example carbamazepine and lamotrigine) are associated with skin rash or Stevens Johnson Syndrome in some individuals, and should thus be used carefully, after weighing benefits exceeding risks in HLA-B 1502 positive Asian population (Food and Drug Administration, 2008).

Antidepressants are also metabolized by hepatic cytochrome enzymes. Genetic differences in the presence or activity of certain cytochrome enzymes can account for substantial interindividual variability in blood levels of certain psychotropic medications and can significantly affect tolerability and effectiveness of any particular medication. The enzymes 2D6, 3A4, 1A2, and 2C are involved in pharmacokinetics of antidepressant drugs and can contribute to wide interpatient and interethnic variability. Cytochrome enzyme 2D6 has low activity in 3–10% of Caucasians and 2% of African Americans and Asian population (Richelson, 1997). It is inhibited by the antidepressants fluoxetine, paroxetine, and sertaline and induced by mood stabilizers such as carbamazepine. A small percentage of African Americans, Asians, and Caucasians are slow metabolizers with respect to cytochrome enzyme 1A2 which is involved in the metabolism of antipsychotic medications such as haloperidol, clozapine, and olanzapine. A study that involved genotyping patients with respect to CYP2C9, CYP2C19, and CYP2D6 alleles indicated significant influence of CYP2D6 genotype and minor influence of CYP2C19 on plasma concentration of patients taking antidepressants (Grasmäder, Verwohlt, & Rietschel, 2004).

Other Psychiatric Disorders

Family studies have demonstrated an increased prevalence of anxiety disorders among first-degree relatives of probands with anxiety disorder. Twin studies of individuals with generalized anxiety disorder have concluded that this order has increased prevalence in monozygotic twins (Kendler, Neale, Kessler, Heath, & Eaves, 1992). The relative risk of inheriting panic disorder among first-degree relative of panic disorder probands ranges from 2.6- to 20-fold, with a median value of 7.8-fold (Knowles & Weissman, 1995). Posttraumatic stress disorder (PTSD) which is caused by environmental factors has not been found to have increased familial prevalence in family studies (Davidson, Smith, & Kudler, 1989).

Family, twin, and adoption studies have demonstrated that genetics may influence the risk of substance use. The types of drugs available dictate which drugs are used when experimentation with drugs begins. Rates of substance abuse vary based on ethnicity, religion, and physical availability of drugs, as well as peer group pressure. Risk of alcoholism is increased 7-fold in first-degree relatives of alcoholic probands (Merinkagas, 1989), hence demonstrating high familial prevalence of alcoholism in family studies. Adoption studies have also provided strong evidence of genetic factors involved in alcoholism, especially alcoholism in biological parents which predicts higher rates of alcoholism in male children. The evidence does not support heritability as strongly in female children of alcoholic parents raised by adoptive parents (Cadoret, Cain, & Grove, 1980). Sons of alcoholic parents, compared to sons of nonalcoholic parents, show that they have decreased intensity of subjective feeling of intoxication, reduced objective signs of intoxication, and earlier and more severe alcohol-related problems with poorer treatment outcomes (Schuckit & Gold, 1988).

Conclusion

The field of psychiatric genetics has witnessed unprecedented efforts over the last two decades to identify the underlying genetic basis of psychiatric disorders. Psychiatric disorders are frequently complex, and patients suffer with comorbidities which limits the clinical classification system, although familial, twin, and adoption studies have strongly favored the genetic basis of psychiatric illnesses. So far, a number of risk genes have been identified, but no single gene has been identified that explains the inheritability of respective psychiatric disorders. It is possible that single genes resulting in major phenotypic manifestations of psychiatric disorders might not exist. However, increased risk for psychiatric disorders could result from additive effects of a large number of small genes and their interaction with environmental effects stressors.

The medication armamentarium for treatment of psychiatric disorders is expanding at an exponential pace. The availability of new genetic information, especially development in the field of pharmacogenetics, will empower health care providers and their patients to make appropriate medication selections, adjust pharmacotherapy on an individual level to maximize tolerability, and ultimately improve health outcomes.

References

American Psychiatric Association. (1994). *Diagnostic and statistical manual of mental Disorders* (4th ed.). Washington, DC: American Psychiatric Press.

Berrettini, W. (2003). Bipolar disorder and schizophrenia: Not so distant relatives? *World Psychiatry, 2*(2), 68–72.

Bersani, G., Taddei, I., Venturi, P., Osborn, J., & Pancheri, P. (1995). Familial occurrence and obstetric complications in siblings discordant for schizophrenia. *Minerva Psychiatrica, 36*, 127–132.

Cadoret, R. J., Cain, C. A., & Grove, W. (1980). Development of alcoholism in adoptees raised apart from alcohol in biologic relatives. *Archives of General Psychiatry, 37*, 561–563.

Calabrese, J. R., Hirschfeld, R. M., Reed, M., Davies, M. A., Frye, M. A., Keck, P. E., Jr., et al. (2003). Impact of bipolar disorder on a U.S. community sample. *Journal of Clinical Psychiatry, 64*, 425–432.

Cardno, A. G., & Gottesman, I. I. (2000). Twin studies of schizophrenia: from-bow-and-arrow concordances to start wars was Mx and functional genomics. *American Journal of Medical Genetics, 97*, 12–17.

Craddock, N., O'Donovan, M. C., & Owen, M. J. (2005). The genetics of schizophrenia and bipolar disorder: dissecting psychosis. *Journal of Medical Genetics, 42*, 193–204.

Davidson, J., Smith, R., & Kudler, H. (1989). Familial psychiatric illness in chronic post traumatic stress disorder. *Comprehensive Psychiatry, 30*, 485–486.

Derenne, J. L., & Baldessarini, R. J. (2005). Clozapine toxicity associated with smoking cessation. *American Journal of Therapy, 12*(5), 469–471.

Food and Drug Administration. (2008). Information for healthcare professionals: Carbamazepine (marketed as Carbatrol, Equetro, Tegretol, and generics). Last revised January 31, 2008; Last accessed May 28, 2008; Available at http://www.fda.gov/cder/drug/InfoSheets/HCP/carbamazepineHCP.htm

Gershon, E. S., Hamovit, J., Guroff, J. J., Dibble, E., Leckman, J..F., Sceery, W., et al. (1982). A family study of schizoaffective, bipolar I, bipolar II, unipolar and normal control probands. *Archives of General Psychiatry, 39*, 1157–1167.

Goes, F. S., Zandi, P. P., Miao, K., McMahon, F. J., Steele, W., Willour, V. L., et al. (2007). Mood-incongruent psychotic features in bipolar disorder: familial aggregation and suggestive linkage to 2p11-q14 and 13q21-33. *American Journal of Psychiatry, 64*(2), 236–47.

Goldstein, J. M., Tsuang, M. T., & Faraone, S. V. (1989). Gender and schizophrenia: Implications for understanding the heterogenicity. *Psychiatry Research, 28*, 243–253.

Gottesman, I. I., & Shields, J. (1982). *Schizophrenia. The epigenetic puzzle.* Cambridge, UK: Cambridge University Press.

Grasmäder, K., Verwohlt, P. L., & Rietschel, M. (2004). Impact of polymorphism of sytochrome-P450 isoenzyme 2C9, 2C19 and 2D6 on plasma concentration and clinical effects of antidepressants in naturalistic clinical setting. *European Journal of Clinical Pharmacology, 60*(5), 329–36.

Kendler, K. S. (1986). Genetics of schizophrenia. In A. J. Frances & R. E. Hale (Eds.). *American Psychiatric Associations Annual Review* (Vol. 5, pp. 25–41). Washington, DC: American Psychiatric Press.

Kendler, K. S., Neale, M. C., Kessler, R. C., Heath, A. C., & Eaves, L. J. (1992). Generalized anxiety disorder in women: a population based twin study. *Archives of General Psychiatry, 49*, 267–272.

Knowles, J. A., & Weissman, M. M. (1995). Panic disorder and agoraphobia. In J. M. Oldham & M. B. Riba (Eds.). *American Psychiatric Press Review of Psychiatry* (Vol. 14, pp. 383–404). Washington, DC: American Psychiatric Press.

Lieberman, J. A., Yunis, J., Egea, E. Canoso, R. T., Kane, J. M., & Yunis, E. J. (1990). HLA-B38, DR4, DQw3 and clozapine- induced agranulocytosis in Jewish patients with schizophrenia. *Archives of General Psychiatry, 47*, 945–948.

McGuffin, P., Rijsdijk, S., Andrew, M., Sham, P., Katz, R., & Cardno, A. (2003). The heritability of bipolar affective disorder and the genetic relationship to unipolar depression. *Archives of General Psychiatry, 60*, 497–502.

Merinkagas, K. R. (1989). Genetics of alcoholism: a review of human studies. In I. Wetterberg (Ed.). *Genetics of neuropsychiatric diseases* (pp. 269–280). London: Macmillan.

Owen, M. J., Craddock, N., & O'Donovan, M. C. (2005). Schizophrenia: genes at last? *Trends in Genetics, 21*, 518–525.

Payne, J. L., Mackinnon, D. F., Mondimore, F. M., McInnis, M. G., Schweizer, B., Zamoiski, R. B., et al. (2008). Familial aggregation of postpartum mood symptoms in bipolar disorder pedigrees. *Bipolar Disorders, 10*(1), 38–44.

Pope, H. G. Jr., & Yurgelun-Todd, D. (1990). Schizophrenic individual with bipolar first-degree relatives: analysis of two pedigrees. *Journal of Clinical Psychiatry , 51*, 97–101.

Potash, J. B., Chiu, Y.-K., MacKinnon, D. F., Miller, E. B., Simpson, S. G., McMahon, F. J., et al. (2003). Familial aggregation of psychosis in a replication set of 69 bipolar pedigrees. *American Journal of Medical Genetics, 116B*, 90–97.

Pulver, A. E., Brown, C. H., Wolyniec, P., McGrath, J., Tam, D., Adler, L., et al. (1990). Schizophrenia: age at onset, gender and familial risk. *Acta Psychiatrica Scandinavica, 82*, 344–351.

Richelson, E. (1997). Pharmacokinetic drug interaction s of new antidepressants: a review of the effects of on metabolism of other drugs. *Mayo Clinic Proceedings, 72*(9), 835–847.

Robins, L. N., & Regier, D. A. (Eds.). (1991). *Psychiatric disorders in America: The Epidemiologic Catchment Area Study.* New York: Free Press.

Sham, P., Jones, P., Russell, A., Gilvarry, K., Bebington, P., Lewis, B., et al. (1994). Age at onset, sex and familial psychiatric comorbidity in schizophrenia: Camberwell Collaborative Psychosis Study. *British Journal of Psychiatry, 165*, 466–473.

Schuckit, M. A., & Gold, E. O. (1988). A simultaneous evaluation of multiple markers of ethanol/placebo challenges in sons of alcoholics and controls. *Archives of General Psychiatry, 45*, 211–216.

Tienari, P. (1991). Interaction between genetic vulnerability and family environment: The Finnish adoptive family study of schizophrenia. *Acta Psychiatrica, 84*, 460–465.

Tozzi, F., Prokopenko, I., Perry, J. D., Kennedy, J. L., McCarthy, A. D., Holsboer, F., et al. (2008). Family history of depression is associated with younger age of onset in patients with recurrent depression. *Psychological Medicine, 13*, 1–9.

Weissman, M. M., Gershon, E. S., Kidd, K. K., Prusoff, B. A., Leckman, J. F., Dibble, E., et al. (1984a). Psychiatric disorders in the relatives of probands with affective disorder: The Yale University-National Institute on Mental Health Collaborative study. *Archives of General Psychiatry, 41*, 13–21.

Weissman, M. M., Wiskramaratne, P., Merikangas, K. R., Leckman, J. F., Prusoff, B. A., Caruso, K. A., et al. (1984b). Onset of major depression in early childhood: increased familial loading and specificity. *Archives of General Psychiatry, 41*, 1136–1143.

Winokur, G., Coryell, W., Keller, M., Endicott, J., & Leon, A. (1995). A family study of manic depressive (bipolar I) disease. Is it a distinct illness separable from primary unipolar depression? *Archives of General Psychiatry, 52*, 367–373.

Zullino, D. F., Delessert, D., Eap, C. B., Preisig, M., & Baumann, P. (2002). Tobacco and cannabis smoking cessation can lead to intoxication with clozapine and olanzapine. *International Clinical Psychopharmacology, 17*(3), 141–143.

Chapter 15
Substance Abuse in Minority Populations

W.A. Vega and A.G. Gil

Introduction

The United States has one of the highest levels of combined licit and illicit substance abuse compared to Western European, Latin American, and Asian nations, and addiction makes a major contribution to the national burden of disease (WHO World Mental Health Survey Consortium, 2004). Alcohol and tobacco use contribute an even higher burden of morbidity and mortality than do illicit drugs in the United States and throughout the world (Rehm, Taylor, & Room, 2006). Therefore the total substance abuse impact on American society is staggering in terms of both financial and human cost because it affects all sectors of the population (McGinnis & Foege, 1999; Rice, Kelman, & Miller, 1991). Moreover, drug problems are frequently accompanied by myriad co-occurring medical conditions and mental health problems (Merikangas et al., 1998). A very strong case can be made that substance use constitutes the most serious health problem facing American society and that it is largely a preventable problem (Erickson, 2001; Mokdad, Marks, Stroup, & Gerberding, 2004).

The use of substances is a culturally influenced behavior; therefore, the likelihood of drug use by individuals is governed in part by access to drugs and by societal and subcultural definitions about the types of substances that are tolerated (e.g. tobacco vs. cocaine), who can use them (e.g. sex, age groups, social position), the circumstances under which their use is accepted (e.g. work, recreation, public vs. private settings), and by whom (e.g. society, family, friends, peers, strangers) (Oetting, 1993; Vega & Gil, 1998). We would expect, and we find, great variability in rates and patterns of substance use, ranging from intolerance to conditional tolerance, across societies and among the subcultures that comprise them.

Ethnic minority populations are not inherently at greater risk of using substances in the United States, or elsewhere, due solely to their social status. There are compelling reasons why ethnic minorities could be *less* likely to abuse substances,

W.A. Vega (✉)
David Geffen School of Medicine, University of California Los Angeles, CA
e-mail: wvega@mednet.ucla.edu

S. Loue, M. Sajatovic (eds.), *Determinants of Minority Mental Health and Wellness*, DOI 10.1007/978-0-387-75659-2_15,
© Springer Science+Business Media, LLC 2009

including adherence to traditional-religious values and mores that are intolerant of intoxication, restrictive gender roles that proscribe substance use by women, perceived vulnerability to criminal sanctions, fear of negative health effects and social ostracism, and prohibitive cost. U.S. minorities reflect these patterns in varying degrees. There are also social factors that influence drug experimentation and addiction. Minorities in the United States are disproportionately residentially segregated and of lower social position. They are often stereotyped and discriminated against, experience frustrated mobility expectations, and reside in areas where access to both legal and illegal drugs is ample and marketing of these substances highly profitable. Drug use and addiction is endemic in the U.S. underclass and represents a potential coping strategy and aversive lifestyle adaptation to harsh conditions (Obot, 1996). However, U.S. substance use is a society-wide problem, and there is no simple formula to identify group or individual vulnerability for drug abuse or to reduce its pernicious effects. The most useful approach followed by researchers is to investigate the life course of those who experiment with drugs and ultimately progress to drug dependence in order to identify biologic, social–structural, and cultural determinants of drug use.

Contemporary Explanatory Models of Drug Use

Contemporary social science and epidemiologic research on drug use has subdivided into broad topic areas. One such topic area has focused on factors associated with drug use initiation and progression during childhood and adolescence, and there is a rich body of theory and epidemiologic data that has tracked patterns and risk factors (Baumrind & Moselle, 1985; Brook, Hamburg, Balka, & Wynn, 1992; Brook, Whiteman, & Gordon, 1983; Chavez & Swaim, 1992; Hawkins, Catalano, & Miller, 1992; Jessor, 1991; Kaplan, Johnson, & Bailey, 1988; Kaplan, Martin, & Robbins, 1985; Newcomb & Bentler, 1986; Oetting & Beauvais, 1991). This tradition has continued through the regular publication of sentinel survey data sponsored by the U.S. public health agencies, and we report some of this information in this chapter.

The second topic area has developed more recently, in part promulgated by the development of more sophisticated methodologies for measuring and categorizing the severity of drug use habituation as a medical disorder. Various protocols have been developed for "case-identification" of alcohol, tobacco, and illicit drug disorders which have utility for estimating the scope of the problem in populations and for treatment studies (Grant et al., 1993; Lucas et al., 2001; Robins et al., 1988; Wittchen et al., 1991). The actual criteria used for determination of "caseness" are continuing to undergo refinements. This second topic area has proven essential as a tool in the rapidly expanding research in neuroscience, which includes imaging and behavioral genetics (Tsuang, Bar, Harley, & Lyons, 2001; Volkow, Fowler, & Wang, 2002). These newer directions are focused on drug effects in brain structure and functioning. Multiple methods of observation are used to identify biologic mechanisms implicated in addiction, and genetic determinants of vulnerability for serious drug problems *as a function of interactions with social environments* (Licinio, 2002). The interview-based case-finding protocols now regularly administered to respondents in epidemiologic and clinical research are considered adequate markers of an addiction *phenotype* for research purposes (Anthony, Warner, & Kessler, 1994). We present information in this chapter about drug disorders using medical criteria of the *Diagnostic and Statistical Manual,*Fourth Edition (American Psychiatric Association [DSM-IV], 1994).

In summary, the current state of substance use research is at a very important point of interdisciplinary integration, and the current emphasis on drug effects in brain functioning and consequent behavior, along with improved understanding of addiction as a chronic relapsing medical disorder, have acted as a stimulus for reorganizing and reinterpreting much of the epidemiologic information about drug use and progression.

The Importance of Social, Cultural, and Environmental Factors in Drug Use

Notwithstanding the fundamental importance of the biologic-genetic substrate in creating a vulnerability to addiction, the best evidence available suggests that environmental factors account for the overwhelming (and essential) influence in the development of substance addictions, as is the case for other complex diseases (Cooper, 2003). Only about 1 in 10 people who use potentially addictive substances become dependent on them. Biologic-genetic factors explain no more than 50% of the potential for addiction of even the most addictive substances and explain far less for most addictive substances. Simply put, biological processes of addiction, even those attributable to genetic propensities, are dependent on environmental stimuli. Therefore, research on personal, cultural, social stress, social-network, and environmental risk and protective factors continues to receive intense scrutiny. Research on drug addiction in recent decades has generated thousands of research papers covering these topics. Yet relatively few scientific papers have focused extensively on the unique features of minority substance use. This is surprising because there is great potential for improved models that provide a foundation for future gene-environment interaction research based on the unique patterns of substance use exhibited by U.S. minority groups (Vega & Gil, 1998).

This chapter briefly summarizes information about African American and Latino drug use, including the presentation of data from regional and national surveys. We focus on three sets of factors in this review: person and family factors, peer and delinquency factors, and educational and community factors. Each of these domains (e.g. pathways) has been shown in the research literature to have important effects (risk and protective) on drug use and collectively form the basis for understanding human development in the first 20 years of life when experimentation, progression, and addiction to drugs reach their peak and negatively influence successful transitions into adult roles. Most "gateway" drug use leading to progression begins during late childhood, initially with rapid increases in use of drugs that are legally available to adults (e.g. alcohol, tobacco, inhalant agents, and over-the-counter medications) followed by abuse of these substances and, for some individuals, progression to marihuana use during early to mid-adolescence (Kandel, 1975; Kandel & Faust, 1975). Temporally the next step in the sequence is increased experimentation with other illicit drugs after mid-adolescence and the progression to drug dependence for a fraction of users.

Tobacco and alcohol (or both) are the customary "starter" drugs, and historically account for the greatest population burden of disease. Abstainers who never use these two substances have extraordinarily low rates of drug use (Vega, Chen, & Williams, 2007). Very few people begin experimenting with drugs after the age of 25; therefore delayed first use of drugs will slow the progression sequence and ultimately reduce population prevalence rates (Vega et al., 2002). Youth that begin the use of "gateway" substances (e.g. alcohol and tobacco) between 11 and 13 years of age have a much greater likelihood of progressing to addiction (Vega & Gil, 2005), and this basic pattern holds for African American and Latino youth as well, albeit with variations primarily in pathways (e.g. persistent vs. irregular use of gateway drugs) before progression to marihuana use (Ellickson, Hays, & Bell, 1992; Vega & Gil, 1998).

Factors Influencing Prevalence Patterns for African American and Latino Youth

The starting point for understanding the similarities and differences in African American and Latino drug use patterns is in childhood and adolescence. This is the formative period of family-social network and environmental influences on youth that affect socialization and social control around substance use. Both ethnic groups have similarly elevated high school drop out rates in high- risk urban areas and similar rates of children living in poverty (Kogan, Luo, Brody, & Murry, 2005). Available research has identified a subset of factors that have important effects on youth drug use. These factors do not have uniform effects in Latinos and African Americans.

African American and Latino Youth

African American youth offer the most dramatic departure from the expected patterns seen in U.S. culture regarding both risk factors and pathways to drug use. Risk factor exposures are excellent predictors of adolescent experimentation with drugs; there is a strong linear correlation between the number of personal, family, peer, and other environmental risk factors experienced and the likelihood of drug use. However, for reasons that are not well understood, African Americans do not have the same reactivity as Latinos when exposed to the same level of risk factors during early adolescence, and their substance use rates for both licit and illicit drugs remain relatively low – below levels of Latino and non-Latino White youth – at this stage of development (Turner & Lloyd, 2003; Vega, Gil, & Zimmerman, 1993). Some researchers believe that differences in African American acculturation within family social networks deter early adolescent drug use by emphasizing anti-drug attitudes and social intolerance in domestic settings. However, the loss of traditions (e.g., deculturation and assimilation) in African American communities may now be having a "weathering" effect – especially in low income communities (Brook, Whiteman, Balka, Win, & Gursen, 1997; De La Rosa, Vega, & Radisch, 2000; Herd, 1987). The protective effects that suppress early substance use in African American communities have been obscured by the intense scrutiny given to female-headed households in poverty and Black male social deviance and incarceration rates. Research studies have shown consistently high levels of African American adolescent male conduct problems, and the expected pattern observed in other ethnic groups (including Latinos) is for conduct problems to co-occur with drug use.

While there is no longer a "typical family" configuration in American society, African Americans and Latinos do differ somewhat in modal family structure. About half of African American children and adolescents live in single parent households, and these families are more likely to be in lower socioeconomic circumstances. Among Latinos, children in immigrant families are more likely (nearly 80%) to reside in two-parent families, but the proportion of children in one-parent households nearly doubles (to nearly 40%) in the 2nd and 3rd generations of U.S.-born Latinos. The U.S. Latino population is undergoing a dynamic cultural shift, as 75% of the population is either foreign-born or children of foreign-born parents (U.S. Bureau of Census, 2002). A good indicator of this shift is increased family instability resulting in female-headed households in poverty, where children are at greater risk of problem behavior and substance use (Griffin, Botvin, Scheier, Diaz, & Miller, 2000).

Among both African Americans and Latinos, social network risk and protective factors are predominantly situated in the immediate family system for children and peer groups for adolescents. Family control of drug use is expressed through, (1) explicit communication of "no-tolerance" attitudes for drug use with children thus preempting "intentions to experiment" from forming and being acted on, (2) by modeling behavior through the presence or absence of substance use/abusing parents or other guardians, and in parenting styles (e.g. conflictive, authoritarian, authoritative, permissive) that reciprocally influence peer-group affiliations of adolescent youth, and (3) the above are reinforced by the strength of bonding emotional support ties in families (Elder et al., 2000; Ellickson, Collins, & Bell, 1999; Gibbons, Gerrard, Cleveland, Wills, & Brody, 2004; Miller-Day, 2008). These processes have been shown to operate in African American and Latino families and to directly affect the anti-drug resilience of children (Belitz & Valdez, 1995; Brook et al., 2001; Cleveland, Gibbons, Gerrard, Pomery, & Brody, 2005; Griffen, Scheier, Botvin, & Diaz, 2000; Jessor, 1993; Lam et al., 2007; Martinez, 2006; McMahon, 2008; Stanton, Xiaoming, Pack, Cottrell, Harris, & Burns, 2002; Xiaoming, Feigelman, & Stanton, 2000).

Historically, African American adults have been characterized by high levels of abstaining from alcohol or illicit drug use. However, there has also been a problematic subgroup experiencing serious alcohol and drug use addiction problems. The situation is partially explained by the disproportionately high rates of abstaining African American female adolescents and adults, contrasted with higher rates of alcohol and illicit drug use among males (and to a lesser extent females) commencing in later adolescence, and progressing to addictive disorders in adulthood (Obot, 1996). This pattern is noteworthy because of the previously mentioned lower rates of substance use initiation in childhood and early adolescence among both boys and girls (Wallace et al., 2002). This delayed progression pattern defies the usual pattern of earlier initiation and progression seen in Latinos and represents a breakdown in protective effects during the critical period when African American adolescents approach important life transitions into adult social roles.

If social controls against drug use operating in indigenous African American and Latino social networks were less effective, we should expect to observe a much higher prevalence of drug use and addiction by 18 years of age in both populations. African American and Latino youth in early adolescence that have already started using alcohol, tobacco, or possibly other drugs are likely to have exceptional family risk factors and higher levels of health, mental health, and behavioral problems (Aktan, Kumpfer, & Turner, 1996; Brook, Adams, Balka, & Johnson, 2002; Gil, Vega, & Biafora, 1997; Gil, Vega, & Turner, 2002; Krohn, Lizotte, Perez, 1997; Vega, Chen, & Williams, 2007).

U.S.-born Latinos of both sexes, have somewhat higher rates than immigrants of drug experimentation and progression to addiction beginning in early childhood onward through adolescence. This trend is accompanied by weaker family cohesiveness and more family conflicts and parental risk factors, such as depression and substance use, than are found in the families of foreign-born Latinos (Gil, Vega, & Dimas, 1994; Martinez, 2006; Vega & Sribney, 2003). Foreign-born Latinos, especially females, who arrived in the United States during later adolescence or in adulthood, carry over from their nations of origin strong protective effects against illicit drug use. The exception is the subgroup of Latino foreign-born arriving in early childhood because they share a heightened propensity for drug experimentation and progression to dependence as do U.S.-born adult Latinos. The differences in rates of drug addiction between foreign- and U.S.-born Latino adults are large, and foreign-born women rarely experience drug addictions. These differences underscore the influential role of culture in drug use-related socialization, and effects of social adaptation to U.S. society in the U.S.-born generations of Latinos. While Latino adolescent drug use rates are similar to those of U.S. non-Latino White rates, drug addiction rates for U.S.-born Latinos are usually higher than rates for immigrant Latino adolescents. Despite very low socioeconomic status and low educational attainment of foreign-born Latinos, their lifetime rates of addictive disorders and problem behaviors remain lower than U.S.-born Latinos (Ebin et al., 2001; Epstein, Botvin, & Diaz, 2000; Ortega, Rosenheck, Alegria, & Rani, 2000).

Neighborhood Effects on Drug Use

Many Latino and African American people live in neighborhoods where exposure to traumatic events, especially involving the witnessing of, participation in, or being a victim of violence, are commonplace (Brody et al., 2001; Sampson, Raudenbush, & Earls, 1997). In addition, both populations experience high levels of daily life hassles and stressors such as problems in provision of education for children, getting health care, employment instability, discrimination, and frustrated personal expectations. These factors have been shown to have long range effects on the drug use problems of both ethnic groups (Lloyd & Taylor, 2006; Turner & Lloyd, 2003). As noted previously, the anti-drug protective effects of some African American families attenuate in mid-to- late adolescence. Among Latinos, lowering exposure to traumatic events reduces problem drug use markedly, especially for females (Turner, Lloyd, & Taylor, 2005).

Geographic, or "place," effects include trauma, drug sales, and other risk factors, but also include assets which have been shown to reduce drug use. There are important regional, rural-urban, and neighborhood differences in drug use rates among all ethnic populations. Recently, attention has been given to neighborhood effects on drug use within urban areas. The fundamental question is "what value added does 'place' have for explaining drug use rates," including addiction and treatment rates, beyond individual, family, and peer risk factors? Secondarily, "how does place interact with ethnicity, or nativity in the instance of Latinos, to affect drug use?"

There are many methodological issues to contend with in sorting out an answer to these questions. Neighborhoods are influenced by similar macroeconomic and social determinants as are individuals, social networks, and organizations. Thus teasing out discrete effects of neighborhoods on drug use is a major challenge; but, the obvious importance of place in human development underscores the importance of overcoming these complex technical challenges (Roux, 2001; Sastry, Ghosh-Dastidar, Adams, & Pebley, 2006).

As an example, Americans change residences frequently, and the types of neighborhoods people reside in are probably more important for the trajectory of their lifetime drug use than where they are living in middle adulthood. Given the current reliance on cross-sectional surveys, it is difficult to "track" individuals and account for the effects of life course geographic mobility. Overall "area" effects have been shown to be statistically significant for different types of health outcomes such as infant mortality, but frequently the magnitude of the effect is not impressive and is mediated by demographic factors such as foreign birth and language use (e.g. Spanish). Moreover, the temporal interdependence of person and place requires new methodological tools to measure and overcome problems of confounding. Logically, neighborhood characteristics are risk factors that would be expressed through limitations to healthy development imposed by the built environment, and social disorganization that fosters (1) access to and social support for drug use and marketing; (2) violence exposures as victim, witness, or perpetrator; and (3) weak social organizations, including families and educational institutions. The quality of current research is rapidly improving with increasing attention being given to methodological strategies that are better equipped to distinguish discrete levels of explanatory factors on human behavior. A foremost challenge to advance the field is collecting respondent information that is not routinely collected in large federal surveys such as data on neighborhood patterns of social networks and communication, social capital, social cohesion, and collective efficacy.

Prevalence Patterns of Substance Use Across Ethnic Groups

In this section, we provide an overview of epidemiologic trends in drug use by ethnicity as documented in recent national data sets. Table 15.1 presents prevalence estimates for cigarette, alcohol, and illicit drug use among youth aged 12–17 years in 2000, 2003, and 2006. White non-Latinos consistently reported the highest prevalence for all three periods. Notable exceptions to this pattern occur with lifetime illicit drug use in 2003, with Latinos reporting the highest rates. Importantly, for lifetime and past year illicit drug use, in 2003 and 2006, the rates for White non-Latinos, Latinos, and African Americans are very similar. Figure 15.1 provides a visual illustration of the trends for the three periods using past year use. Note the similarity among the three groups in 2006 (Fig. 15.1C). Finally, gender differences within Latino and Black subgroups are relatively minor. For example, for past year cigarette use, the rates are almost identical for males and females within these groups in 2003 and 2006. For past year alcohol use, the rates are also very similar in 2000 and 2006. However, it is important to note that the prevalence of past year alcohol use was higher for Black females than males for both 2000 and 2006, which is a countertrend to the long-standing patterns of abstinence.

Table 15.2 presents similar data for individuals aged 18–25 years. Note that the National Household Survey on Drug Abuse (NHSDA) does not provide gender-specific data for this age group. Findings for this age group are similar in that White non-Latinos reported the highest rates, followed by Latinos. However, there are several important differences. First, White non-Latinos are "ahead" by much

Table 15.1 Prevalence of cigarette smoking, alcohol use and illicit drug use among White, Black and Hispanic youth aged 12–17 years old in the United States (NHSDA)

	Whites	Asians	Blacks	Latinos	Latino		Black	
					Male	Female	Male	Female
2000								
Lifetime cigarette smoking (%)	38.1	23.6	24.4	31.2	32.7	29.6	25.3	23.4
Past year cigarette smoking (%)	23.6	13.9	11.6	18.7	19.3	18.1	13.0	10.2
Lifetime alcohol use (%)	44.3	30.5	32.1	41.8	42.2	41.4	32.9	31.4
Past year alcohol use (%)	36.3	21.4	21.2	32.4	33.0	31.8	20.8	21.6
Lifetime any illicit drug use (%)	27.6	17.3	24.5	27.3	28.9	25.6	25.5	23.5
Past year any illicit drug use (%)	19.7	11.6	15.3	18.2	18.6	17.7	16.3	14.2
2003								
Lifetime cigarette smoking (%)	33.3	17.7	24.3	31.0	31.4	30.6	24.5	24.1
Past year cigarette smoking (%)	19.3	07.8	11.9	17.4	17.3	17.5	11.9	11.8
Lifetime alcohol use (%)	44.8	27.7	36.1	45.3	43.4	47.3	36.2	36.0
Past year alcohol use (%)	37.2	20.9	24.5	35.1	32.9	37.4	22.5	26.5
Lifetime any illicit drug use (%)	30.8	20.1	30.4	31.5	31.7	31.2	32.1	28.6
Past year any illicit drug use (%)	22.9	12.6	19.2	21.6	21.3	21.8	20.3	18.2
2006								
Lifetime cigarette smoking (%)	28.5	14.7	20.0	24.3	25.4	23.1	19.8	20.2

Table 15.1 (continued)

	Whites	Asians	Blacks	Latinos	Latino Male	Latino Female	Black Male	Black Female
Past year cigarette smoking (%)	19.5	11.0	10.8	15.1	15.2	15.0	11.0	10.5
Lifetime alcohol use (%)	43.1	27.4	34.4	39.5	39.7	39.2	33.2	35.6
Past year alcohol use (%)	36.7	20.2	24.1	31.3	31.4	31.2	22.7	25.6
Lifetime any illicit drug use (%)	27.7	24.2	28.5	26.4	26.8	26.0	30.0	26.9
Past year any illicit drug use (%)	20.2	13.7	18.6	18.8	18.0	19.6	19.7	17.3

Source: SAMHSA, Office of Applied Studies, National Household Survey on Drug Abuse, 2000; National Survey on Drug Use and Health, 2003, 2006.

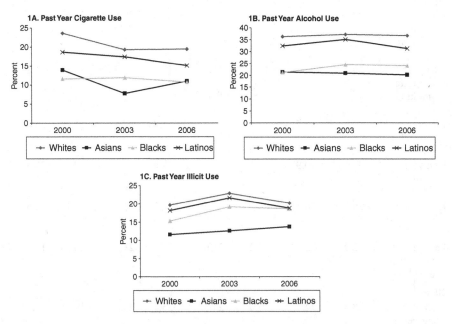

Fig. 15.1 Prevalence of past year use by Ethnic group among youth 12–17 years old (NHSDA)

Table 15.2 Prevalence of cigarette smoking and illicit drug use among White, Black, and Hispanic youth aged 18 to 25 years in the United States (NHSDA)

	Whites	Asians	Blacks	Latinos
2000				
Lifetime cigarette smoking (%)	74.1	41.9	50.2	57.6
Past year cigarette smoking (%)	51.9	27.4	31.5	34.5
Lifetime alcohol use (%)	88.2	66.2	76.2	76.7
Past year alcohol use (%)	80.1	58.4	62.5	63.9
Lifetime any illicit drug use (%)	56.1	27.9	44.5	39.2
Past year any illicit drug use (%)	30.7	14.0	24.7	20.2
2003				
Lifetime cigarette smoking (%)	75.6	52.4	55.8	66.2
Past year cigarette smoking (%)	53.3	33.4	33.0	41.9
Lifetime alcohol use (%)	90.7	79.0	78.6	82.9
Past year alcohol use (%)	83.4	67.6	67.9	70.2
Lifetime any illicit drug use (%)	65.1	43.1	54.6	52.2
Past year any illicit drug use (%)	38.2	22.1	30.6	27.5
2006				
Lifetime cigarette smoking (%)	73.2	47.2	51.4	59.4
Past year cigarette smoking (%)	53.4	33.1	33.0	38.3
Lifetime alcohol use (%)	90.9	76.5	77.4	80.4
Past year alcohol use (%)	85.1	67.3	66.7	69.4
Lifetime any illicit drug use (%)	64.7	37.3	51.9	48.7
Past year any illicit drug use (%)	38.9	20.5	29.2	25.0

Source: SAMHSA, Office of Applied Studies, National Household Survey on Drug Abuse, 2000; National Survey on Drug Use and Health, 2003, 2006.

larger margins. For example, the difference between White non-Latinos and Latinos was almost nonexistent for 12- to 17-year olds, but ranges from 9 to as much as 29 percentage points for those aged 18 to 25 years. This is likely to be influenced by the fact that many Latinos in this age group migrated to the U.S. postadolescence. Second, in this age group there are higher comparative rates of illicit drugs among Blacks, with rates that are second to those of White non-Latinos. This trend is also evident with the younger age group (Table 15.1), with the rates for Blacks approximating those of Latinos. Third, the rate of cigarette use among White non-Latinos is strikingly higher than that of all other groups. All these differences are visually better illustrated in Figs. 15.1 and 15.2.

Long-Term Impact of Early and Mid-adolescence Factors on Substance Use Disorders in Early Adulthood

The following longitudinal analyses utilize data from a cohort study of adolescents conducted in South Florida from 1990 to 2002 (Gil et al., 2002; Lloyd & Taylor, 2006; Turner & Lloyd, 2003; Turner, Lloyd, & Taylor, 2005; Vega &

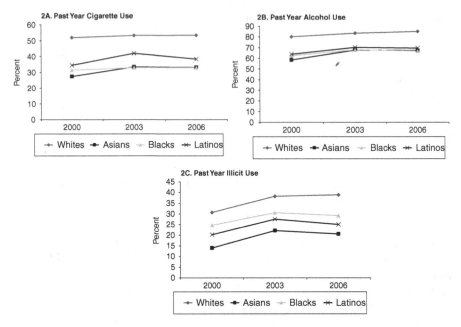

Fig. 15.2 Prevalence of past year use by Ethnic group among youth 18–25 years old (NHSDA)

Gil, 1998). We examine the changing effects of risk factors from early- to mid-adolescence, including the effects of U.S. census-based neighborhood poverty on drug addiction occurring in early adulthood, as determined using DSM-IV alcohol abuse/dependence, and drug abuse/dependence criteria. The risk factors are grouped in six domains: family environment, family structure, drug-use modeling, psychosocial factors, school factors, and delinquency factors. These domains are derived from an extensive empirical research literature, and details regarding these risk domains can be found in Gil et al. (2002). The *family environment* domain contains measures of familism, family communication, family cohesion, and parental derogation. The *drug use modeling* domain contains measures of parental smoking and drug use, as well as peer substance use. The *psychosocial factors* domain included self-esteem, depression, history of suicidality, and perceptions of life chances. *School factors* included perceived teacher derogation, official records in absenteeism and behavior problems and grades. Finally, *delinquency factors* consisted of perceived delinquency and delinquent behavior.

Table 15.3 presents unadjusted odds ratios for early and mid-adolescence. Table 15.4 presents adjusted risk factors during early adolescence in order to determine the impact of 1990 census neighborhood family poverty, while controlling for all the other risk factors. In Table 15.3, it is important to highlight the increase in the impact of all risk factors from early adolescence to mid-adolescence

Table 15.3 Unadjusted Odds Ratios of early and mid-adolescence risk domains for early adulthood DSM-IV Substance Disorders

	U.S. Latino		Foreign Latino		African American		European American	
	Alcohol Ab/Dep	Drug Ab/Dep	Alcohol Ab/Dep	Drug Ab/Dep	Alcohol Ab/Dep	Drug Ab/Dep	Alcohol Ab/Dep	Drug Ab/Dep
Early Adolescence								
Family Environment	1.3*	1.1	1.1	1.4*	1.5*	1.1	1.0	1.3*
Family Structure	1.3*	1.1	.89	.92	.72	.98	1.1	1.3*
Drug-Use Modeling	1.2	1.4**	1.2	1.2	1.3	1.2	1.2	1.5**
Psychosocial Factors	1.2	1.2	.99	1.1	2.0**	1.6**	1.0	1.6**
School Factors	1.3*	1.3*	1.1	1.2	1.5**	1.4*	1.2	1.7***
Delinquency Factors	1.4	2.0*	1.7*	2.1*	2.0*	2.4**	1.2	2.5***
Neighborhood Family								
Poverty	1.7*	1.6*	.95	1.1	1.8**	1.2	.58*	.75
Mid-Adolescence								
Family Environment	1.5*	1.3*	1.4*	1.2	1.9***	1.3*	1.3*	1.4*
Family Structure	1.2	1.2	.92	1.1	.81	.91	1.1	1.4*
Drug-Use Modeling	1.8***	1.5**	1.5*	1.2	1.1	1.2	1.4*	2.2***
Psychosocial Factors	1.2	1.3	1.1	1.1	1.9**	1.2	1.2	1.4*
School Factors	1.4*	1.6*	1.5*	1.7*	1.6*	1.4*	1.4*	1.3*
Delinquency Factors	2.8***	3.4***	4.2***	4.0***	1.6*	2.9***	2.6***	3.0***

Table 15.4 Adjusted Odds Ratios of mid- adolescence risk domains for early adulthood DSM-IV Substance Disorders

	U.S. Latino		Foreign Latino		African American		European American	
	Alcohol Ab/Dep	Drug Ab/Dep	Alcohol Ab/Dep	Drug Ab/Dep	Alcohol Ab/Dep	Drug Ab/Dep	Alcohol Ab/Dep	Drug Ab/Dep
Mid- Adolescence								
Family Environment	1.2	.91	1.2	1.4*	1.2	.87	.98	1.0
Family Structure	1.2	1.0	.80	.84	.67	.89	.94	1.1
Drug-Use Modeling	1.1	1.2	1.2	1.2	1.3	1.1	1.2	1.1
Psychosocial Factors	.97	.95	.80	.67	1.4*	1.3	.95	1.3
School Factors	1.3*	1.3*	.99	1.0	1.5*	1.2	1.2	1.5**
Delinquency Factors	1.0	1.8*	1.7*	1.9*	1.3	2.0**	1.0	1.5*
Neighborhood Family								
Poverty	1.9**	1.8*	.91	1.0	1.7*	1.2	.60*	.86

among U.S. Latinos. Among foreign Latinos, the delinquency factors are the most influential, particularly during mid-adolescence with equally high odds of 4.2 and 4.0 for alcohol abuse/dependence and drug/use dependence. It is also notable that the delinquency factors are influential for all ethnic groups and at both time periods. Finally, neighborhood poverty was significant for U.S. Latinos for alcohol and drugs, for African Americans for alcohol, and for European Americans for alcohol, but in the opposite direction, indicating that European Americans growing up in neighborhoods with less poverty were *more* likely to develop alcohol abuse/dependence.

Finally, Table 15.4 illustrates that neighborhood family poverty remained significant for U.S. Latinos even after controlling for all the other risk domains. Importantly, after the introduction of neighborhood family poverty into the model, only school factors remained significant for alcohol abuse/dependence, and only school and delinquency remained significant for drug abuse/dependence among U.S.-born Latinos. Among African Americans, neighborhood poverty remained significant for alcohol abuse/dependence, and delinquency factors were no longer significant. The neighborhood family poverty reduces or eliminates the effects of other salient psychosocial risk factors for both Latino and African American adolescent drug use.

Conclusion

Population drug use patterns are cyclical (Gfroerer & Brodsky 1992). Drug epidemics occur and penetrate into various minority communities idiosyncratically, and it is difficult to predict how rapidly they will spread across regions or the country, or how long they will endure. Generally, the secular trend has been toward decreases in the overall use of illicit drugs following a peak in the 1970s across all ethnic groups, albeit with occasional and stunning reversals such as crack cocaine and methamphetamine epidemics. The current epidemic of methamphetamine use is an interesting example of selectivity, with high impact on non-Latino Whites contrasted with less impact thus far on African Americans. Another example is the long-standing problem of inhalant abuse among Latinos and American Indians, with no comparable impact on African Americans (Mathew, Balster, Cottler, We, & Vaugh, 2008; Wallace et al., 2002). Inhalant abuse offers an illuminating comparison because substances used for inhalation are inexpensive and accessible to virtually all youth, which decreases the likelihood that access explains differences in use levels.

Despite the history of cyclical drug use patterns in the United States, there has been a consistent trend during the past 10 years regarding lifetime drug use among Latinos and African Americans. Despite somewhat lower prevalence of use among foreign-born Latinos, U.S.-born Latinos continue "catching-up" with White non-Latino adolescents and are starting experimentation at earlier ages. While African Americans continue to exhibit lower rates during early adolescence, they are also "catching-up" with White non-Latinos during the period from mid- to later-adolescence. Gender differences, whereby females reported lower lifetime rates of substance use, are narrowing for both Latino and African American youth; however, alcohol and drug "disorder" (as differentiated from lifetime use) rates remain higher for males. These trends are illustrated by the national data presented in this chapter.

Recognizing that the peak period for developing drug dependence occurs between 15 and 29 years of age, a critical issue with Latinos is the very youthful structure of the population, since 40% of the population is younger than 21 years of age. This fact, combined with the facts that Latinos have high poverty rates, rapid population expansion, and increasing numbers of female-headed households living in poverty, underscores the need for broad public policy initiatives to decrease the burden of drug use for the entire population. There is increased evidence of trends toward higher lifetime and past year rates of drug use among Latinos similar to recent trends for African American adults, albeit not yet attaining the prevalence rates of White non-Latinos for licit or illicit drug use (National Institute on Drug Abuse, 1995). Although not specially addressed in this chapter, we also presented some data on Asians, who have consistently demonstrated lower rates for all substances except past year alcohol and cigarette use. For ethnic groups there are important variations in internal population characteristics that affect drug use levels.

While environmental factors influence drug use and misuse, there are complex reciprocal relationships between drug use and factors associated with the disproportionate residential patterns of ethnic minorities, whereby they are segregated into high-risk, high-stress environments where families in poverty, or nearly in poverty, are concentrated. While the risk factors domains utilized in the longitudinal studies presented in this chapter are broad in the sense that they involve family, school, peer, and psychosocial domains, the reality is that these risk exposures do not occur in isolation but are frequently accompanied by residential status in neighborhoods with many aversive features such as social disorganization, widespread violence, and substance abuse. Public policy must focus on reducing economic inequality, and public health and urban planners must focus on eliminating these environmental conditions, if meaningful changes in ethnic health disparities are to be accomplished (Robinson, 2008). This requires attention to the interactions that exist between multiple social and interpersonal levels in the causation of health disparities, including negative outcomes such as higher addiction rates (Gehlert et al., 2008).

The social conditions for minority children and their families which result in health disparities are numerous. Both Latino and Black children in the United States are more than 12 times as likely as White children to be poor and to live in poor neighborhoods (Acevedo-Garcia, Osypuk, McArdle, & Williams, 2008). The situation for a large proportion of Latino and African American children (20.5% and 17%, respectively) has been described as "double jeopardy," that is, circumstances of living in poor families and poor neighborhoods (Nicotera, 2008). Additionally, the conditions for poor Black and Latino children are more severe than those of their White counterparts, with the typical poor Black and Latino child more likely to reside in neighborhoods of concentrated poverty than their low income White counterparts. For example, while the typical poor White child lives in a neighborhood where the poverty rate is 13.6%, the rate for Latino children is about twice as high (26%), and for Black children it is even higher (30%), reflecting *de facto* segregation patterns (Acevedo-Garcia, Osypuk, McArdle, & Williams, 2008). Adequate educational attainment is another important factor which has been identified as a marker for health disparities. Importantly, increases in life expectancies between the 1980s and 2000 appear to have been concentrated among highly educated groups (Meara, Richards & Cutler, 2008).

The health disparities found among minority populations in the United States are clearly connected to tobacco, alcohol, and other drug use (Spiegler, Tate, Aitken, & Christian, 1989; U.S. Department of Health and Human Services 1998). Similarly, drug use is related to disruptions in life span transitions, school achievement, employment, and family stability, and leads to lower socioeconomic status and involvement in the justice system (Blumstein & Beck, 1999). These problems exist within the context of detrimental social and economic conditions, and thus interventions and prevention efforts must occur within a larger policy context of addressing these root social conditions.

References

Acevedo-Garcia, D., Osypuk, T. L., McArdle, N., & Williams, D. R. (2008). Toward a policy-relevant analysis of geographic and racial/ethnic disparities in child health. *Health Affairs, 27*(2), 321–333.

Aktan, G. B., Kumpfer, K. L., & Turner, C. W. (1996) Effectiveness of family skills training program for substance use prevention with inner city African American families. *Substance Use & Misuse, 31*, 157–175.

American Psychiatric Association. (1994). *Diagnostic and statistical manual of mental disorders* (4th ed.). Washington, DC: Author.

Anthony, J. C., Warner, L. A., & Kessler, R. C. (1994). Comparative epidemiology of dependence on tobacco, alcohol, controlled substances, and inhalants: Basic findings from the National Comorbidity Survey. *Experimental and Clinical Psychopharmacology, 2*, 244–268.

Baumrind, D., & Moselle, K. A. (1985). A developmental perspective on adolescent drug use. *Advances In Alcohol and Substance Use, 5*, 41–67.

Belitz, J., & Valdez, D. M. (1995). Clinical issues in the treatment of Chicano male gang youths. In A. M. Padilla (Ed.). *Latino Psychology: Critical issues in theory and research* (pp. 148–165). Thousand Oaks, CA: Sage.

Blumstein, A., & Beck, A. J. (1999). Population growth in U.S. prisons, 1980–1996. In M. Tonry & J. Petersilia (Eds.). *Prisons: Crime and justice, a review of research* (Vol. 26., pp. 16–71). Chicago, IL: University of Chicago Press.

Brody, G. H., Ge, X., Conger, R., Gibbons, F. X., Murry, V., M., Gerrard, M., et al. (2001). The influence of neighborhood disadvantage, collective socialization, and parenting on African American children's affiliation with deviant peers. *Child Development, 72*, 1231–1246.

Brook, J. S., Adams, R. E., Balka, E. B., & Johnson, E., (2002). Early adolescent marijuana use: Risks for transition to young adulthood. *Psychological Medicine, 32*, 79–91.

Brook, J. S., Brook, D. W., De La Rosa, M., Whiteman, M., Johnson, E., & Montoya, I. (2001). Adolescent illegal drug use: The impact of personality, family, and environmental factors. *Journal of Behavioral Medicine, 24*, 183–203.

Brook, J. S., Hamburg, B. A., Balka, E. B., & Wynn, P. S. (1992). Sequences of drug involvement in African-American and Puerto Rican adolescents. *Psychology Reports, 71*, 179–182.

Brook, J. S., Whiteman, M., Balka, E., Win, P., & Gursen, M. (1997). African American and Puerto Rican drug use: A longitudinal study. *Journal of American Childhood and Adolescent Psychiatry, 36*, 1260–1268.

Brook, J. S., Whiteman, M., & Gordon, A. S. (1983). Stages of drug use in adolescence: Personality, peer, and family correlates. *Development Psychology, 19*, 269–277.

Chavez, E. L., & Swaim, R. C. (1992). An epidemiological comparison of Mexican-American and White non-Latino 8th and 12th grade students' substance use. *American Journal of Public Health, 82*, 445–447.

Cleveland, M. J., Gibbons, F. X., Gerrard, M., Pomery, E. A., & Brody, G. H. (2005) The impact of parenting on risk cognitions and risk behavior: A study of mediation and moderation in a panel of African American adolescents. *Child Development, 76*, 900–916.

Cooper, R. S. (2003). Gene-environment interactions and the etiology of common complex disease. *Annals Internal Medicine, 139*, 437–440.

De La Rosa, M., Vega, R., & Radisch, M. A. (2000). The role of acculturation in the substance abuse behavior of African American and Latino adolescents: Advances, issues, and recommendations. *Journal of Psychoactive Drugs, 32*, 33–42.

Ebin, V. J., Sneed, C. D., Morisky, E. D., Rotheram-Borus, M. J., Magnusson, A. M., & Malotte, C. K. (2001). Acculturation and interrelationships between problem and health-promoting behaviors among Latino adolescents. *Journal of Adolescent Health, 28*, 62–72.

Elder, J. P., Campbell, N. R., Litrownik, A. J., Ayala, G., Slymen, D. J., et al. (2000). Predictors of cigarette and alcohol susceptibility and use among Latino migrant adolescents. *Preventive Medicine, 31*, 115–123.

Ellickson, P. L., Collins, R. L., & Bell, R. M. (1999). Adolescent use of illicit drugs other than marijuana: how important is social bonding and for which ethnic groups? *Substance Use and Misuse, 34*, 317–346.

Ellickson, P. L., Hays, R. D., & Bell, R. M. (1992). Stepping through the drug use sequence: Longitudinal scalogram analysis of initiation and regular use. *Journal of Abnormal Psychology, 101*, 441–451.

Epstein, J. A., Botvin, G. J., & Diaz, T. (2000). Alcohol use among Latino adolescents: Role of linguistic acculturation and gender. *Journal of Alcohol and Drug Education, 45*, 16–32.

Erickson, N. (2001). *Substance abuse: The nation's number one health problem. Office of Justice Programs, Office of Juvenile Justice and Delinquency Prevention-OJJDP Fact Sheet # 17.* Washington, DC: U.S. Department of Justice.

Gehlert, S., Sohmer, D., Sacks, T., Mininger, C., McClintock, M., & Olopade, O. (2008). Targeting health disparities: A model linking upstream determinants to downstream interventions. *Health Affairs, 27*(2), 339–349.

Gfroerer, J., & Brodsky, M. (1992). The incidence of illicit drug use in the United States, 1962–1989. *Addiction, 87*, 1345–1351.

Gibbons, F. X., Gerrard, M., Cleveland, M. J., Wills, T. A., & Brody, G. (2004). Perceived discrimination and substance use in African American parents and their children: A panel study. *Journal of Personality and Social Psychology, 86*, 517–529.

Gil, A. G., Vega W. A., & Biafora, F. (1997). Temporal influences of family structure, and family risk factors on drug use initiation in a multi-ethnic sample of adolescent boys. *Journal of Youth and Adolescence, 23*, 373–393.

Gil, A. G., Vega, W. A., & Dimas, J. (1994). Acculturation stress and personal adjustment among Latino adolescent boys. *Journal of Community Psychology, 22*, 43–54.

Gil, A. G, Vega, W. A., & Turner, R. J. (2002.) Early adolescent risk factors for African American and European American DSM-IV substance abuse disorders in adulthood. *Public Health Reports, 117*, 15– 29.

Grant, B. F., Dawson, D. A., Stinson, F. S., Chou, P. S., Kay, W., & Pickering, R. (1993). The Alcohol Use Disorder and Associated Disabilities Interview Schedule-IV (AUDADIS-IV): reliability of alcohol consumption, tobacco use, family history of depression and psychiatric diagnostic modules in a general population sample. *Drug Alcohol Dependency, 71*, 7–16.

Griffin, K. W., Botvin, G. J., Scheier, L. M., Diaz, T., & Miller, N. L. (2000). Parenting practices as predictors of substance use, delinquency, and aggression among urban minority youth: Moderating effects of family structure and gender. *Psychology of Addictive Behavior, 14*, 174–84.

Hawkins, D. J., Catalano, R. F., & Miller, J. Y. (1992). Risk and protective factors for alcohol and other drug problems in adolescence and early adulthood: Implications for substance abuse prevention. *Psychological Bulletin, 112*, 64–105.

Herd, D. (1987). Rethinking black drinking. *British Journal of Addiction, 82*, 219–223.

Jessor, R. (1991). Risk behavior in adolescence: A psychosocial framework for understanding and action. *Journal of Adolescent Health, 12*, 597–605.

Jessor, R. (1993). Successful adolescent development among youth in high-risk settings. *American Psychologist, 48*, 117–126.

Kandel, D. B. (1975). Stages of adolescent drug involvement in drug use. *Science, 190*, 912–914.

Kandel, D. B., & Faust, R. (1975). Sequence in stages and patterns of adolescent drug use. *Archives of General Psychiatry, 32*, 923–932.

Kaplan, H. B., Martin, S., & Robbins, C. (1985). Toward an explanation of increased involvement in illicit drug use: Application of a general theory of deviant behavior. In J. R. Greenley (Ed.), *Research in community and mental health* (Vol. 5, pp. 205–252). Greenwich, CT: JAI Press.

Kaplan, H. B., Johnson, R. J., & Bailey, C. A. (1988). Applications of a general theory of deviant behavior: Self-derogation and adolescent drug use. *Journal of Health and Social Behavior, 23*, 274–294.

Kessler, R. C., & Walters, E. E. (2002). The National Comorbidity Survey. In M. T. Tsaung & M. Tohen, M. (Eds.), *Textbook in psychiatric epidemiology* (2nd ed., pp. 343–362). New York: John Wily & Sons.

Kogan, S. M., Luo, Z., & Brody, G. H. (2005). The influence of high school drop out on substance use among African American youth. *Journal of Ethnicity in Substance Use, 4*, 35–51.

Krohn, M. D., Lizotte, A. J., & Perez, C. M. (1997). The interrelationship between substance use and precocious transitions to adult statuses. *Journal of Health and Social Behavior, 38*, 87–103.

Lam, W. K. K., Cance, J. D., Eke, A. N., Fishbein, D. H., Hawkins, S. R., & Williams, J. C. (2007). Children of African-American mothers who use crack cocaine: Parenting influences on youth substance use. *Journal of Pediatric Psychology, 32*, 877–887.

Licinio, J. (2002). Gene-environment interactions. *Molecular Psychiatry, 7*, 123–124.

Lloyd, D. A., & Taylor, J. (2006). Lifetime cumulative adversity, mental health and the risk of becoming a smoker. *Health: An Interdisciplinary Journal for the Social Study of Health Illness and Medicine, 10*, 95–112.

Lucas, C. P., Zhang, H., Fisher, P. W., Shaffer, D., Regier, D. A., Narrow, W. E., et al. (2001). The DISC predictive scales (DPS): Efficiently screening for diagnoses. *American Academy of Child and Adolescent Psychiatry, 40*, 443–449.

Martinez, C. (2006). Effects of differential family acculturation on Latino adolescent substance use. *Family Relations, 55*, 306–317.

Mathew, O. H., Balster, R. L., Cottler, L. B., Wu, L., & Vaughn, M. G. (2008). Inhalant use among incarcerated adolescents in the United States: Prevalence, characteristics, and correlates of use. *Drug and Alcohol Dependence, 93*, 197–209.

McGinnis, J. M., & Foege, W. H. (1999). Mortality and morbidity attributable to use of addictive substances in the United States. *Proceedings of the Association for American Physicians, 111,* 109–118.

McMahon, T. J. (2008). Drug abuse and responsible fathering: A comparative study of men enrolled in methadone maintenance treatment. *Addiction, 103,* 269–283.

Meara, E. R., Richards, S., & Cutler, D. M. (2008). The gap gets bigger: Changes in mortality and life expectancy, by education, 1981–2000. *Health Affairs, 27*(2), 350–360.

Merikangas, K. R., Mehta, R. L., Molnar, B. E., Walters, E. E., Swendsen, J. D., Aguilar-Gaxiola, S., et al. (1998). Comorbidity of substance use disorders with mood and anxiety disorders: Results of the International Consortium in Psychiatric Epidemiology. *Addictive Behaviors, 23,* 893–907.

Miller-Day, M. (2008). Talking to youth about drugs: What do late adolescents say about parental strategies? *Family Relations, 57,* 1–12.

Mokdad, A. H., Marks, J. S., Stroup, D. F., & Gerberding, J. L. (2004). Actual causes of death in the United States, 2000. *Journal of the American Medical Association, 291,* 1238–1245.

National Institute on Drug Abuse. (2003). *Drug use among ethnic racial minorities.* NIH Publication No. 03-3888. Washington, DC: Author.

Newcomb, M. D., & Bentler, P. M. (1986a). Substance abuse and ethnicity: Differential impact of peer and adult models. *Journal of Psychology, 120,* 83–95.

Newcomb, M. D., & Bentler, P. M. (1986b). Frequency and sequence of drug use: A longitudinal study from early adolescence to young adulthood. *Journal of Drug Education, 16,* 101–120.

Nicotera, N. (2008) Children speak about neighborhoods: Using mixed methods to measure the construct neighborhood. *Journal of Community Psychology, 36,* 333–351.

Obot, I. S. (1996). Problem drinking, chronic disease, and recent life events. In H. W. Neighbors & J. S. Jackson (Eds.), *Mental health in Black America* (pp. 45–61). Thousand Oaks, CA: Sage.

Oetting, E. R. (1993). Orthogonal cultural identification: Theoretical links between cultural identification and substance use. In M. R. De La Rosa & J. L. Recio Adrados (Eds.), *Drug abuse among minority youth: Methodological issues and recent advances* (NIH Publication No. 93-3479) (pp. 32–56). Washington, DC: National Institute of Drug Abuse.

Oetting, E. R., & Beauvais, F. (1991). Adolescent drug use: Findings of national and local surveys. *Journal of Consulting and Clinical Psychology, 34,* 205–213.

Ortega, A., Rosenheck, R., Alegria, M., & Rani, D. (2000). Acculturation and lifetime risk of psychiatric and substance use disorders and Latinos. *Journal of Nervous Mental Disease, 188,* 728–735.

Rehm, J., Taylor, B., & Room, R. (2006). Global burden of disease from alcohol, illicit drugs and tobacco. *Drug Alcohol Review, 25,* 503–13.

Rice, D. P., Kelman, S., & Miller, L. S. (1991). Estimates of economic costs of alcohol and drug use and mental illness, 1985–1988. *Public Health Reports, 106,* 280–292.

Roux, A. V. D. (2001). Investigating neighborhood and areas effects on health. *American Journal of Public Health, 91,* 1783–1789.

Robins, L. N., Wing, J., Wittchen, H. U., Helzer, J. E., Babor, T. F., Burke, J., et al. (1988). The Composite International Diagnostic Interview: An epidemiologic instrument suitable for use in conjunction with different diagnostic systems and in different cultures. *Archives of General Psychiatry, 45,* 1069–1077.

Robinson, J. (2008). Disparities in health: Expanding the focus. *Health Affairs, 27*(2), 318–319.

Sampson, R. J., Raudenbush, S. W., & Earls, F. (1997). Neighborhoods and violent crime: A multilevel study of collective efficacy. *Science, 277,* 918–924.

Sastry, N., Ghosh-Dastidar, B., Adams, J., & Pebley, A. R. (2006). The design of a multilevel survey of children, families, and communities: The Los Angeles Family and Neighborhood Survey. *Social Science Research, 35,* 1000–1024.

Spiegler, D., Tate, D., Aitken, S., & Christian, C. (Eds.). (1989). *Alcohol use among U.S. ethnic minorities*. Research Monograph 18. Rockville, MD: National Institute on Alcohol Abuse and Alcoholism, 1989.

Stanton, B., Xiaoming, L., Pack, R., Cottrell, L., Harris, C., & Burns, J. M. (2002). Longitudinal influence of peer and parental factors on African American risk involvement. *Journal of Urban Health, 79*, 536–548.

Tsuang, M. T., Bar, J. L., Harley, R. M., & Lyons, M. J. (2001). Genetic and environmental influences on transitions in drug use. *Behavioral Genetics, 29*, 473–479.

Turner, R. J., & Lloyd, D. A. (2003). Cumulative adversity and drug dependence in youth adults: Racial/ethnic contrasts. *Addiction, 98*, 305–316.

Turner, R. J., Lloyd, D. A., & Taylor, J. (2005). Stress burden, drug dependence, and the nativity paradox among U.S. Latinos. *Drug & Alcohol Dependency, 83*, 79–89.

U.S. Bureau of Census. (2002). *Current population survey (CPS)*. Washington, D.C.: Government Printing Office.

U.S. Department of Health and Human Services. (1998). *Tobacco use among U.S. racial/ethnic minority groups—African Americans, American Indians, and Alaska Natives, Asian Americans and Pacific Islanders, and Hispanics: A report of the Surgeon General*. Atlanta, Georgia: U.S. Department of Health and Human Services, Centers for Disease Control and Prevention, National Center for Chronic Disease Prevention and Health Promotion, Office on Smoking and Health.

Vega, W. A., Aguilar-Gaxiola, S., Andrade, L., Bijl, R., Borges, G., Caraveo-Anduaga, J. J., et al. (2002). Prevalence and age of onset for drug use in seven international sites: Results from the International Consortium of Psychiatric Epidemiology. *Drug and Alcohol Dependence, 68*, 285–297.

Vega, W. A., Chen, K. W., & Williams, J. (2007). Smoking, drugs, and other behavioral health problems among multiethnic adolescents in the NHSDA. *Addictive Behaviors, 32*, 1949–1956.

Vega, W. A., & Gil, A. G. (1998). *Ethnicity and drug use in early adolescence*. New York.: Plenum.

Vega, W. A., & Gil, A. G. (2005). Revisiting drug progression: Long range effects of early tobacco use. *Addiction, 100*, 1358–1369.

Vega, W. A., Gil, A. G., & Zimmerman, R. S. (1993). Patterns of drug use among Cuban Americans, African Americans, and White non-Latino boys. *American Journal of Public Health, 83*, 257–259.

Vega, W. A., & Sribney, W. (2003). Parental behavioral risk factors and social assimilation in alcohol dependence of Mexican Americans. *Journal of Studies on Alcohol, 64*, 167–175.

Volkow, N. D., Fowler, J. S., Wang, G. J., et al. (2002). Role of dopamine, the frontal cortex and memory circuits in drug addiction: Insight from imaging studies. *Neurobiology of Learning and Memory, 78*, 610–624.

Wallace, J. M., Bachman, J. G., O'Malley, P. M., Schulenberg, J. E., Cooper, S. M., & Johnson, L. D. (2002). Gender and ethnic differences in smoking, drinking, and illicit drug use among American 8th, 10th, and 12th, grade students 1976–2000. *Addiction, 98*, 225–234.

Wittchen, H. U., Robins, L. N., Cottler, L. B., Sartorious, N., Burke, J. D., & Regier, D. (1991). Cross-cultural feasibility, reliability, and sources of variance of the Composite Diagnostic Interview (CIDI). *British Journal of Psychiatry, 195*, 645–653.

WHO World Mental Health Survey Consortium. (2004). Prevalence, severity, and unmet need for treatment of mental disorders in the World Mental Health Organization World Mental Health Surveys. *Journal of the American Medical Association, 291*, 2581–2590.

Xiaoming, L., Feigelman, S., & Stanton, B. (2000). Perceived parental monitoring and health risk behaviors among urban low-income African American children and adolescents. *Journal of Adolescent Health, 27*, 43–48.

Chapter 16
Neurocognitive Testing of Minorities in Mental Health Settings

Amir Poreh and Alya Sultan

Introduction

The U.S. Census Bureau has recently noted that about one third of the U.S. population is made up of minorities, and this proportion will grow given that at present, 45% of American children under the age of five are minorities (United States Census Bureau, 2008). Changes in the population composition are reminiscent of the great migration of Irish and Eastern Europeans in the past century and call for the reexamination of current practices in general medicine and mental health. To address this latest challenge, the National Institute of Neurological Disorders and the National Institute of Mental Health (2002) have published plans to conduct studies and develop new measures that will assist in addressing the needs of ethnic minority populations.

Addressing these issues in the fields of neuropsychiatry and neurology has been relatively slow-moving. Since there is agreement that the presenting symptoms of neurological and psychiatric disorders are disturbances of brain functions, some researchers and clinicians have not seen any need to reexamine the prevailing diagnostic and treatment methodologies. In this chapter, we will examine how immigration affects the validity of neurocognitive evaluations and provide guidelines for addressing these shortcomings.

The neurocognitive technique dates back to studies conducted at the turn of the 20th century. Such studies typically involved the administration of cognitive and motor tasks that have been shown to correlate with damage to particular brain structures or have implications regarding daily activity. Measures that are used to evaluate neurocognitive functions include standardized measures of memory, intelligence, visual spatial abilities, problem solving, and planning (Lezak, Howieson, & Loring, 2004).

A. Poreh (✉)
Cleveland State University, Cleveland, OH
e-mail: aporeh@yahoo.com

S. Loue, M. Sajatovic (eds.), *Determinants of Minority Mental Health and Wellness*, DOI 10.1007/978-0-387-75659-2_16,
© Springer Science+Business Media, LLC 2009

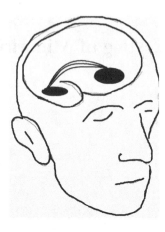

Figure 16.1 demonstrates, for example, the structures associated with language abilities. One sees that two main areas are associated with language abilities. These areas, which were originally discovered in the late 19th century, are responsible for speech production (Broca's area) and comprehension (Wernicke's area). Using very simple tasks such as asking a patient to say the names of as many animals as they can, or repeat sentences, a trained neuropsychiatrist or neuropsychologist has the potential to identify the type of disorder a patient is suffering from and the location of the brain injury. Language assessment also allows a clinician, for example, to evaluate whether a patient is exhibiting early signs of Alzheimer's disease, which is typically characterized by word finding difficulties. When neurocognitive measures are appropriately

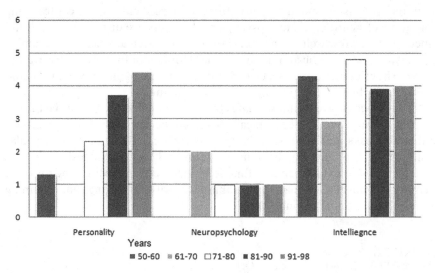

Fig. 16.1 Relative number of cross-cultural publications in three major psychology disciplines across five decades

used, they can provide important information to caregivers and patients. In the case of Alzheimer's disease, a proper neurocognitive assessment can provide valuable information regarding treatment planning and the ability of the patient to function independently and can even predict the course of the disease. However, as we will see in the remainder of this chapter, when clinicians who employ neurocognitive measures ignore cultural differences, they are at risk of making significant mistakes. To understand the pitfalls for neurocognitive assessment, the origins of these measures will be reviewed and then guidelines of how to employ such measures will be provided.

Historical Background on Psychological Assessment and Special Populations

The roots of psychological assessment can be traced to the work of Sir Francis Galton. Galton, who was influenced by the theory of evolution, decided to apply hereditary logic to the assessment of mental attributes and conceptualized intelligence as "man's natural abilities (that) are (exclusively) derived by inheritance." He then proposed that humans' abilities could be enhanced through selective breeding, "eugenics," from the Greek for "wellborn" (Galton, 1869). Galton's call for the improvement of human heredity led him to develop the first standardized measures of cognitive functions, or "intelligence," along with the development of modern techniques for assessing the relationships between variables, which he termed "correlations" (Holt, 2005). After a considerable amount of research, it was determined that Galton's measures of intelligence were not valid in predicting professional academic success (Whipple, 1910).

A decade after the publication of Galton's book, *The Hereditary Genius*, Binet and Simon (1905) developed the first modern intelligence test. This test was commissioned by the French government to assist in the development of programs for children with special needs. Alfred Binet and Théodore Simon rejected the primary role of heredity in the formation of intelligence and defined intelligence as "reasoning, judgment, memory, and the power of abstraction" that is shaped, at least in part, by the environment. Binet and Simon's test allowed for the tailoring of programs for the mentally retarded and for providing objective criteria that allowed governments throughout the world to provide assistance to children who are in need. Some researchers and clinicians, however, started to apply the Binet-Simon intelligence tests for the screening of "bad" genes. Henry Goddard for example, translated the Binet-Simon intelligence scale into English and used the Binet-Simon Test to compare the "intelligence" of different ethnic groups. In 1912, he published a book entitled *The Kallikak Family: A Study in the Heredity of Feeble-mindedness* (Goddard, 1912). In this book, he purportedly demonstrated that a parent, two generations removed, provided the genes for the feeblemindedness of some of its members. Based on his findings, Goddard advocated the practice of sterilization of the feeble minded, a notion that was later supported by the U.S. Supreme court in the landmark case of Buck v. Bell, 274 U.S. 200 (1927). In 1913, Henry Goddard established an intelligence testing program at Ellis Island. The data collected in this program estimated that 83% of the Jews, 80% of the Hungarians, 79% of the Italians, and 87% of the Russians were feeble minded (Goddard, 1915). These so-called objective findings reflected the general attitude among many Americans regarding the mental inferiority of southern and eastern European immigrants (Gelb, Allen, Futterman, & Mehler, 1986).

When the United States entered World War I, millions of army recruits were conscripted. Since the United States did not have a career army or a well-defined social class hierarchy, as in most European countries, the American Psychological Association (APA) was assigned to develop screening measures designed to not only reject feeble minded and mentally ill recruits but also served to identify the recruits who were fit to serve as officers. Three test batteries of the Army tests were developed. These included the Army Alpha for literate recruits, the Army Beta for the illiterates, and an individual exam for those who failed both. Yerkes's (1921) final report on these test batteries showed that the average mental age of Caucasian Americans was slightly above those of Eastern European immigrants, and African Americans scored the lowest on mental age. Yerkes's data led to the adoption of the Immigration Act of 1924, which restricted the number of immigrants from "undesirable" racial groups.

A decade later, in the late 1930s, the theory of eugenics served as the basis for the Nazis's implementation of a series of programs designed to "improve" their genetic makeup. These programs initially included the killing of disabled children and adults through "euthanasia" programs and later served as the basis for the Holocaust, the systematic killing of millions of "undesirable" people including Jews, Gypsies, homosexuals, and "Slavs." The legacy of mental testing and eugenics was still evident in the early 1970s, when intelligence and aptitude testing was used for the discrimination of minorities in the workplace. The use of such measures in the work place was eventually curtailed following the landmark case of Griggs vs. Duke Power Company (1971). In this case, the U.S. Supreme Court ruled against the use of measures that are not a "reasonable measure of job performance," regardless of the absence of actual intent to discriminate.

Parallel to the Civil Rights Act of 1962, an increasing number of psychologists became interested in studying the role of cross-cultural differences in psychological assessment. Torrance (1962) and Gowan and Torrance (1965) were the first to publish studies on this topic. These studies were followed by studies that advocated the development of culture-specific norms for psychological measures. The research of Torrance and his associates was later followed by studies that emphasized development of minority-specific norms for various personality and intelligence measures. In the 1970s, researchers incorporated these studies into a more cohesive theoretical framework which they termed Cross Cultural Psychology. Noteworthy during that period was the work of

Anthony Marsella (see Marsella, 1987, for a review of this topic) on the cross-validation of self-report measures of depression among Asians as opposed to Europeans. Also of importance is the work of Gay and Abrahams (1973) that compared the assessment procedures of African Americans and Caucasian children. Lonner (1980) reviewed 347 articles that were published in the *Journal of Cross Cultural Psychology* between 1970 and 1979. He concluded that most of the articles were in the areas of personality and intellectual assessment. He also noted that 662 of the authors were from the United States and that the next two leading contributing countries were Israel (9%) and Canada (8%). These countries accounted for 52% of the publications. As many as 514 cultural groups were studies during this period. The most frequently studied minorities were made up of individuals from the following origins: Canadian and U.S. Caucasians, Eastern and Central Europeans, African American, Indians, Israelis, U.S. Hispanics, Australian Aborigines, New Zealand Caucasians, and Japanese.

Cross-Cultural Neurocognitive Assessment

Since the 1960s, the area of cross-cultural psychological assessment has flourished, while the role of ethnicity and cultural differences in the assessment of neurocognitive functions has received little interest (see Fig. 16.1). This lack of interest reflects the general notion within the neuroscience community that ethnicity and culture play a limited role in the evaluation of cognitive functioning (Cuellar, 1998). In the late 1980s, this notion was challenged by researchers, as it became clear that some minorities perform poorly on neurocognitive tasks, even in the absence of neurological impairment. Hence, it was concluded that minorities might be often misdiagnosed by clinicians who employ standardized neurocognitive measures. Moreover, with the rapid change in the demographics of the United States, it was clear that this issue needed to be adequately addressed (Ferraro, 2002; Fletcher-Janzen, Strickland, & Reynolds, 2002).

Minorities and Neurocognitive Assessment

To address the multifaceted impact of cultural factors, Poreh (2002) adapted the Brunswick Lens Model (Cuèller, Arnold, & Gonzalez, 1995) to conceptualize the role of cultural elements in neurocognitive assessment (see Fig. 16.2). He described the importance of the following factors in neuropsychological assessment of minorities and bilinguals: (a) ethnicity significantly affects the validity of neuropsychological testing; (b) many tests have not been adequately adapted and translated to particular cultures. For example, tests that have been translated to Arabic might not include items that are typical to Egyptians, Lebanese,

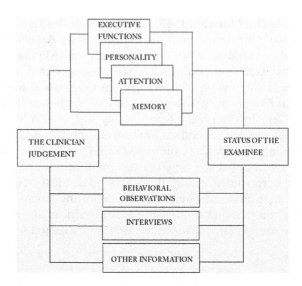

Fig. 16.2 Brunswick's Lens Model applied to cross-cultural neuropsychological assessment (adapted from Poreh, 2002)

or Saudi Arabians, each having their own dialect; (c) scant research has been conducted on bilingualism and the effects of immigration on neurocognitive test performance; and (d) localization of injury as it pertains to language areas is not yet well understood.

In addition to the adaptation of tests to various cultures, many of the existing neuropsychological tests have not been validated on certain ethnic groups and often provide norms that are the result of pooling the data of mainstream and minorities (Stanczak, Stanczak, & Awadalla, 2001). To address these psychometric limitations, various methodologies have been devised. Anastasi (1988), for example, suggested that when developing new measures, test developers take into account the role of education, language, and performance speed within homogeneous minority group performance. She recommended the selection of test items that are common in all cultures and the validation of these items against multiple criteria. Examples of studies that employed this methodology include Ostrosky, Ardila, and Rosselli's (1997) translation into Spanish of the Mini Mental Status Exam, one of the most widely used screening tools for the assessment of cognition. Another example is Ponton et al.'s (1996) publication of Spanish norms for commonly used neurocognitive tests. The latter norms were stratified by age, education, and gender.

Anastasi (1988) also emphasized the role of nomenclatural variations in the performance of minorities on standardized tests. Such factors included differences in the tempo of life, as is evident when comparing rural and urban subcultures. After applying these ideas to neurocognitive assessment, Ackerman and Banks (2001) noted that ethnicity cannot fully describe test performance differences, particularly when using categorical classification systems. For example, Lyketsos, Garrett, Liang, & Anthony (1999) examined the neurocognitive decline of African Americans suffering from Cerebral Vascular Accident (CVA) and symptoms of Parkinson's disease. They reported greater cognitive decline in patients with less formal education. In this study, having more than 8 years of formal education was associated with greater reserve of cognitive capacity. Manly, Schupf, Tang, and Stern (2005) reported that literacy level and not years of education appeared to be an important mediator of the interactions of biological and environmental factors. Hence, these studies illustrate that even subtle cultural and educational differences may play an important role in the assessment of minorities.

Some clinicians have advocated for the development of cultural free tests. This methodology has been extensively applied to the assessment of neurocognitive deficits in minorities, including in the study of illiteracy (Ardila, Rosselli, & Puente, 1994; Ardila, 1995; Cole & Engestroem, 1997), aging (Crook et al., 1993), memory (Mayfield & Reynolds, 1997), learning disabilities (Duane & Leong, 1985), and awareness of illness (Prigatano, Ogano, & Amakusa, 1997).

In sum, the multiplicity of variables that affect the performance of minorities on neurocognitive measures necessitate not only the development of both new tests and norms, but in many cases, a general awareness of practitioners regarding the important role of subtle variables on neurocognitive test performance. Enhancing such awareness and outlining the hazards that are involved when conducting such evaluations will be addressed in the next section of the chapter.

The Hazards of Neurocognitive Assessment of Minorities

Poreh (2002) outlines several hazards associated with the assessment of minorities. These include the following: (a) assessment of minorities does not advocate the deviation from standardized procedures; (b) "testing the limits" should be done only after the entire test has been administered under standard conditions; (c) psychologists need to gather information about the examinee's cultural background and motivation prior to the assessment. Additional guidelines adopted from other sources, suggest the following: (d) whenever the tests are unable to control specific culture variables such as language or acculturation, one should consider evaluating the patient using measures that have been specifically adapted and standardized to the given population; and (e) attempts should be made to distinguish between various levels of acculturation.

According to Dana (1996), a distinction between four levels of acculturation is recommended: (a) traditional, (b) marginal, (c) bicultural, and (d) assimilation. Such levels can be determined subjectively or by using standard scales such as the Acculturation Rating Scale for Mexican Americans (Cuèller, Harris, & Jasso, 1980).

A particular area that is perilous when conducting assessments is evaluations in forensic settings. Such evaluations are often used to assess the effects of brain injury secondary to motor vehicle accidents, exposure to toxins, and posttraumatic stress disorder, as well as assess one's competency to stand for trial (Table 16.1). In such evaluations, the level of motivation of the examinee is typically addressed in order to rule out malingering. According to the APA (1994), malingering is "the intentional production of grossly exaggerated physical or psychological symptoms, motivated by external incentives such as avoiding military duty, avoiding work, obtaining financial compensation, evading criminal prosecution, or obtaining drugs." Techniques for assessing such

Table 16.1 Tests that provide minority specific norms for commonly used neurocognitive tests (Portions of this table were adapted from Poreh, 2002)

Areas of cognition and tests	African Americans	Hispanic Americans
General Cognitive Ability		
Mini Mental Status Exam	Ripich, Carpenter, & Ziol, 1997	Taussig & Ponton, 1996
Wechsler Intelligence Test	Lucas et al., 2005	Psychological Corporation
Achievement Tests		
Woodcock–Johnson Battery	Payette & Clarizio, 1994	Prewitt-Diaz & Rievera, 1989
Executive Functions		
Design fluency Wisconsin Card Sorting		Delago, Guerrero, Goggin, & Ellis, 1999
Trail Making Test	Steinberg et al., 2005	Artiola & Mullaney, 1998
Attention		
Paced Auditory Serial Addition Test	Diehr, Heaton, Miller, & Grant, 1999	Diehr et al., 1999
Stroop	Steinberg, Bieliauskas, Smith, & Ivnik, 2005	
Memory		
Rey Auditory-Verbal Learning Test	Ripich et al., 1997 Manly et al., 1998b	Demsky, Mittenberg, Quintar, Katell, & Golden, 1988
Wechsler Memory Scale	Ferman et al., 2005	Ponton et al., 1996
Language Tests		
Boston Naming Test	Manly et al., 1998b	Kohnert, Hernandez, & Bates, 1998
Verbal Fluency Test	Gladsjo et al., 1999 Ripich et al., 1997 Steinberg et al., 2005	Manly et al., 1998a Portocarrero, Burright, & Donovick, 2007 Psych Corp.
Visual Perceptual Tests		
Hooper Visual Organization Test	Lewis et al., 1997 Manly et al., 1998b	– Rosseli & Ardila, 1996

behaviors have been reviewed by Spreen and Strauss (1998). The authors distinguished between conventional measures like self-report inventories and specific tests that were devised to detect malingering, such as the Portland Digits Recognition Test. Current use of malingering tests is considered to be the mainstream in forensic neuropsychological testing and has been incorporated into decision-making trees in neuropsychological assessment (Lucas, 1998; Lishman 1998; Faust, 1996).

The role of malingering in minorities undergoing forensic evaluation is complex. This issue has rarely been addressed in the forensic literature. However, cultural differences with regard to the judicial system do exist. In some cultures the tendency to "make oneself be heard" is accepted as the only way to get proper compensation. Such a behavior is characteristic of what Dana (1996) would have defined as "traditional" for "marginally assimilated" individuals. This is particularly true for individuals who have often experienced discrimination and feel alienated from the mainstream of society. It is also applicable to individuals who grew up in totalitarian regimes where "honest" behavior is rarely reported as a concept of justice. Whenever one encounters such an examinee, particularly immigrants, it is important to take into account their test performance within the cultural context of their illness, along with the interaction between the patient and clinician.

The author of this chapter has encountered a number of patients with well-documented neurological conditions who "failed" malingering tests. An example of such a case is a woman with a North African background who suffered from an ACOM (Anterior Communicating Artery) aneurysm and underwent neurosurgery. A few days post-surgery, she was evaluated by the author, who quickly noticed that she was failing on the most rudimentary neurocognitive tasks. Her performance on a task that requires visual-scanning, for example, was more than 8 standard deviations below the mean. Since these findings did not correspond with her neurological condition, she was administered a series of malingering tests. Her performance on all these tasks confirmed the fact that she was attempting to present herself as significantly disabled.

While it would be foolish to determine the degree of her disability on the basis of her medical history alone, it would also be equally foolish to completely discard the possible neurocognitive deficits that have resulted from the aneurysm and subsequent neurosurgery. In fact, studies show that patients with ACOM aneurysms are often unaware of their deficits. Hence, in such cases, a careful review of the neuroradiological studies, and particularly the interaction of the patients' cultural background and type of injury, is essential before making a final conclusion. In addition, a consultation with a specialist regarding the immigrants' culture and how it relates to a patient's health along with test taking attitudes are recommended. In the above example, the woman later confided to the surgeon that she purposely malingered. She explained that when she immigrated to Israel she lost both her parents, grew up as an orphan, and was extremely concerned regarding the future and well-being of her children. Hence, she decided to exaggerate her symptoms in order to obtain the largest possible compensation. She noted that she realized her behavior was wrong but felt that she could not trust the "system" to properly compensate her. Following her discussion with the neurosurgeon, the patient was re-evaluated. Her deficits were accurately documented.

Service Delivery Guidelines

The significant role of cultural variables in the manifestation of neurocognitive symptoms suggests that one should be aware of existing service delivery guidelines. The American Psychiatric Association suggests that one should take into account several factors when conducting psychiatric evaluations: (1) the cultural identification of the individual, (2) the cultural explanations of the individual's illness, (3) the cultural elements impacting the relationship between the individual and the clinician, and (4) overall culture assessment for diagnoses and care. The APA (1991) provides similar guidelines.

Dana (1996) introduced the concept of "culturally competence assessment." This concept tends to clarify the application of service delivery to multicultural populations and includes four components: (a) culturally specific service delivery in the first language of the client, (b) evaluation of cultural orientation, (c) appropriate assessment methodology and tests, and (d) guidelines for providing feedback to clients and their significant others.

Beyond the delivery of appropriate services, some argue that clinicians bring with them a particular interaction style. This interaction style shapes her/his cultural and personal service style (Artiola, Fortuny & Mullaney, 1998). Keeping this in mind, neuropsychiatrists and neuropsychologists should alter their expectations of individuals from other cultures and adapt their evaluation process accordingly. Various articles addressing the expectations of different cultural groups regarding medical service delivery are available. These include the work of Gibbs (1985) among American Indians. In addition, reading and familiarizing oneself with the attitudes and morals of the patients being cared for by the practitioner is likely to assist in the assessment process, particularly when evaluating "traditional" or "marginally assimilated" patients.

Summary and Conclusions

The psychological and neuropsychological assessment of minorities has come of age, particularly in the United States, due to the extensive work of researchers, clinicians, and professional organizations. However, literature reviews show that much work is still needed to adapt and norm neurocognitive measures for certain populations. These include immigrants who are neither fluent in their host country language nor are as fluent in their mother tongue as those who did not leave their country of origin. Thus, even when norms are available for various minorities, these norms fail to distinguish between levels of cultural orientation and acculturation.

It is essential to adopt guidelines for each cultural group when considering cognitive assessment for minorities. For example, when assessing Hispanics, one should take into consideration both the general guidelines published by the APA and those published for this particular group (Ardila et al., 1994). Another important guideline is, whenever possible, to refer clients for whom English is a second language to a colleague who is fully fluent in their native language and familiar with their culture. Unfortunately, however, neurologists, neuropsychiatrists, and neuropsychologists from different cultural backgrounds are not always available.

The increase in bi-cultural or even tri-cultural populations complicates the evaluation of minorities. For example, Poreh (2002) examined elderly Israelis from more than 30 cultural backgrounds who immigrated at different times to their host country. The results of the study showed that native Hebrew speakers produced higher raw phonemic fluency than nonnative peers. Non-native speakers, however, produced longer words that were based on Latin sources.

In conclusion, understanding both the culture and psychosocial functioning of patients who are referred for neuropsychological assessment is of great importance for both diagnostic and care-planning purposes. Although it is often assumed that the performance on cognitive tasks, personality measures, and measures of malingering and motivation offer an adequate estimation of functioning of daily living activities, little research has addressed these assumptions. Thus, continued research is needed to clarify these relationships. This will lead to an increase in reliable information concerning the application of techniques that are best suited for multicultural patients. Such research should aim at creating mega databases that allow for not only the creation of ethnic specific general population norms but also clinical norms, specifically for various patient populations based on homogeneous ethnic and cultural background. In this way, the diagnostic and predictive capability of neurocognitive measures will be enhanced. To achieve such a goal, existing neurocognitive tests need to be moved to the web. In this manner, multiple sites can collect data on underrepresented ethnic groups, who tend to be concentrated in particular parts of the country. Web-based assessment and data collection would also allow clinicians to employ complex algorithms to predict the rate of cognitive decline (actuarial models), taking into account multiple variables including age, education, and ethnicity.

References

Ackerman, R. J., & Banks, M. E. (2001). Looking for threads – Commonalties and Differences. In R. Ferraro (Ed.), *Minority and cross-cultural aspects of neuropsychological assessment* (pp. 329–343). Lisse, Netherlands: Swets & Zeitlinger Publishers.

American Psychological Association. (1991). *Service guidelines for ethnic, linguistic and culturally diverse populations.* Washington DC: American Psychological Association.

American Psychiatric Association. (1994). *Diagnostic and statistical manual of mental disorders* (DSM-IV 1st ed.). Washington DC: American Psychiatric Association.

Anastasi, A. (1988). *Psychological testing*. New York: Macmillan.

Ardila, A. (1995). Directions of research in cross cultural neuropsychology. *Journal of Clinical and Experimental Neuropsychology, 17*, 143–150.

Ardila, A., Rosselli, M., & Puente, A. E. (1994). *Neuropsychological assessment of the Spanish speaker*. New York: Plenum Press.

Artiola, I., Fortuny, L., & Mullaney, H. (1998). Assessing patients whose language you do not know: Can the absurd be ethical. *Clinical Neuropsychologist, 12 (1)*, 113–126.

Binet, A., & Simon, T. (1905). Méthodes nouvelles pour le diagnostic du niveau intellectuel des anormaux. *L'Année psychologique, 11*, 191–244.

Cole, M., & Engestroem, Y. (1997). A cultural-historical approach to distributed cognition. In G. Salomon (Ed.), *Distributed cognitions: Psychological and educational considerations* (pp. 1–46). New York: Cambridge.

Crook, T. H., Lebowitz, B. D., Pirozzolo, F. J., Zappala, G., Cavarzeran, F., Measso, G., & Massari, D. C. (1993). Recalling names after introduction: Changes across the adult life span in two cultures. *Developmental Neuropsychology, 9*, 103–113.

Cuellar I. (1998). Cross-Cultural Clinical Psychological Assessment of Hispanic Americans. *Journal of Personality Assessment, 70*, 71–86.

Cuellar, I., Hairis, I., C., & Jasso, R. (1980). An acculturation scale for normal Mexican American and clinical populations. *Hispanic Journal of Behavioral Sciences, 3*, 199–217.

Cuellar, I., Arnold, B., & Gonzalez, G. (1995). Cognitive referents of acculturation: Assessment of cultural constructs in Mexican Americans. *Journal of Community Psychology, 23*, 339–356.

Dana, R. H. (1996). Culturally competent assessment practice in the United States. *Journal of Personality Assessment, 66*, 472–487.

Delago, P., Guerrero, G., Goggin, J. P., & Ellis, B. B. (1999). Self-assessment of linguistic skills by bilingual Hispanics. *Hispanic Journal of Behavioral Sciences, 21*, 31–46.

Demsky, Y. I., Mittenberg, W., Quintar, B., Katell, A. D., & Golden, C. J. (1998). Bias in the standard American norms with Spanish translations of the WMS-R. *Assessment, 5*, 115–121.

Diehr, M. C., Heaton, R. K., Miller, W., & Grant, I. (1999). The Paced Auditory Serial Addition Task (PASAT): Norms for age, education, and ethnicity. *Assessment, 6*, 101.

Duane, D. D., & Leong, C. K. (1985). *Understanding learning disabilities: International and multidisciplinary views*. New York: Plenum Press.

Faust, D. (1996). Assessment of brain injuries in legal cases. In Fogel, B. S., Schiffer, R. M., & Rao, S. M. (Eds.), *Neuropsychiatry*. Baltimore: Williams & Wilkins.

Ferman, T. J., Lucas, J. A., Ivnik, R. J., Smith, G. E., Willis, F. B., Petersen, R. C., et al. (2005). Mayo's older African American normative studies: Auditory verbal learning test norms for African American elders. *Clinical Neuropsychology, 19*, 214–228.

Ferraro, R. F. (2002). Minority and cross-cultural aspects of neuropsychological assessment. Lisse, Netherlands: Swets & Zeitlinger Publishers.

Fletcher-Janzen, E., Strickland, T., & Reynolds, C. R. (2002). *Handbook of Cross-Cultural Neuropsychology*. Springer, New York.

Galton, F. (1869). *Heredity of genius – the law and consequences*. New York: Macmillan and Co.

Gay, G., & Abrahams, R. D. (1973). Does the pot melt, boil, or brew? Black children and white assessment procedures. *Journal of School Psychology, 11*, 330–340.

Gelb, S., Allen, G., Futterman, A., & Mehler, B. (1986). Rewriting mental testing history: The view from the American Psychologist. *Sage Race Relations Abstracts, 11*, 18–31.

Gibbs, J. T. (1985). Establishing a treatment relationship with black clients: Interpersonal vs. instrumental strategies. In C. Germain (Ed.), *Advances in clinical social work* (pp. 184–195). Silver Spring, MD: National Association of Social Work, Inc.

Gladsjo, J. A., Schuman, C. C., Evans, J. D., Peavy, G. M., Miller S. W., & Heaton, R. K. (1999). Norms for letter and category fluency: Demographic corrections for age, education, and ethnicity, *Assessment, 6*, 147–178.

Goddard, H. H. (1912). *The Kallikak Family: A study in the heredity of feeble-mindedness*. New York: Macmillan.

Goddard, H. H. (1915). *Feeble mindedness: Its causes and consequences*. New York: MacMillan Company.

Gowan, J. C., & Torrance, E. P. (1965). An intercultural study of non-verbal ideational fluency. *Gifted Child Quarterly, 9*, 13–15.

Holt, J., (2005). *Measure for measure*. (Book Review) *The New Yorker, 24/31*, 84–90.

Kohnert, K. J., Hernandez, A. E., & Bates, E. (1998). Bilingual performance on the Boston Naming Test: Preliminary norms in Spanish and English. *Brain and Language, 65*, 422–440.

Lewis, S., Campbell, A., Takushi, C., Ruby, B. A., Dennis, G., Wood, D., & Weir, R. (1997). Visual organization test performance in an African American population with acute unilateral cerebral lesions. *International Journal of Neuroscience, 91*, 295–302.

Lezak, M. D., Howieson, D. B., & Loring, D. W. (2004). *Neuropsychological assessment* (4th ed.). New York: Oxford University Press.

Lishman, W. A. (1998). *Organic psychiatry: The psychological consequences of cerebral disorder* (3rd ed.). Oxford, UK: Blackwell Science Ltd.

Lonner, W. J. (1980). A decade of cross-cultural psychology: JCCP, 1970–1979. *Journal of Cross-Cultural Psychology, 11*, 7–34.

Lucas, J. A. (1998). Traumatic brain injury and post concussive syndrome. In P. J. Synder & P. D. Nussbaum (Eds.), *Clinical neuropsychology* (pp. 67–95). Washington, DC: American Psychological Association.

Lucas, J. A., Ivnik, R., Smith, G., Ferman, T., Willis, F., Peterson, R., et al. (2005). Brief report on WAIS-R normative data collection in Mayo's Older African Americans Normative Studies. *The Clinical Neuropsychologist (Neuropsychology, Development and Cognition), 19*(2), 184–188.

Lyketsos, C. G., Garrett, E., Liang, K. Y., & Anthony, J. C. (1999). Cannabis use and cognitive decline in persons under 65 years of age. *American Journal of Epidemiology, 149*, 794–800.

Manly, J. J., Jacobs, D. M., Sano, M., Bell, K., Merchant, C.A., Small, S.A., et al. (1998a). Cognitive test performance among nondemented elderly African Americans and Whites. *Neurology, 50*, 1238–1245.

Manly, J. J., Miller, S. W., Heaton, R. K., Byrd, D. D., Reilly, J., Velasquez, R. J., et al. (1998b). The effect of African-American acculturation on neuropsychological test performance in normal and HIV- positive individuals. *Journal of the International Neuropsychological Society, 4*, 291–302.

Manly, J. J., Schupf, N., Tang, M. X., & Stern, Y. (2005). Cognitive decline and literacy among ethnically diverse elders. *Journal of Geriatric Psychiatry & Neurology, 18*(4), 213–217.

Marsella, A. (1987). The measurement of depressive experience and disorder across cultures. In A. J. Marsella, R. M. A. Hirschfeld, & M. M. Kratz (Eds.), *The measurement of depression* (pp. 376–397). New York: Guilford Press.

Mayfield, J. W., & Reynolds, C. R. (1997). Black-White differences in memory test performance among children and adolescents. *Archives of Clinical Neuropsychology, 12*, 111–122.

National Institutes of Health (2002). Strategic Research Plan and Budget to Reduce and Ultimately Eliminate Health Disparities. Volume I – Fiscal Years 2002–2006. U.S. Department of Health and Human Services.

Ostrosky, F., Ardila, A., & Rosselli, M. (1997). *NEUROPSI: Una. batera neuropsicològica breve [NEUROPSI; A brief neuropsychological test battery]*. Mexico: D.F. Laboratories Bayer.

Payette, K. A., & Clarizio, H. F. (1994). Discrepant team decisions: The effects of race, gender, achievement, and IQ on LD eligibility. *Psychology in the Schools, 31*, 40–48.

Ponton, M., Satz, P., Herrera, L., Ortiz, F., Urrutiia, C., Young, R., et al. (1996). Normative data stratified by age and education for the Neuropsychological Screening Battery for Hispanics (NeSBHIS): Initial report. *Journal of the International Neuropsychological Society, 2*, 96–104.

Poreh, A. (2002). Neuropsychological and psychological issues associated with cross-cultural and minority assessment. In R. Ferraro (Ed.), *Minority and cross-cultural aspects of neuropsychological assessment* (pp. 329–343). Lisse, Netherlands: Swets & Zeitlinger Publishers.

Portocarrero, J. S., Burright, R. G., & Donovick, P. J. (2007). Vocabulary and verbal fluency of bilingual and monolingual college students. *Archives of Clinical Neuropsychology, 22*(3), 415–422.

Prewitt-Diaz, J., & Rivera, R. (1989). Correlations among scores on the Woodcock-Johnson achievement subtest (Spanish), WISC-R (Spanish) and Columbia Mental Maturity Scale. *Psychological Reports, 64*, 987–990.

Prigatano, G. P., Ogano, M., & Amakusa, B. (1997). A cross-cultural study on impaired self-awareness in Japanese patients with brain dysfunction. *Neuropsychiatry, Neuropsychology, and Behavioral Neurology, 10*, 135–143.

Ripich, D. N., Carpenter, B., & Ziol, E. (1997). Comparison of African-American and white persons with Alzheimer's disease on language measures. *Neurology, 48*, 781–783.

Rosseli, M., & Ardilla, A. (1996). Cognitive effects of cocaine and polydrug abuse. *Journal of Clinical and Experimental Neuropsychology, 18*, 122–135.

Spreen, O., & Strauss, E. (1998). *A compendium of neuropsychological tests: Administration, norms, and commentary* (2nd ed.). New York: Oxford University Press.

Stanczak, D., Stanczak, E., & Awadalla, A. (2001). Development and initial validation of an Arabic version of the Expanded Trail Making Test: Implications for cross-cultural assessment. *Archives of Clinical Neuropsychology, 16*, 141–149.

Steinberg, B. A., Bieliauskas, L. A., Smith, G. E., & Ivnik, R. J. (2005). Mayo's older Americans normative studies: Age- and IQ-adjusted norms for the Trail-Making Test, the Stroop Test, and MAE Controlled Oral Word Association Test. *Clinical Neuropsychologist, 19*, 329–377.

Taussig, M., & Ponton, M. (1996). Issues in neuropsychological assessment for Hispanic older adults. Cultural and linguistic factors. In G. Yeo, & T. D. Gallagher (Eds.), *Ethnicity and the dementias* (pp. 45–58). Washington DC: Taylor and Francis.

Torrance, E. P. (1962). Cultural discontinuities and the development of originality of thinking. *Exceptional Children, 29*, 2–13.

United States Census Bureau. (April 2008). United States – Age and Sex. 2006 American Community; S0101. Available at www.census.gov/popest/estimates.php.

Whipple, M. G. (1910). Manual of Mental and Physical Tests. Warwick & York Inc., Baltimore, U.S.A.

Yerkes, R. (1921) *Psychological examining in the United States Army. Memoirs of the National Academy of Sciences* (Vol. 25). Washington, DC: U.S. Government Printing Office.

Chapter 17
Stress and Resilience

AnnaMaria Aguirre McLaughlin, Lisa Stines Doane, Alice L. Costiuc
and Norah C. Feeny

It has long been recognized that the experience of "stress" can have detrimental effects on both physical and mental health. Yet, only in the past several decades have models been developed to explain the pathways through which stress impacts health. More recently, these early models have been expanded to include cultural variables, including the role of culture on the experience of stress. Empirical investigations have begun to examine differences in the experience and associated outcomes of stress across racial/cultural groups, and these studies have illuminated the processes at work in the perception, experience, and impact of stress. A newly emerging body of literature has focused on resilience—that is, the successful adaptation to stressful experiences, and several culturally relevant variables have been proposed as potential protective factors that foster resilience among racial/ethnic minorities. This chapter will provide a brief overview of the major theories of stress and resilience and the impact of stress on mental health, with an emphasis on those models that incorporate culture. We will also review the major, unique contributors to stress in racial/ethnic minority populations, with a particular focus on women. Finally, the chapter will review the literature on resilience in racial/ethnic minorities, summarizing the factors that foster resilience in these groups, and conclude with recommendations for further areas of study.

Theories of Stress

Early notions of stress and its impact on humans arose from Walter Cannon (1932) and Hans Selye (1936), and their seminal works on systemic stress and adaptation. In these theories, stress was conceptualized as a response, as opposed to a stimulus event or an interaction between the stimulus and response. Selye proposed that stress occurs when the body is exposed to

A.A. McLaughlin (✉)
Case Western Reserve University, Cleveland, OH
e-mail: annamaria.aguirre@case.edu

S. Loue, M. Sajatovic (eds.), *Determinants of Minority Mental Health and Wellness*, DOI 10.1007/978-0-387-75659-2_17,
© Springer Science+Business Media, LLC 2009

potential threats (e.g., exposure to cold temperatures, surgery) and results in a nonspecific, physiological response to these stimuli. According to Selye's theory, this response is described as nonspecific, as the physiological reaction is assumed to be consistent regardless of the stimulus. Selye suggested that, during stress, the body experiences three phases of adaptation: a "general alarm reaction", in which the body prepares itself for "fight or flight" (building upon Cannon's work), resistance to the stress, and exhaustion.

These early stress theories have been criticized for several reasons. First, these theories assume that the human response to stress is universal, without considering individual variation in response to events based on factors such as personality and appraisal (e.g., Hobfoll, 1989). Further, these frameworks do not incorporate the role of stress associated with being a member of a minority group, thereby rendering them less culturally relevant and generalizable (Hobfoll, 2001). Finally, some have argued that these theories, with a focus on stress as an outcome, lack predictive validity as it is difficult to identify predictors prospectively (Hobfoll, 1989). In response to these criticisms, newer theories have been developed that expand upon Cannon and Selye's theories to include psychological constructs such as perception, cognitive appraisal, and resources.

Psychological Theories of Stress

Lazarus and Folkman (1984) developed a cognitive transactional theory of stress, incorporating the interaction between the environment and the individual. They proposed that stress occurs when the demands of the environment exceed the resources the individual has available for coping with the stress. An important component of this theory is the notion of appraisal, which they define as "the process of categorizing an encounter, and its various facets, with respect to its significance for well-being" (Lazarus & Folkman, 1984, p.31). They suggest that there are two forms of such appraisals: *primary appraisal*, in which an individual evaluates the potential consequences of the stressor, and *secondary appraisal*, which involves identifying steps that can be taken to deal with the stressor, if any, based on one's available resources and coping abilities. Further, they proposed that this process of evaluative appraisal mediates the stress response, such that those events that are appraised as positive or challenging may not lead to a stress response, whereas those that are perceived as negative or threatening will lead to the stress response.

While clearly more nuanced than early stress theories, one criticism of appraisal models of stress is that they define stress as an outcome based only on appraisal of the stress-evoking situation without a focus on objective demands. Further, appraisal theories suggest an idiographic evaluation of potentially stressful events, which neglects the potential influence of a cultural-collectivist perspective on the experience of stress (Hobfoll, 2001). Hobfoll's (1989) Conservation of Resources (COR) theory is a model of stress that is adaptable to considering the impact of racial/cultural factors in the experience of and response to stress. COR theory is based on the notion that loss (or threat of loss) of resources is the principal component in the stress process and that loss of resources is more powerful than resource gain. Hobfoll categorized four domains of resources: objects (e.g., home, car), personal characteristics (e.g., optimism), conditions (e.g., seniority, financial security) and energies (e.g., time, knowledge). Although COR theory does focus on individual appraisal of loss, to some degree it differs from traditional appraisal theories in that COR theory proposes that perceptions of loss are often socially learned or culturally common and based on real, objective observations of resources (Hobfoll, 2001). In the following paragraphs, we expand upon the notion that stress must be considered within a cultural context. Though not comprehensive, we hope to shed light on three significant areas of stress affecting minority mental health: acculturation, racism, and poverty.

Acculturation

As opposed to early research, which assumed that acculturation occurred as a series of steps in a single direction (Gordon, 1964), Berry (1980, 1997) proposed one of the most widely utilized theories of acculturation, a bidimensional approach, which he defined as "the dual process of cultural and psychological change that takes place as a result of contact between two or more cultural groups and their individual members" (Berry, 2005, p. 698). Acculturating individuals are confronted with two central issues: their preference for preserving their culture and identity and their preference for interacting and participating within the larger, dominant society alongside other racial/ethnic cultural groups. Multiculturalism or integrating both the culture of origin and the dominant culture has been shown to be the least stressful acculturative strategy (Berry, 1997; Berry, Phinney, Sam, & Vedder, 2006). In contrast, marginalization or not taking part in the dominant culture and, simultaneously, either inability or choosing not to preserve the culture of origin has been shown to be most stressful (Berry, 1997; Berry et al., 2006).

Several studies have examined the relationship between acculturation and stress in racial/ethnic minorities. Overall, there are conflicting results: many studies have found that greater acculturation is associated with higher levels of stress (Bratter & Eschbach, 2005; Buddington, 2002; Mak, Chen, Wong, & Zane, 2005; Pillay, 2005), whereas others have found no such relationship (Castillo, Conoley, & Brossart, 2004; Franzini & Fernandez-Esquer, 2004) or actually have identified acculturation as a protective factor against stress (Cho, Hudley, & Back, 2003; Lee, Koeske, & Sales, 2004). Stress from the acculturation process has been linked to mental health outcomes including elevated levels of anxiety and depression (Crockett et al., 2007; Hwang & Ting, 2008), suicidal ideation (Hovey, 2000; Walker, Wingate, Obasi, & Joiner, 2008), vulnerability to bulimic symptoms in women (Perez, Voelz, Pettit, & Joiner, 2001), and higher overall psychological distress (Hwang & Ting, 2008).

As previously mentioned, some investigations have shown that acculturation can serve as a protective factor against stress. The more an individual engages in the dominant society, or the more acculturated they become, while retaining preferred aspects of the original culture, the lower the levels of perceived distress (Berry, 1997; Berry et al., 2006). Lee and colleagues (2004) speculate that at higher levels of acculturation, more opportunities for social support are available from the host culture and original culture, providing a stress-buffering effect. Various other studies suggest that highly acculturated individuals acclimate more successfully to the ways of the mainstream culture, which eases the day-to-day interactions thereby potentially decreasing the likelihood of psychological distress (Cho, Hudley, & Back, 2003; Kim & Omizo, 2006; LaFromboise, Coleman, & Gerton, 1993).

Perhaps the inconsistencies found across acculturation studies stem from the absence of uniform definitions of key constructs such as culture or acculturation and instruments used to measure acculturation. As Koneru, Weisman de Mamani, Flynn, and Betancourt (2007) assert in their review of the literature, studies that use a single variable (e.g. place of birth, language, length of residence) to represent acculturation fail to measure important aspects of acculturation such as "specific values, beliefs, expectations, roles, norms, or cultural practices" (p. 77). At the same time, using numerous and diverse instruments to measure acculturation can account for the discrepancies found between studies, making it difficult to glean meaning from the different findings. Additionally, results are often not generalizable because the sample size was not sufficiently large (Buddington, 2002; Lee, Koeske, & Sales, 2004) or representative (Franzini & Fernandez-Esquir, 2004; Lee, Koeske, & Sales, 2004). While the current methodology has some limitations, we may conclude that the process of acculturation does pose significant challenges but that these challenges can be successfully navigated. Optimal outcome is fostered in a culture that values diversity and fosters the minority individual's integration of cultures. By cultivating multiculturalism, the host culture enhances the mental health of its diverse members, thereby contributing to the growth of the larger society.

Racism

The experience of racial/ethnic discrimination is a major source of stress for many racial/ethnic minority women (Borrell, Kiefe, Williams, Diez-Roux, & Gordon-Larsen, 2006; Hassouneh & Kulwiki, 2007; Murry, Brown, Brody, Cutrona, & Simons, 2001; Schulz et al., 2006; Wadsworth et al., 2006). An individual can encounter racism/discrimination in interpersonal, collective, symbolic, societal, or political contexts (Harrell, 2000), and the associated stress can be acute or chronic (Clark, Anderson, Clark, & Williams 1999). It is when race-related stressors are "perceived to tax or exceed existing individual and collective resources or threaten well-being" (Harrell, 2000, p. 44) that negative outcomes may transpire. Psychological distress including depressive symptomatology (Brown et al., 2000; Gee, Spencer, Chen, Yip, & Takeuchi, 2007; Karlson, Nazroo, McKenzie, Bhui, & Weich, 2005; Prelow, Mosher, & Bowman, 2006; Schulz et al., 2006), symptoms of anxiety (Gee, Spencer, Chen, Yip, & Takeuchi, 2007; Karlson et al., 2005), and psychosis (Karlsen & Nazroo, 2002) have been linked to stress and racism/discrimination.

Clark and colleagues (1999) put forth a biopsychosocial model which, proposes that several factors moderate or mediate the relationship between stress and mental health outcomes. Internal mechanisms through which racism is thought to lead to stress have been explored including choice of coping techniques (Clark et al., 1999; Liang, Alvarez, Juang, & Liang, 2007; Noh & Kaspar, 2003; Thompson, 2006), level of self-esteem (Moradi, & Risco, 2006; Harrell, 2000), nature of racial identity (Jones, Cross, & DeFour, 2007), and level of cognitive ability (Utsey, Lanier, Williams, Bolden, & Lee, 2006). External mechanisms such as social isolation (Smith, 1985; Utsey et al., 2006), pressure to assume racial roles (Smith, 1985), socioeconomic status (Harrell, 2000), and past racism-related experiences can also contribute to heightened stress from racism/discrimination (Clark, Anderson, Clark, & Williams, 1999; Harrell, 2000). Racism is a significant stressor too often experienced by many racial/ethnic minority group members. While negative repercussions of racism are well established, there are important variables at social and individual levels that interact and influence how one endures and manages such stressors. It is essential that mental health endeavors focus on fostering the individual attributes that have been outlined here as mediators of outcome.

The negative psychological impact of racism warrants continued attention. As this country continues to evolve in its demographic makeup and as racism continues despite these demographic changes, it is necessary for primary mental health initiatives to focus on those individual variables that mediate between racism/discrimination and mental health outcome. That is, given what we know about individual mediators of health, early and long-term interventions that focus on adaptive coping techniques, development of racial identity, and self-esteem are likely to buffer against the ill effects of racism/discrimination. It is imperative that continued research focus on these mediating variables and that we use this data to inform and advance mental health initiatives for individuals from diverse backgrounds.

Poverty

Given that low-income neighborhoods are characterized by disproportionately high rates of minority group members, it follows that these individuals are at risk for increased stress and decreased mental health (O'Hare & Mather, 2003).

The literature on poverty has established a consistent relationship between poor mental health outcomes and low socioeconomic status (SES) (Bogard, Trillo, Schwartz, & Gerstel, 2001; Chapman, Hobfoll, & Ritter, 1997; Gyamfi, Brooks-Gunn, & Jackson, 2001). Indeed, in one national study, impoverished individuals were at a three times greater risk for depression compared to nondepressed individuals (Kessler et al., 2003). While poverty has been frequently tied to depression, factors associated with poverty are frequently stressful in and of themselves. Such factors associated with impoverished neighborhoods include high rates of unemployment, crime and violence, and social isolation (Massey, 2005).

While poverty is tied to unfavorable mental health outcomes and minority group status, the relationship is not entirely clear. That is, it appears that research has not ascertained a direct relationship between minority group status, poverty, and poor mental health outcomes. Some studies have suggested that African Americans experience greater levels of stressors even after controlling for SES, suggesting that racial/ethnic minorities are at increased risk of experiencing stress despite economic status (Kessler, 1979; Kessler, Mickelson, & Williams, 1999). Leventhal, Fauth, and Brooks-Gunn (2005) conducted a randomized experiment in which children in impoverished neighborhoods were provided vouchers to move to low-poverty neighborhoods. Their findings indicated that, even after moving into low-poverty areas, children did not sustain educational improvements and they demonstrated lower engagement compared to youths in high-poverty neighborhoods (Leventhal, Fauth, & Brooks-Gunn, 2005). Leventhal and colleagues (2005) posit that this may have been due to continued poverty after the move (the families moved but did not move up in SES), which contributed to continued stress. Additionally, poor outcome despite moving to low-poverty areas may have been associated with a lack of intervention following the move, which in and of itself can sometimes be a stressor. There are important, not clearly understood factors that may influence the role of poverty on mental health for minority group members. While attempts have been made to understand what can happen when minorities are provided the opportunity to relocate to a higher SES neighborhood, it is clear that questions remain about what factors link poverty to poor outcomes.

In contrast to the research on acculturation and racism, which have included a wide range of racial/ethnic groups, most research on poverty and stress among racial/ethnic minorities has focused on African Americans. Thus, it may be difficult to generalize these findings to other minority group members. Research that explores the relationship between SES and mental health outcomes across diverse racial and ethnic groups is greatly needed to enhance our understanding in this area. Specifically, research that controls for confounding variables such as decreased access to health care, poorer quality schooling, and increased neighborhood violence may help elucidate the manner in which poverty contributes to depression and other poor mental health outcomes in minorities.

Resilience

It is critical to resist pathologizing the racial/ethnic minority experience and outcome. While there are clear and significant stressors linked to the minority experience in this country, it is simultaneously evident that most individuals survive and thrive despite these stressors. One way in which research has attempted to understand how individuals thrive despite stressful circumstances is through the study of resilience.

The study of psychological resilience has focused predominantly on youth populations and arose from a need to understand why some children demonstrate adaptation despite experiencing many risk factors associated with the development of psychopathology. Across age groups, definitions of resilience vary, yet most definitions converge on two fundamental tenets. That is, resilience occurs in the face of *heightened vulnerability*, and it involves *adaptation* or *typical development* in spite of this risk. Resilience is differentiated from recovery in that the latter denotes initial symptoms that gradually subside versus the ability to remain asymptomatic following potentially stressful circumstances or traumatic events (Bonanno, 2004). Importantly, a recent body of research emphasizes that adaptation following a highly stressful or potentially traumatic event (e.g. death of a spouse, exposure to September 11 terrorist attack) is more likely to occur than symptoms of pathology and that some individuals, in the face of these stressful events, may even demonstrate thriving or posttraumatic growth (Bonanno, Galea, Bucciarelli, & Vlahov, 2006; Bonanno et al., 2002). While resilience has been less studied with respect to minority populations, this section will provide an overview of the research, which is primarily qualitative, as it pertains to resiliency factors in different minority groups.

Theories of Resilience

Garmezy, Masten, and Tellegen (1984) identified three primary models of resilience including the compensatory model, protective factor model, and challenge model. These models overlap yet emphasize different important personal characteristics or attributes (e.g., reliance on faith, high intelligence) that may operate in adaptation to stressful circumstances. The compensatory model posits that exposure to stressors decreases competence and that certain personal attributes function additively to raise competence. The compensatory factors, or personal attributes, work independently on the outcome to bring about adaptation, and those without this personal variable will experience lower adaptation compared to those with it. The second model highlighted by Garmezy and colleagues (1984) is the protective factor model, which emphasizes the interaction between stress and personal attributes. Here a given attribute mediates as a protective effect, buffering the effects of the stress. The third model, the challenge model, is based on the notion that some stress actually augments the potential for adaptation. That is, the challenge of moderate levels of stress, when overcome by the individual, serves to inoculate (Rutter, 1987) the individual, preparing him or her to face subsequent challenges or stressors.

It is not well-understood how these models function for racial/ethnic minorities given a dearth of research involving minorities and resilience. Since there is no cultural model that helps us understand resilience in minorities, we must do our best to extend the existing models to what we know about minority health outcomes. We may surmise, given information presented earlier in this chapter, that at least protective factors seem to function to bring about positive outcomes. That is, certain individual-level characteristics (Garmezy would deem "protective" factors) appear to buffer against the effects of racism (e.g., self-esteem, racial identity, coping strategies). It is imperative that current research efforts attempt to clarify how models of resilience function for racial/ethnic minorities. We do not intend to expand theoretically upon this topic in this chapter. We hope, rather, to shed light on the current research that examines broadly resilience in different minority groups.

As mentioned earlier in this chapter, it is well-established that the racial/ethnic minority experience in the U.S. is characterized by many stressors, including but not limited to, acculturation, discrimination, socioeconomic hardship, and marginalization. Resilience in adult racial/ethnic minorities has been examined by only a handful of investigators. Qualitative research has been used frequently to describe the experience of resilience in minority groups. A qualitative investigation conducted by Johnson (1995) studied resilience in culturally diverse families asking, "...what strengths did you feel contributed to your ability to cope with and overcome the difficulties you faced?" His findings underscore two main themes, which were consistent across families of American Indian, African American, Latino, and Asian background. These two themes were the perception of the family as a "sacred vessel" for maintenance of the culture, and acknowledgement of the importance of extended kinship as a source of emotional and economic support. These themes of family as central in terms of tradition and social support are echoed in other studies examining resiliency among diverse cultural groups. Here, resilience appears to be tied to non-Western ideals and is characterized by collectivism. While Johnson's study (1995) uniquely highlights commonality among different racial/ethnic groups, most research in this area focuses on racial/ethnic minority groups by themselves, seldom making more wide-reaching inferences across groups. Thus, following the state of literature, we will examine resilience as it pertains to individual minority groups such as African Americans, American Indians (or, Native Americans), Asians, and Latinos.

African Americans

As with empirical examinations of differences in the impact of stress on mental health, most research conducted on resilience in specific racial/ethnic minority groups has utilized African American samples. In a study examining quality of life as a resiliency outcome, traditional and culturally specific factors associated with coping were found to predict more favorable outcome (Utsey, Bolen, Lanier, & Williams, 2007). Family cohesiveness believed to be a "traditional" protective factor (Utsey et al., 2007) positively predicted quality of life, while culture-specific factors such as spirituality and collectiveness were also positively predictive of quality of life (Utsey et al., 2007).

Somewhat in contrast, using a qualitative approach, Brodsky (2000) found that the influence of religion on resilience varied on a case-by-case basis. That is, in her interviews of 10 resilient African American single mothers living in poverty and stressful environments, some women cited religion/spirituality as a protective factor, others did not note a role of religion in their resiliency. For those expressing the importance of spirituality in their resilience, differences were found in how this influence came to be (Brodsky, 2000). While individual differences in protective factors differed among the women, Brodsky (1999) found that some commonalities emerged. Specifically, resilient individuals were able to appreciate, locate, and utilize resources from supportive domains (for some it was family, while for others a significant other or church) and reframe some stressors as contributing to their contentment with their situation and motivation (lack of economic security as a way of teaching children importance of work ethic). Brodsky's (1999, 2000) rich illustrations of resilience in urban, African American, single-mothers highlights resilience of this cultural group, while emphasizing differences in how protective factors appear and function in adaptation. This research on resilience helps us to begin to understand the importance of social resources for racial/ethnic minorities. As we continue to examine adaptive outcomes for other racial/ethnic groups, we will see further support for the importance of social resources in bringing about adaptive outcomes.

American Indians

Very few studies have investigated resilience among American Indians, and those that have, have used varying definitions of the concept. For example, one study operationalized resilience in American Indians as enrollment or graduation from college (Montgomery, Miville, Winterowd, Jeffries, & Baysden, 2000). Using qualitative methods, the participants in this study emphasized that their ability to attain a higher level of education was a function of their integration of American Indian culture and family values in their learning, in the university setting, in their self-talk, and in their perception of social support systems. For example, one participant noted that her self-talk included the following: "the important thing for me is to remember where I am from, and to remember the people who helped me." Another student described the social support she sought out from other members of the American Indian community: "I made those connections with other tribal members, because that was my home away from home...." These comments underscore an integrationist approach to acculturation while also highlighting the importance of social support in adaptation to the stress experienced as a minority.

In another study, resilience in American Indians was examined in former prison inmates and defined as no recidivism over a 3-year period following release from incarceration (Angell & Jones, 2003). Comparing outcomes of Caucasians and American Indians of the Lumbee tribe, results indicated that Lumbee individuals were resilient against recidivism in terms of violent and drug-related crimes compared to the Caucasians. This finding did not hold when looking at property and miscellaneous offenses. Angell and Jones (2003) followed up with a case presentation of a Lumbee woman who stopped abusing drugs following her release from incarceration. The authors emphasized the role of her grandmother and a large network of other Lumbee, including a healer, that helped her overcome her substance abuse. Again, the role of social support and importance of maintaining strong ties to the culture of origin is further supported as integral to adaptation. While only a couple of studies have looked at resilience in American Indians, and these studies have been qualitative in nature, we can nonetheless conclude that adaptation is cultivated for this minority group when individuals are encouraged to stay close to their cultural roots and seek out the support of friends and family.

Asian Americans

Investigations of resilience in Asian American populations are few and far between. Nonetheless, the research that does exist underscores the importance of collectivism when defining and examining resilience in this group. In a recent study conducted by Bonanno, Galea, Bucciarelli, and Vlahov (2007), ethnicity was studied as a possible predictor of resilience. After controlling for SES and prior trauma, Asians were found to be 3 times more likely to be resilient (defined as no psychopathology) compared to Caucasians. This is in contrast to other studies, which have focused more on refugee populations, demonstrating decreased resilience in Asians (Lee, Lei, & Sue, 2001). One possibility for the divergence in findings is the greater rate of prior traumas experienced by refugee populations.

Phan (2006) interviewed Vietnamese refugee mothers with resilient children (resilience was defined as academically successful children) and gathered qualitative data about what the mothers felt fostered their child's resilience. According to the mothers, this resilience resulted from parental sacrifice for the greater good of their children. Phan (2006) posits that this notion of sacrifice for children is in line with an Eastern perspective, in which a collective view is emphasized over the individual. In this case, the child's and family's needs are put forth before the parents' individual needs. While there are conflicting findings regarding rates of resilience for Asian Americans, with some research showing decreased and other research documenting increased resilience, it appears that adaptation in this group may be best examined from a non-Western perspective. It is difficult to make broad inferences about Asian Americans based on this small amount of research. However, it appears that familial functioning may be an important aspect that future research endeavors ought to investigate further.

Latinos

Given the high rate of growth and large numbers of Latinos in this country, it is surprising that adaptation is understudied for this ethnic group. The small body of research that does exist makes it difficult to derive inferences, yet helps provide the beginnings of, hopefully, a growing literature. Research on exposure to stress and trauma documents lower resilience, or greater likelihood of development of PTSD, among Latinos (Perilla, Norris, & Lavizzo, 2002). However, in one recent study, when SES was controlled, Latino ethnicity was not predictive of decreased resiliency (Bonanno et al., 2007). Spencer-Rodgers and Collins (2006) examined resilience among Latino adults, operationalized as high self-esteem and found that, overall, high levels of global self-esteem were evident. A primary objective of this study was to examine the influence of perceived group (Latino) disadvantage on lower self-esteem. Contrary to hypotheses, perceived group disadvantage had only indirect effects on self-esteem outcome and was buffered by self-protective processes. These self-protective processes such as attachment to group and holding a personal high regard for one's group were more strongly related to higher self-esteem than was perceived disadvantage.

These findings highlight that affiliation with one's cultural group can foster resilient outcome. Though studied among Latin Americans living in violence-stricken areas of Colombia, the value of cultural solidarity was echoed in accounts of resilient coping in the face of political upheaval (Hernandez, 2002). While there is a dearth of research examining resilience in Latinos, the existing qualitative accounts point to the importance of cultural ties and valuing one's culture of origin in adaptation.

Summary

This chapter focused on the notion that stress and resilience must be considered within a cultural context. Until recently, theories of stress and its impact have not incorporated cultural factors potentially important to mental health in racial/ethnic minorities. We focused on three significant areas of stress particularly relevant to minority mental health – acculturation, racism, and poverty.

Each of these factors in and of themselves is associated, in varying degrees, with negative mental health outcomes in minorities.

It is also the case that both individual and broader cultural factors can help mitigate their negative impact. Within the context of the broader culture, the sometimes stressful process of acculturation and its negative impact can be lessened by a "multicultural" stance, that is, one that accepts and values the richness and diversity brought by all of its members. Similarly, at the individual level, outcomes for racial/ethnic minorities can be maximized by establishing connections to the dominant culture, while maintaining the traditions, values, and supports of the culture of origin.

With regard to racism, there is a well-established association with a range of mental health difficulties among minorities. However, we are just beginning to understand factors that may mediate the negative impact of racism, including such things as racial identity, self-esteem, and coping skills. Of course, ultimately, the goal is to eliminate racist attitudes and behaviors. Until then, we should devote considerable work to better understanding factors that buffer the impact of racism.

Lastly, while poverty has been consistently linked to poor mental health outcomes, and racial/ethnic minorities experience poverty at disproportionately high rates, the relationship between poverty, minority status, and mental health problems warrants further attention. Indeed, it is unclear if specific stressors (e.g., exposure to crime/violence, social isolation) are confounding the relationship between poverty and mental health problems and whether certain individual-level protective factors may shield the ill-effects of poverty. Clearly, there are many significant stressors contributing to poor mental health faced by racial/ethnic minorities, a few of which we touched upon above. It is imperative, however, that we recognize that most individuals do persevere despite these significant stressors.

In addition to the impact of stress on ethnic and racial minorities, the lens has recently begun to shift toward examining resilience among such populations. Overall, this area of research is in its early stage and thus far relies primarily on qualitative accounts of protective factors associated with resiliency. Though differences exist among the diverse racial/ethnic minority groups, a few common themes emerge, including the essential role of social support in bringing about adaptation in the face of significant stressors. Another theme that can be discerned from this research is the utility of reframing stressful events and circumstances (demonstrated in the Lumbee and African American accounts of their protective factors). Armed with knowledge of the individual experience of the members of minority groups provided by the rich accounts highlighted above, research endeavors can aim to address important yet understudied areas. Specifically, the need for continued research with larger groups is needed so that qualitative views of individual experiences may be supplemented by an understanding for group differences and factors associated with resilience. Large-scale investigations examining the role of social support and culturally specific cognitive reframing could greatly enhance the development of culturally relevant and sensitive interventions. Clearly the qualitative research provides great depth of study, while highlighting the need for continued research examining resilience in minority populations.

References

Angell, G. B., & Jones, G. M. (2003). Recidivism, risk, and resiliency among North American Indian parolees and former prisoners: An examination of the Lumbee First Nation. *Journal of Ethnic & Cultural Diversity in Social Work*, *12*(2), 61–77.

Berry, J. W. (1997). Immigration, acculturation and adaptation. *Applied Psychology: An International Review*, *46*, 5–34.

Berry, J. W. (1980). Acculturation as varieties of adaptation. In A. Padilla (Ed.), *Acculturation: Theory, models and findings* (pp. 9–25). Boulder: Westview.

Berry, J. W. (2005). Acculturation: Living successfully in two cultures. *International Journal of Intercultural Relations*, *29*, 697–712.

Berry, J. W., Phinney, J. S., Sam, D. L., & Vedder, P. (2006). Immigrant youth: Acculturation, identity, and adaptation. *Applied Psychology: An International Review*, *55*(3), 303–332.

Bogard, C. J., Trillo, A., Schwartz, M., & Gerstel, N. (2001). Future employment among homeless single mothers: The effects of full-time work experience and depressive symptomatology. *Women & Health*, *32*(1–2), 137–157.

Bonanno, G. A. (2004). Loss, trauma, and human resilience: Have we underestimated the human capacity to thrive after extremely aversive events? *American Psychologist*, *59*(1), 20–28.

Bonanno, G. A., Galea, S., Bucciarelli, A., & Vlahov, D. (2006). Psychological resilience after disaster: New York City in the aftermath of the September 11th terrorist attack. *Psychological Science*, *17*(3), 181–186.

Bonanno, G. A., Galea, S., Bucciarelli, A., & Vlahov, D. (2007). What predicts psychological resilience after disaster? The role of demographics, resources, and life stress. *Journal of Consulting and Clinical Psychology*, *75*(5), 671–682.

Bonanno, G. A., Wortman, C. B., Lehman, D. R., Tweed, R. G., Haring, M., Sonnega, J., et al. (2002). Resilience to loss and chronic grief: A prospective study from preloss to 18-months postloss. *Journal of Personality and Social Psychology*, *83*(5), 1150–1164.

Borrell, L. N., Kiefe, C. I., Williams, D. R., Diez-Roux, A. V., & Gordon-Larsen, P. (2006). Self-reported health, perceived racial discrimination, and skin color in African Americans in the CARDIA study. *Social Science & Medicine*, *63*, 1415–1427.

Bratter, J. L., & Eschbach, K. (2005). Race/ethnic differences in nonspecific psychological distress: Evidence from the National Health Interview Survey. *Social Science Quarterly*, *86*(3), 620–644.

Brodsky, A. E. (1999). "Making it": The components and process of resilience among urban, African-American, single mothers. *American Journal of Orthopsychiatry*, *69*(2), 148–160.

Brodsky, A. E. (2000). The role of religion in the lives of resilient, urban, African American, single mothers. *Special Issue: Spirituality, Religion, and Community Psychology*, *28*(2), 199–219.

Brown, T. N., Williams, D. R., Jackson, J. S., Neighbors, H. W., Torres, M., Sellers, S. L., et al. (2000). "Being black and feeling blue": The mental health consequences of racial discrimination. *Race & Society*, *2*(2), 117–131.

Buddington, S. A. (2002). Acculturation, psychological adjustment (stress, depression, self-esteem) and the academic achievement of Jamaican immigrant college students. *International Social Work*, *45*(4), 447–464.

Cannon, W. (1932). *Effects of strong emotions*. Oxford, England: University of Chicago Press.

Castillo, L. G., Conoley, C. W., & Brossart, D. F. (2004). Acculturation, White marginalization, and family support as predictors of perceived distress in Mexican American female college students. *Journal of Counseling Psychology, 51*(2), 151–157.

Chapman, H. A., Hobfoll, S. E., & Ritter, C. (1997). Partners' stress underestimations lead to women's distress: A study of pregnant inner-city women. *Journal of Personality and Social Psychology, 73*(2), 418–425.

Cho, S., Hudley, C., & Back, H. J. (2003). Cultural influences on ratings of self-perceived social, emotional, and academic adjustment for Korean American adolescents. *Assessment for Effective Intervention, 29*(1), 3–14.

Clark, R., Anderson, N. B., Clark, V. R., & Williams, D. R. (1999). Racism as a stressor for African Americans. *American Psychologist, 54*(10), 805–816.

Crockett, L. J., Iturbide, M. I., Stone, R. A. T., McGinley, M., Raffaelli, M., & Carlo, G. (2007). Acculturative stress, social support, and coping: relations to psychological adjustment among Mexican American college students. *Cultural Diversity and Ethnic Minority Psychology, 13*(4), 347–355.

Franzini, L., & Fernandez-Esquer, E. (2004). Socioeconomic, cultural, and personal influences on health outcomes in low income Mexican-origin individuals in Texas. *Social Science & Medicine, 59*, 1629–1646.

Garmezy, N., Masten, A. S., & Tellegen, A. (1984). The study of stress and competence in children: A building block for developmental psychopathology. *Child Development, 55*(1), 97–111.

Gee, G. C., Spencer, M., Chen, J., Yip, T., & Takeuchi, D. T. (2007). The association between self-reported racial discrimination and 12-month DSM-IV mental disorders among Asian Americans nationwide. *Social Science & Medicine, 64*, 1984–1996.

Gordon, M. M. (1964). *Assimilation in American life: The role of race, religion, and national origins.* New York: Oxford University Press.

Gyamfi, P., Brooks-Gunn, J., & Jackson, A. P. (2001). Associations between employment and financial and parental stress in low-income single black mothers. *Women & Health, 32*(1–2), 119–135.

Harrell, S. P. (2000). A multidimensional conceptualization of racism-related stress: Implications for the well-being of people of color. *American Journal of Orthopsychiatry, 70*(1), 42–57.

Hassouneh, D. M., & Kulwiki, A. (2007). Mental health, discrimination, and trauma in Arab Muslim women living in the US: A pilot study. *Mental Health, Religion, and Culture, 10*(3), 257–262.

Hernandez, P. (2002). Resilience in families and communities: Latin American contributions from the psychology of liberation. *The Family Journal, 10*(3), 334–343.

Hobfoll, S. E. (1989). Conservation of resources: A new attempt at conceptualizing stress. *American Psychologist, 44*(3), 513–524.

Hobfoll, S. E. (2001). The influence of culture, community, and the nested-self in the stress process: Advancing conservation of resources theory. *Applied Psychology: An International Review, 50*(3), 337–369.

Hovey, J. D. (2000). Acculturative stress, depression, and suicidal ideation in Mexican immigrants. *Cultural Diversity and Ethnic Minority Psychology, 6*(2), 134–151.

Hwang, W., & Ting, J. (2008). Disaggregating the effects of acculturation and acculturative stress on the mental health of Asian Americans. *Cultural Diversity and Ethnic Minority Psychology, 14*(2), 147–154.

Johnson, A. C. (1995). Resiliency mechanisms in culturally diverse families. *The Family Journal, 3*(4), 316–324.

Jones, H. L., Cross, Jr., W. E., & DeFour, D. C. (2007). Race-related stress, racial identity attitudes, and mental health among Black women. *Journal of Black Psychology, 33*(2), 208–231.

Karlsen, S., & Nazroo, J. Y. (2002). Relation between racial discrimination, social class, and health among ethnic minority groups. *American Journal of Public Health, 82*(4), 624–631.

Karlson, S., Nazroo, J. Y., McKenzie, K., Bhui, K., & Weich, S. (2005). Racism, psychosis and common mental disorder among ethnic minority groups in England. *Psychological Medicine, 35*(12), 1795–1803.

Kessler, R. C. (1979). Stress, social status, and psychological distress. *Journal of Health & Social Behavior, 20*, 100–108.

Kessler, R. C., Berglund, P., Demler, O., Jin, R., Koretz, D., Merikangas, K., et al. (2003). The epidemiology of major depressive disorder: Results from the National Comorbidity Survey Replication (NCS-R). *JAMA: Journal of the American Medical Association, 289*(23), 3095–3105.

Kessler, R. C., Mickelson, K. D., & Williams, D. R. (1999). The prevalence, distribution, and mental health correlates of perceived discrimination in the United States. *Journal of Health and Social Behavior, 40*(3), 208–230.

Kim, B. S. K., & Omizo, M. M. (2006). Behavioral acculturation and enculturation and psychological functioning among Asian American college students. *Cultural Diversity and Ethnic Minority Psychology, 12*(2), 245–258.

Koneru, V. K., Weisman de Mamani, A. G., Flynn, P,M., & Betancourt, H. (2007). Acculturation and mental health: Current findings and recommendations for future research. *Applied and Preventative Psychology, 12*, 76–96.

LaFromboise, T., Coleman, H. L. K., & Gerton, J. (1993). Psychological impact of biculturalism: Evidence and theory. *Psychological Bulletin, 114*(3), 395–412.

Lazarus, R. S, & Folkman, S. (1984). *Stress, appraisal, and coping.* New York: Springer.

Lee, J., Koeske, G. F., & Sales, E. (2004). Social support buffering of acculturative stress: a study of mental health symptoms among Korean international students. *International Journal of Intercultural Relations, 28*, 399–414.

Lee, J., Lei, A., & Sue, S. (2001). The current state of mental health research on Asian Americans. *Journal of Human Behavior in the Social Environment, 3*, 159–178.

Leventhal, T., Fauth, R. C., & Brooks-Gunn, J. (2005). Neighborhood poverty and public policy: A 5-year follow-up of children's educational outcomes in the New York City moving to opportunity demonstration. *Developmental Psychology, 41*(6), 933–952.

Liang, C. T. H., Alvarez, A. N., Juang, L. P., & Liang, M. X. (2007). The role of coping in the relationship between perceived racism and racism-related stress for Asian Americans: Gender differences. *Journal of Counseling Psychology, 54*(2), 132–141.

Mak, W. W. S., Chen, S. X., Wong, E. C., & Zane, N. W. S. (2005). A psychosocial model of stress-distress relationship among Chinese Americans. *Journal of Social and Clinical Psychology, 24*(3), 422–444.

Massey, D. S. (2005). Racial discrimination in housing: A moving target. *Social Problems, 52*(2), 148–151.

Montgomery, D., Miville, M. L., Winterowd, C., Jeffries, B., & Baysden, M. F. (2000). American Indian college students: An exploration into resiliency factors revealed through personal stories. *Cultural Diversity & Ethnic Minority Psychology, 6*(4), 387–398.

Moradi, B., & Risco, C. (2006). Perceived discrimination experiences and mental health of Latina/o American persons. *Journal of Counseling Psychology, 53*(4), 411–421.

Murry, V. M., Brown, P. A., Brody, G. H., Cutrona, C. E., & Simons, R. L. (2001). Racial discrimination as a moderator of the links among stress, maternal psychological functioning, and family relationships. *Journal of Family and Marriage, 63*, 915–926.

Noh, S., & Kaspar, V. (2003). Perceived discrimination and depression: Moderating effects of coping, acculturation, and ethnic support. *American Journal of Public Health, 93*, 232–238.

O'Hare, W., & Mather, M. (2003). *The growing number of kids in severely distressed neighborhoods: Evidence from the 2000 census.* Washington, DC: Anne E. Casey Foundation.

Perez, M., Voelz, Z. R., Pettit, J. W., & Joiner, Jr., T. E. (2001). The role of acculturative stress and body dissatisfaction in predicting bulimic symptomatology across ethnic groups. *International Journal of Eating Disorders, 31*(4), 442–454.

Perilla, J. I., Norris, F. H., & Lavizzo, E. A. (2002). Ethnicity, culture, and disaster response: Identifying and explaining ethnic differences in PTSD six months after Hurricane Andrew. *Journal of Social and Clinical Psychology, 21*, 20–45.

Phan, T. (2006). Resilience as a coping mechanism: A common story of Vietnamese refugee women. In P. T. P. Wong & L. C. J. Wong (Eds.), *Handbook of multicultural perspectives on stress and coping* (pp. 427–437). Dallas, TX: Spring Publications.

Pillay, Y. (2005). Racial identity as a predictor of the psychological health of African American Students at a predominantly White university. *Journal of Black Psychology, 31*(1), 46–66.

Prelow, H. M., Mosher, C. E., & Bowman, M. A. (2006). Perceived racial discrimination, social support, and psychological adjustment among African American college students. *Journal of Black Psychology, 32*(4), 442–454.

Rutter, M. (1987). Psychosocial resilience and protective mechanisms. *American Journal of Orthopsychiatry, 57*(3), 316–331.

Schulz, A. J., Gravlee, C. C., Williams, D. R., Israel, B. A., Mentz, G., & Rowe, Z. (2006). Discrimination, symptoms of depression, and self-rated health among African American women in Detroit: Results from a longitudinal analysis. *American Journal of Public Health, 96*(7), 1265–1270.

Selye, H. (1936). A syndrome produced by diverse nocuous agents. *Nature, 138*(4), 32.

Smith, E. M. J. (1985). Ethnic minorities: Life stress, social support, and mental health issues. *The Counseling Psychologist, 13*(4), 537–579.

Spencer-Rodgers, J., & Collins, N. L. (2006). Risk and resilience: Dual effects of perceptions of group disadvantage among Latinos. *Journal of Experimental Social Psychology, 42*(6), 729–737.

Thompson, V. L. S. (2006). Coping responses and the experience of discrimination. *Journal of Applied Social Psychology, 36*(5), 1198–1214.

Utsey, S. O., Bolden, M. A., Lanier, Y., & Williams, O. (2007). Examining the role of culture-specific coping as a predictor of resilient outcomes in African Americans from high-risk urban communities. *Journal of Black Psychology, 33*(1), 75–93.

Utsey, S. O., Lanier, Y., Williams, III, O., Bolden, M., & Lee, A. (2006). Moderator effects of cognitive ability and social support on the relation between race-related stress and quality of life in a community sample of Black Americans. *Cultural Diversity and Ethnic Minority Psychology, 12*(2), 334–346.

Wadsworth, E., Dhillon, K., Shaw, C., Bhui K., Stansfeld, S., & Smith, A. (2006). Racial discrimination, ethnicity and work stress. *Occupational Medicine, 57*, 18–24.

Walker, R. L., Wingate L. R., Obasi, E. M., & Joiner, T. E., Jr. (2008). An empirical investigation of acculturative stress and ethnic identity as moderators for depression and suicidal ideation in college students. *Cultural Diversity and Ethnic Minority Psychology, 14*(1), 75–82.

Chapter 18
Methodological Challenges in Research on the Determinants of Minority Mental Health and Wellness

Peter Guarnaccia

Introduction

Over the last decade, there has been an increasing focus on "health disparities" at the National Institutes of Health, the Institute of Medicine, and more broadly in society (Smedley, Stith, & Nelson, 2003; USDHHS, 2001). This attention to racial and ethnic disparities has raised a number of issues concerning how we define and document a range of concepts in minority mental health and wellness research. If we are going to assess the level of health disparities, and more importantly, intervene to address them, we need to be sure that we have clearly measured those disparities, identified the groups where they occur, understood the sources of the disparities, and assessed the health care services issues that underlie them. This is no small task. The research record to date has been more effective at defining the disparities that exist than at assessing the sources of those disparities or, even less so, of developing interventions to ameliorate them.

This chapter is directed at both reviewing and providing guidance on research approaches in assessing minority mental health and wellness. The chapter will first address issues in defining race and ethnicity. If racial and ethnic disparities in mental health are to be studied, clearly a first step is to define what we mean by racial and ethnic groups and which groups are the "minorities" who experience the disparities. The next section will examine the area of language in research. This section will particularly focus on methodological issues in translating measures for studying mental health disparities.

The following sections will examine how to assess mental health and wellness with minority populations. While methods for assessing mental health, really mental health problems and disorders, are quite well developed for a range of ethnic and racial minority groups, the assessment of wellness is less well

P. Guarnaccia (✉)
Institute for Health, Health Care Policy, and Aging Research, Rutgers University, New Brunswick, NJ
e-mail: pguarnaccia@ifh.rutgers.edu

S. Loue, M. Sajatovic (eds.), *Determinants of Minority Mental Health and Wellness*, DOI 10.1007/978-0-387-75659-2_18,
© Springer Science+Business Media, LLC 2009

developed. This is equally true for European American populations. A key issue will be how much to adapt existing measures to include content relevant to ethnic minority groups. Another issue is bringing a stronger focus on religion and spirituality into the research. The last section of this part of the chapter will look at social and cultural issues that are intimately tied to mental health and wellness, including acculturation processes, discrimination, and the processes and impacts of immigration.

The final sections will examine issues in building a research program on minority mental health and wellness. One key set of issues focuses on the integration of qualitative and quantitative methods. Given that much of the research in this area still involves a significant amount of discovery of new knowledge about the extent and nature of differences among minority groups and with the European American population, there is a large role for qualitative methods. At the same time, establishing reliable patterns of mental health problems and their solutions requires larger scale and more generalizable quantitative research. Maintaining a balance among research methods so that both cultural particularities and cross-cutting generalities can be identified continues to be a major challenge. For minority mental health research to succeed, there is a compelling need for the building of teams that are themselves culturally diverse. The final section of this chapter will provide some guidance and approaches to working in bilingual/bicultural research teams, largely based on my own 20-year career in minority mental health research.

Defining Race and Ethnicity

One of the most vexing problems in minority mental health research is defining the racial and ethnic groups to study. Many epidemiological and services researchers choose to and/or are constrained to use the Census categories developed by the U.S. Census Bureau and the Office of Management and the Budget (American Anthropological Association, 1997; U.S. Census Bureau, 2000; Office of Management and Budget, 1997). I argue that these categories confuse the issue of what is race and ethnicity and are also difficult to implement in community research. They force respondents into categories that they often feel do not represent them. For these reasons these categories can distort the research process. I argue that we need to move beyond the Census categories if we want to do research that reflects the experience of minority communities.

The current Census definitions only recognize Hispanic as an ethnicity [see Form D-61A of the U.S. Bureau of the Census]. The Census asks first "Is this person Spanish/Hispanic/Latino?" The responses are: "No, Not Spanish/Hispanic/Latino," "Yes, Mexican, Mexican American, Chicano," "Yes, Puerto Rican," "Yes, Cuban," and "Yes, Other Spanish/Hispanic/Latino." There are a number of peculiar and problematic features of this definition, not the least of which is that only Hispanic is recognized as an ethnicity. This would come as a great surprise to a variety of other "ethnics" who have strong cultural identities in the U.S. The second feature is that the first identity mentioned is "Spanish," yet few people who identify as Hispanic are from Spain and those from Spain rarely would use the ethnic identifier of Hispanic. In fact, the contentions among the use of the global terms Hispanic and Latino revolve significantly around the issue of whether only the European origin of Latinos in the U.S. is being recognized (Hayes-Bautista & Chapa, 1987). The European prejudice of the Census by listing Spanish first is highly problematic in research with U.S. Latino communities.

Another issue is the listing of multiple identifiers for Mexican, including the cultural and political label of "Chicano," but only single listings for Puerto Rican and Cuban (Hazuda et al., 1986). Many political Puerto Ricans, especially those born in the U.S., use the term "Boricua" as a parallel identity to "Chicano" for Mexicans. Cubans also refer to themselves as Cuban Americans when they want to highlight their affinity with the politics of the U.S. over that of Cuba. Clearly the selective listing of these different terms for specific Latino groups reflects a political process more than a scientific approach to categorization (Gaboda, Tsikiwa, Warner, & Guarnaccia, 2000).

Finally, the lumping of all other Latinos in one big group obscures the incredible diversity and growing populations of these groups in the U.S. The Census does provide a space for filling in the specific Hispanic group for those in the other category. The rapidly rising populations of Ecuadorians and Peruvians in the Northeast, the large Central American populations in California and Washington, D.C., and the growing Dominican communities along the Eastern seaboard all argue that the older focus on only 3 Latino groups is outdated. As the second generation of Latinos grows dramatically, having only one group identifier will no longer be sufficient as many young Latinos have parents from different Latino groups.

Following the Hispanic ethnicity question is the race question, which asks "What is this person's race?" The categorizations are revealing of the conflation of race and ethnicity in the Census and lack of clarity of when it matters to further define the respondent's "race." "White" is presented as an unmarked category; the instructions in the Census identify the following groups as White: people having their origins in Europe, the Middle East, and North Africa (Office of Management and Budget, 1997). There is no instruction to specify the group – the "White" category is assumed to be homogenous and undifferentiated.

Similarly, people of African origin are expected to check the box for "Black, African American or Negro." Again, no option is provided to allow for further specification. The results of the National Survey of American Life make clear that the experiences of Black immigrants, particularly from the Caribbean, are quite different from Black Americans, in spite of their shared history of forced relocation and slavery (Jackson et al., 2004). Also the categories show minimal sensitivity to the continued use of "Negro" as a term.

The Asian groups and Pacific Islander groups are treated quite differently. For both groups, several specific national origins are listed – Asian Indian, Chinese, Filipino, Korean and Vietnamese for Asians; Native Hawaiian, Guamanian, Chamorro, and Samoan for Pacific Islanders. For both groups there is an "Other" category with instructions to fill in the specific group. The Asian groups appear to represent the largest population groups in the U.S. The Pacific Islanders reflect those groups that were colonized by the U.S. and are therefore the most numerous groups eligible to be counted in the U.S Census.

American Indians and Alaska Natives are asked to write in their enrolled or principal tribe if they check this racial category. It is not clear whether the contentious status of tribes as legally recognized or not should be reflected in the Census.

While Asians and Pacific Islanders are asked to fill in their **race**, an interesting shift in language occurs for American Indians and Alaska Natives who are asked to fill in their **tribe**; for Hispanic ethnicity, respondents are asked to write in their **group**. The differences in detail of categorization (being asked to fill in a specific group or not) and the differences in language (group, race, tribe) are not trivial. They reflect real confusion on the part of the designers of the Census about what is being measured. Long ago, the notion that Italians, for example, were a sub-race of Whites went out of fashion as prejudicial, even racist. So the White category is no longer differentiated. But is it any clearer that Koreans, again as an example, are a sub-race of Asians? The Census does note that the race category mixes questions about race and national origin (U.S. Bureau of the Census, 2001). And the 2000 Census allows people to identify themselves as multiracial. But one has to ask what is the purpose of this categorization and what analytic purposes does it serve? How can categories that mix so many different statuses be useful as research tools?

Another strange feature of the separation of Hispanic ethnicity and race is the emergence of the categories of Non-Hispanic White and Non-Hispanic Black; note there is no category of Non-Hispanic Asians or American Indians. It is striking to note this shift so that Hispanics are the reference category against which Whites and Blacks are compared – that is the implication of this terminology. Is this simply a result of the ordering of the questions or is there some other conceptual issue being marked here?

This issue gets further confused because Hispanics/Latinos are supposed to choose a race category. On the basis of extensive personal research experience in Latino communities, and direct discussion of this issue with Latinos in focus groups, most Latinos find this approach bizarre (Alegria et al., 2004). They ask why no Hispanic/Latino category exists among the race and national origin questions. They argue forcefully and convincingly that given the histories of their countries, the majority of Hispanics are a mix of races – combining American Indian, African and European, as well as Asian, roots in different mixtures depending on the particular country. The result is that many Latinos leave the race question blank or they check the Other Race box. However, the Census reflects its commitment to these categorizations by developing an algorithm for assigning Latinos to racial categories when they do not fill them out. Thus, Puerto Ricans, Cubans, and Mexicans are coded as White, but Dominicans are coded as Black, regardless of their own identities or physical appearances. Guatemalans and Hondurans are coded as Other for reasons that are not clear (Gaboda et al., 2000).

Anthropological and sociological work on race makes quite clear that racial categories are social, and not biological, categories (Hahn & Mulinare, 1992; Stroup & Hahn, 1994; Williams, Lavisso-Mourney, & Warren, 1992; see also American Anthropological Association RACE Project, 2007). This approach received further support from the Human Genome Project that showed that genetic variability within groups labeled as races was as great or greater than genetic differences between what are typically referred to as races. All categorization systems are social systems of grouping people.

From my perspective the term **ethnic group** is a better term to mark the various social and cultural groups in the U.S. American Indians, Asians, Blacks, Latinos, Pacific Islanders and Whites are all large groupings of ethnicity which in practice break up into more specific ethnic groupings. For purposes of this chapter, I am going to define ethnic groups as cultural groups interacting in a multicultural context. Ethnic groups arise out of a need to define oneself and one's group in comparison to other cultural groups who may be co-residing, cooperating and/or competing within a particular social and political context. Ethnic groups not only share cultural features but also histories, migrations, and political and economic processes, which define them both to themselves and to others. In my two decades of community research experience, I have found that people use these broad terms, such as Asian, largely for political purposes to ally with a particular group, but these terms do not capture who people think they are. My experience is that people think in much more specific identities having to do with national origins and cultural practices of their families. These local conceptions should be reflected in our research categorizations.

The research implications of this are that we should be asking people to self identify their ethnic origins and to provide multiple boxes for people to put themselves in (Waters, 1990). It is both valid and useful to ask people to highlight their primary ethnic identity when they mention more than one. My experience is that this is generally not a difficult task when explained properly. The research team can then aggregate up as needed. The research starts with the definition of the person being studied. In health research with those who cannot respond for themselves – young children, people with certain disabilities, the deceased – then family members should be queried. Last names are often unreliable and appearance is even less so. Yet in research on how mortality is coded, one of the key areas for disparities research, physician, or funeral director judgment is used to a startling extent (Gaboda et al., 2000). This has resulted in people being born one ethnicity and dying a second one (Hahn & Mulinare, 1992).

Specificity is important in coding people's ethnicity in mental health and wellness research. Results of the recent national studies of mental health across a range of ethnic groups indicate that the important differences are at the level of specific ethnic groups, as well as across broad group comparisons (Alegria et al., 2004; Jackson et al., 2004). It is important not to lose this initial specificity in the data-collection process. Aggregating up through recoding of the ethnicity variables is highly feasible. If the data is not collected with specificity in mind, it is not possible to disaggregate these broad categories.

Role of Language in Research

According to the National Latino and Asian American mental health study (NLAAS), more than 50% of Latinos and Asian Americans in the United States speak languages other than English as their primary language (Guarnaccia et al., 2007). The complexity of questions about mental health and wellness require that questions be asked in people's most fluent languages, even when minorities may be functional in English for everyday activities. This means that questions about mental health status, mental health services utilization, and wellness issues will need to be translated from English, the language in which the overwhelming majority of questions are developed and available, into a range of other languages.

Translation should be viewed as an integral part of the research process (Brislin, 1986; Brislin, Lonner, & Throndike, 1973; Matias-Carrelo et al., 2003). It is not just the deceptively simple process of rephrasing questions in English into another language. Writing effective questions to assess mental health and wellness in other languages requires not only fluency in both languages but understanding of the cultural frameworks surrounding the languages to be used. Translation allows the researchers to examine the cultural and clinical assumptions embedded in English phrasings of questions, as well as how those questions translate into another language. The world is shaped through our cultural understandings of it, and these understandings are embedded in the terms, categories, and grammar we use (Good, 1994; Jenkins & Karno, 1992). Thus, the process of developing and translating research instruments is fundamentally a cultural process, as well as a scientific and technical one.

Some of the challenges of translation are created by the fact that research instruments are implicitly cultural documents even when researchers do not realize that they are. A simple and widely known example is the use of the feelings of "down and blue" to describe depression. These terms are found in many widely used measures of depression because they are so colloquial and so frequently used by American English speakers to describe the feelings of depression. They are powerful descriptors in English exactly because they embed a range of feelings and experiences of depression in a couple of simple and widely understood words. Yet these dimensions of these words make them very difficult to translate in any straightforward way. If one translated these directly into Spanish, or another widely spoken language in the U.S., they would make no sense as signs of depression. So the first task is to "translate" these idiomatic expressions in English into less colloquial English terms so that they can then be effectively rendered in a second language. This simple example indicates that effective translation of measures requires a team of researchers who are widely fluent in both English and the other language they will be translating the measure into (Matias-Carrelo et al., 2003).

The experience of developing the instruments for the NLAAS and related research projects has provided enhanced guidelines for translation of mental health and wellness measures (Alegria et al., 2004). These go beyond, but still incorporate, the usual processes of translation and back translation. But newer approaches add additional steps to test the measures in community contexts similar to the ones to be studied. They also engage the researchers in a more in-depth process of review and discussion than was typically the case in earlier efforts at translation. This process is most fully described and developed in Matias-Carrelo et al. (2003) and summarized below.

The first stage in the translation process is to develop an expert committee of mental health researchers who are fully bilingual and also fully understand the concepts and issues of measurement involved in the research. This group will oversee the entire translation process and will ultimately make the final decisions on the research instruments in all the languages to be used in the study. This committee brings in a professional translator who is bilingual/bicultural and whose first language is the language that the measures will be translated into. One of the key issues is to be sure the translator does not do a literal translation of the questions from English to the second language, but rather a colloquial translation. The goal is to have the meaning of the question remain the same even if the structure of the question (word order, for example) and the length of the question changes to adapt to the second language. The translator should keep running notes on questions that were difficult to translate or where the equivalence of words was not easy to achieve.

Once the instrument is fully translated, a second back translator is brought in whose first language is English and is fluent in the second language. This person should be blind to the original English interview and should be given the new second language interview without commentary to translate back into English. The back translator should note questions that were difficult to interpret and express in English.

The two translated versions are then given to the expert committee to review. The first step is to compare the original English version to the back-translated English version to identify discrepancies in wording and meaning that appear significant for equivalence between the questions. Where the two English versions are different in important ways, the expert committee reviews the translated version to see where the problems arose from. This process centrally uncovers issues in accurate translation. It also identifies other issues in the original English version of the questions. I have already noted the issues raised by colloquial use of English in phrasing questions. This may not be a problem in the original English interview, but can pose a major issue for translation. A second issue that often emerges is that the original question is too long, has too many phrases, and in other ways is expressed in a complex way that makes translation difficult and may result in awkward phrasings.

These issues raise questions about whether the original English version should be modified as well or whether it is acceptable to have the translated question be somewhat different. Following on the "down or blue" example above, often the translated word refers to "sad" in the second language (at least that is my experience in Spanish). This raises questions of whether the original English should be changed to sad as well or whether sad is an appropriate equivalent for down or blue.

Other issues that have emerged in Spanish translation of measures are that the Spanish words have additional meanings that the word in English did not have. An example here is the translation of attack, as in panic attack, as *ataque* in Spanish. The research group in Puerto Rico recognized more than 20 years ago that *ataque* referred not just to a sudden episode of panic as understood in American psychiatry, but might also be interpreted as an *ataque de nervios*, a cultural syndrome in Puerto Rico and other Latino groups that share symptoms with panic attacks but have a very different meaning, phenomenology, and association with a psychiatric disorder (Guarnaccia, Angel, & Worobey, 1989; Guarnaccia, Canino, Rubio-Stipec, & Bravo, 1993; Lewis-Fernandez et al., 2005). In fact, this recognition by the Puerto Rico group of a possible area of misunderstanding launched my two-decade research career on *ataques de nervios* in Latino culture and their relationship to mental health issues.

Another problematic area has been symptoms of psychoticism, especially hearing voices or visual hallucinations. Given the prominence of spiritual experiences in Latino and other cultures, for example South Asian cultures, these questions need to be contextualized quite differently to avoid their yielding false positive responses. This is especially true of lay-administered or self-administered questionnaires, where there is no opportunity for rephrasing or explaining the meaning of the questions (Guarnaccia, Guevara-Ramos, Gonzales, Canino, & Bird, 1992; Lewis-Fernandez et al., in press).

Once the bilingual/bicultural expert committee has resolved the issues that emerge from comparing the English versions of the interview, they then review the translation itself for clarity, grammatical issues, and to be sure that it captures the mental health concepts accurately. It is valuable to have the expert committee reflect diversity in national origin of speakers (at least this is the case for Spanish-speaking countries) as the ways of phrasing questions is different in different places. For example, in translating the Composite International Diagnostic Interview (CIDI) for use in multiple Latin American and Latino contexts, the simple and oft-used phrase "how often" was expressed in at least three different ways across Latin America (Canino & Bravo, 1994). Thus, the interview embedded these alternate wordings, and the interview training manual included instructions to interviewers on which form of the phrase to use in which countries.

A newer addition to the process of translation has proven to be very useful in the final phase of adapting the instruments for use in the community. This involves taking all or parts of the interview to community focus groups for discussions of the language and meaning of the questions (Matias-Carrelo et al., 2003). Having led several of these groups for the NLAAS and other studies, I can attest to their usefulness. I have consistently been impressed with the level of engagement of community participants, properly oriented and motivated for the task, in the process of adaptation and translation of research measures.

The focus groups are highly useful for several reasons. A key one is that the measures should be designed for the communities to be studied, and there is no substitute for members of those communities assessing the language and structure of the questions. Skilled translators are university trained and often use a formal version of the language different from what community respondents use. Even when the reading level of the questions is set ahead of time, it is still important to check that the translation is appropriate for the community to be studied. Some of these issues may start with the language used in the original English language version of the instrument. Another issue emerges from the diversity within minority communities in the U.S. in terms of ethnic origin, migration experience, and level of acculturation to U.S. society and English. All these factors affect language use.

Language embeds the values of a culture (Good, 1994). An accurate translation may still mean something different in another culture because of different values. There are many excellent examples of these issues in the work of Matias-Carrelo and colleagues (2003), but I will select one here. This had to do with the translation of the concept of family burden, a widely used measure for assessing the impact on families of caring for a relative with serious mental illness (Reinhard, Gubman, Horwitz, & Minsky, 1994). The expert committee felt that the Spanish word *carga* was an equivalent translation of the word "burden." But the focus groups' reaction to *carga* was that it carried a negative connotation of caring for an ill relative, which went against the Latino families' notions that it is the role of the family to care for someone in the home when they are sick. The families suggested that the term *responsabilidades* ("responsibilities") was a more appropriate term. This is a good example of how the cultural definitions of the role of family and its role in caregiving gets expressed differently in ways that are critical to understand in the process of translation.

It is also important to review the response formats typical of questions in mental health questionnaires to be sure that they translate across languages and cultures. One issue is the format of Likert scales, Cantrell ladders and 0–100 scales that are very familiar to most people in the U.S. because of their high exposure to these formats through schooling, testing, and other media exposures. One issue is the sheer number of points and whether it is easy for people to distinguish among them.

The other issue with respect to such scales arises in the anchoring terms that are used to help people assess where they are on the scale. As an example, one ubiquitous wellness measure is the self-assessed health question, which is typically scaled on a 5-point Likert scale with the anchoring words being "excellent," "very good," "good," "fair," and "poor," with "good" being the middle category. In work I did with Ron Angel on these questions from the Hispanic Health and Nutrition Examination Survey (HHANES) (Angel & Guarnaccia, 1989), we found that Hispanics tended to self-assess their health as worse than the physicians in the study did, and also worse than European Americans had done in previous versions of the HANES studies. Among several reasons for these differences, we hypothesized that the translation of the scale may have affected responses. In Spanish, the scale was translated as: *excelente, muy bueno, bueno, regular* and *malo*. The category of *regular* is not as negative a category as "fair" is in English and would indicate average health. One of our concerns was that this translation shifted the midpoint of the scale lower in Spanish than in English. While there were also important social reasons why Hispanic respondents' health would be worse than other groups, this linguistic and cultural issue likely contributed somewhat to the differing assessments.

Once the results of the focus groups are available, the bilingual/bicultural expert committee reviews the instrument one more time to further refine the questions and assure that the measures will be fully understandable by participants in the study. At this point, the expert committee must not only take into consideration issues of language and translation, but also the broader context of the study. If the study is meant to be comparable to other studies, as the NLAAS was with the National Comorbidity Study (NCSR) and the NASL, then changes suggested by the translation process and the focus groups may not be implemented if they would affect comparability with the other studies (Alegria et al., 2004). For example, the race/ethnicity questions in the NLAAS were kept as comparable to the other studies and the Census, even though focus group participants made the criticisms I mentioned earlier of these questions. At the same time, an additional set of items were added later in the demographic section of the interview that allowed respondents a much wider range of self-identifiers for race and ethnicity that reflected the team's knowledge of the diversity of ways these statuses were referenced across the Americas (Alegria et al., 2004).

While some may view this process as overly time consuming and cumbersome, in practice it is essential if researchers are serious about doing minority and cross-cultural mental health research. Particularly, if these processes are viewed as integral to the research, rather than a phase to get through so the real research can start, the team will gain important insights into issues of mental health and wellness of the communities to be studied.

Measuring Mental Health

The measurement of mental health problems among multicultural populations has advanced considerably. The development of various translations and adaptations of the Composite International Diagnostic Interview (CIDI) for use in the WHO World Mental Survey Initiative, as well as with the National Latino and Asian American Study (NLAAS) and the National Survey of American Life (NSAL) in the U.S., means that there is a well translated psychiatric diagnostic interview for use with people from many of the major cultures and language groups in the world (Alegria et al., 2004; Jackson et al., 2004; Kessler & Ustun, 2004). This is no small accomplishment and reflects major advances in the understanding of how to culturally adapt standardized psychiatric research instruments for multicultural populations.

The publications of these studies, as well as the release of these data sets for public access, means that investigators have much better information on the state of mental health among the diverse populations of the world. Many of these studies also incorporate a range of questions on the use of mental health services. These studies provide invaluable data for comparing more local studies to a range of national and international samples of relevance to those interested in the mental health of multicultural populations.

The overwhelming focus of these instruments and studies is on psychiatric disorders defined by the major nosological systems: the ICD-10 and DSM-IV. This means that mental health is still largely framed within Euro-American conceptualizations and categorizations of psychiatric disorders. The NLAAS did incorporate screeners for and more detailed questions about neurasthenia among Asian, particularly Chinese communities, and *ataque de nervios* among Latino populations (Alegria et al., 2004). Both of these cultural syndromes have long research histories which examine their cultural meanings and experiences, as well as their relationship to psychiatric disorders (Chang et al., 2005; Kleinman, 1982; Zheng et al., 1997; Guarnaccia et al., 1993; Guarnaccia, Rivera, Franco, & Neighbors, 1996; Guarnaccia & Rogler, 1999; Lewis-Fernandez et al., 2002, 2005). The investigators who developed questions on these syndromes for the NLAAS have contributed to much of this recent literature. At the same time, the development of these modules within a CIDI framework means that the data on these syndromes is quite limited for in-depth study of these experiences. Rather these data provide a starting place for future research on these syndromes in the U.S. (Guarnaccia & Rogler, 1999).

Another limitation of the broad range of CIDI measures is that they define mental health as mental disorder within fixed categories. For those who want to study mental health problems in a more dimensional way, there are several widely used scales that assess mental health status in a continuous fashion. Several of these have a long track record in multicultural populations in the U.S. and elsewhere and have been well translated into a number of languages. The Center for Epidemiological Studies – Depression scale is one of the most widely used measures of depressive affect and more general demoralization. The CES-D was used in the Hispanic Health and Nutrition Study (HHANES), a major study of the health and mental health of the U.S. Latino population in the mid-1980s. The translation into Spanish was found to be effective across major Latino groups. There have also been several studies of the factor structure of the CES-D in the HHANES and in other studies with Latinos

(Guarnaccia et al., 1989). The HHANES also provides comparative national data for the Latino population, though now fairly dated.

For more clinical research, the Hamilton and Beck Scales of depression and anxiety have been widely used across cultural groups and are available in a variety of translations. These scales are more sensitive indicators of clinical improvement when used repeatedly over the course of treatment. There is also ample data on the performance of these measures in multicultural populations in the U.S.

Measuring Wellness

Across all groups, the measurement of wellness is less developed than the measurement of mental disorder. Thus, a major challenge is the availability of good wellness measures for any population. One area of methodological development is Quality of Life (QOL) measurement. QOL has emerged as an important measure for the study of the impact of both pharmacological and psychosocial treatments (Spilker, 1996). QOL measures tend to focus on general health assessments, physical and social functioning, limitations on daily activities, pain, and, in some cases, spirituality.

Because of the importance of Quality of Life as an outcome measure for clinical trials, the National Cancer Institute initiated a major program for the development of QOL measures for multicultural populations (Guarnaccia, 1996). These projects involved both the translation and adaptation of measures for different cultural groups. QOL measures exist both for specific diseases and for more general assessment of QOL.

Lehman's (1995) measure of QOL is widely used in studies of people with serious mental illness. It incorporates assessments of a wide range of domains of life, including social relationships, housing, and work. Matias-Carrelo et al. (2003) provide details on the translation of this measure into Spanish.

One area that has proven particularly challenging in cross-cultural research is the measurement of social functioning. One of the key challenges for minority populations is assessing the extent to which limitations in social functioning are a result of the person's problems and mental health status or the ways that broader societal contexts limit the opportunities for healthy social functioning. In assessing social functioning of those with mental illness, researchers need to examine in a comparative way measures of social functioning in the broader community. Problems such as unemployment or sporadic employment may be as determined by larger economic forces as by a person's mental health status. Practically, talking with family about the different contexts of social functioning is essential to both assessing which dimensions of social functioning are most critical within the family and community and how the person with mental illness compares to others in the community.

As part of the WHO World Mental Health Survey, the WHO developed its own Disability Assessment Scale (WHO-DAS II), which was tested in 19 countries and translated for use in those settings (Vazquez-Barquero et al., 2000). The WHO-DAS II is a promising measure that incorporates assessments of interactions with the broader social world as well as evaluations of self-care and functioning.

Spirituality is another challenging area for assessment. The adaptation of QOL measures for minority communities brought issues of spirituality to the fore. Spirituality is generally distinguished from religious practice and attendance at meetings; it focuses more on connection with some higher power that provides a sense of purpose and meaning in a person's life. The Fetzer Institute has been a major institution that has developed measures of spirituality (Fetzer Institute, 1999).

Incorporating Social and Cultural Issues

There are several key correlates of mental illness and wellness that are important to the field of multicultural mental health research. The assessment of these areas has been furthered by the NLASS and NSAL studies. These studies made a concerted effort to assess social and cultural issues that are associated with mental health but not as frequently incorporated into epidemiological research. At the same time, there is considerable room for development and refinement of these measures, particularly as they relate to specific study populations and the dynamics of local contexts.

Measuring Acculturation

Acculturation has been widely discussed and used in minority mental health research (Chun, Organista, & Marin, 2003; Guarnaccia et al., 2007). Acculturation refers to the processes of adaptation and adjustment that occur when people move from one social and cultural context to another. It involves complex processes of learning the new culture, maintaining or dropping aspects of the culture of origin, and developing new cultural formations. A full discussion of the complexities and issues in acculturation research are well beyond the scope of this chapter, but there are a number of excellent reviews of the issue, including a recent book published by the American Psychological Association (Chun, Organista, & Marin, 2003).

The measurement of acculturation has been a major focus of Latino mental health researchers (Rogler, Malgady, & Cortes, 1991); but has also been discussed in Asian American (Suinn-Lew, 1987) and African American (Landrine & Klonoff, 1996) mental health research. Language based measures have been the most widely used; that is measures that examine fluency in and social use of a native language and English in different contexts. Other key measures of acculturation have included nativity, migration history, and involvement with cultural practices (food, music, and media) from both the home and host country.

The key issue for assessing the relationship of acculturation processes to mental health outcomes is conceptualizing which different measures are relevant and why they are relevant for those outcomes (Guarnaccia et al., 2007). There is considerable overlap of which measures are frequently used to assess acculturation. The larger issue is how to interpret these variables as windows into more complex processes of acculturation. While much of the research has been focused on scale development, the diversity of measures and, more importantly of experiences and contexts of acculturation, suggest that strategies that more fully and systematically assess acculturation through multivariate modeling approaches may be a more productive strategy (Guarnaccia et al., 2007). Analyses from the NLAAS make clear that different dimensions of the acculturation experience are important for different kinds of mental health outcomes (Alegria et al., 2007a,b). One of the key issues in moving acculturation research forward is to develop stronger conceptual frameworks that link key variables and measures to broader social, historical and cultural processes. At the same time, the conceptual work also involves new methodological approaches to linking measures of culture change to mental health outcomes. Multivariate approaches by ethnic group show more promise in analyzing these processes than further scale development.

Immigration

Assessing the impact of immigration experiences on mental health and wellness is an area closely related to, but separable from acculturation measures. The different aspects of the migration process can have differential effects on mental health and wellness (Guarnaccia, 1997; Portes, & Rumbaut, 2001). The motivations for leaving the home country as well as the manner of exit set the stage for the process. Some people are forced to leave due to violence and threats to their well-being. They may have little opportunity to plan and are already traumatized to some extent before even starting their journey. At the other extreme are those who fully plan to leave their home country and have great optimism for the new opportunities they hope to find in their new home.

The process of the migratory journey has great potential for affecting mental health and wellness. The ease or difficulty of the trip plays a major role. Some journeys are quite long and fraught with danger. Single women travelers are at particularly high risk of sexual abuse during trips where they are very vulnerable. Other journeys can be quite easy and pose few challenges in and of themselves.

The context of reception also plays a key role. Some immigrants arrive as refugees and receive extensive services and supports from the governments of their new home. These can include assistance in finding a place to live, food subsidies, assistance with medical care, and help in transferring educational and professional credentials in their new home. Others arrive with no supports and, if they are undocumented, live in considerable fear in addition to having to figure out all the practical aspects of living. Informal support networks often fill in where government programs are not available, as well as being adjuncts to more formal programs.

Social Supports

Community supports are also important to the adaptation and adjustment of new immigrants, as well as to the health and well-being of long term residents of a community. Social supports may come from several levels of social organiza-tion. Family supports are usually central to mental health and well-being. Families play a key role in nurturing their members, providing material and emotional supports, and dealing with illnesses and misfortunes of many kinds.

Members of social organizations such as churches, social clubs, and schools often develop programs that promote community wellness and provide support to those going through mental health problems. The extensiveness of these resources and their ability to mobilize support in times of need are greatly shaped by broader social, economic and political forces.

Ethnic enclaves (Portes & Jensen, 1987; Nee & Sanders, 1987) play a complex role in the adaptation of immigrants to a new society. They often contain not only co-ethnics, but people from the same regions or communities of members' countries of origin. Thus they provide a sense of familiarity so important to the beginning stages of adjustment. Enclaves also provide networks to key social services as well as connections for jobs. They buffer language issues as longer term members of the community often are bilingual and can help new arrivals negotiate the broader society. At the same time, enclaves can isolate recent arrivals from the broader society and slow their processes of adjustment. Again, the resources of ethnic communities vary widely depending on the social and cultural capital within the community and the relationships of the community with broader society.

Role of Discrimination

One key dimension of the broader society that has been the focus of research on minority mental health and wellness has been the role of discrimination. In this area, the most developed work has come from researchers of the African American experience in the U.S. (Krieger, 1999; Williams, Neighbors, &

Jackson, 2003), but research on the role of discrimination in minority mental health has been expanding for other ethnic groups as well. Discrimination can occur at a structural level in terms of laws and policies that disadvantage some groups over others. It also occurs at the individual level in more overt and subtle forms.

All forms of discrimination are relevant to the mental health and wellness of minority communities. Research is in the early stages in terms of identifying the relative impacts of different levels and types of discrimination on mental health status and also access to mental health resources. Structural discrimination exists in the form of differential availability of and access to health and mental health services and insurance and other resources needed to access those services. More individual forms of discrimination are mediated through the attitudes and values of helping organizations and professionals. And much discrimination occurs at the level of day-to-day interactions among people.

The assessment of discrimination is complex as well. One level of assessment is on measuring different forms of discrimination – denial of services, disrespectful treatment, and lack of access. A dimension of these measures is the extent of both perceived and concrete discrimination. Another dimension involves assessing why the person thinks they were discriminated against, which may involve race, language, gender, social class, and sexual orientation among a number of features. A further dimension is whether the discrimination was directed at the group a person belongs to, at someone close to the person or the person themselves (Williams, Neighbors, & Jackson, 2003). The consequences of the discrimination are also important to assess. In terms of impact on mental health and wellness, frequency of discrimination and specific types of discrimination may have independent or cumulative effects. Assessing the methodological and substantive aspects of the impact of discrimination on mental health and wellness is an active area of research that promises to provide a much clearer sense of its consequences.

Combining Qualitative and Quantitative Methods

There has been a growing interest in mixed methods research in minority mental health and wellness research. This interest has particularly involved integrating more qualitative research methods into minority mental health research because of concerns that concepts, methods and approaches to mental health research are not well adapted for multicultural populations. Mixed methods approaches that engage qualitative methods more fully are viewed as one solution to how to adapt standard research approaches for multicultural communities and clients. The development of the NLAAS measures provides good examples of how to achieve this kind of integration (Alegria et al., 2004).

Qualitative research is specifically designed for exploring a topic in an open-ended way and gaining understanding of a new or little explored area (Bernard,

2006). Because qualitative research seeks to examine a topic from the perspective of those interviewed, it allows researchers to examine whether their conception of a mental health issue or treatment intervention makes sense within the cultural group under study. Qualitative research is not the same as ethnography. Ethnography is a comprehensive approach to community research that involves active and long-term engagement in a community of a different culture from that of the researcher. It typically begins with an extended period of participant observation by the researcher. This involves observation of and engagement with key aspects of life of the community, with detailed fieldnotes on what is observed along with questions and hypotheses about the observations being noted on a daily basis. This emphasis on observation allows the ethnographer to become engaged with the community, to hear how key issues are discussed on an everyday basis, and to observe behavior directly as a grounding for later interviewing about the motivations for and meaning of those behaviors. Following this period of participant observation, the researcher engages in a series of more structured research activities, including a range of interviews and other data-gathering techniques. By now it should be clear that doing a few focus groups is not the same as ethnography!

While focus groups are not the same as ethnography, they are very useful research tools in minority mental health research. Focus groups can be used throughout the research process to explore ideas about mental illness, wellness and treatment resources; to translate and adapt research interviews; and to assess treatment intervention manuals and other aspects of intervention programs. Focus groups involve small group interviews with about 8–10 participants each from the groups under study (Morgan & Kreuger, 1988). The key aspect of making a focus group effective is to transform the participants into the experts on the topic under investigation and the researcher into their student. There are a growing number of examples of the use of focus groups in minority mental health and wellness research (Cabassa et al., 2007; Martinez & Guarnaccia, 2007).

There are a number of types of qualitative interview approaches, including key informant interviewing, informal, open-ended interviews, semi-structured and structured interviews, domain exploration techniques (Spradley, 1979), life history interviews and interviews using responses to a vignette, photograph, or event to gain insights into cultural issues of concern. Some more structured techniques include free lists and pile sorts, as well as sentence completion tasks, which are very useful to assess categorizations of illnesses and health care resources (Weller et al., 2002). Detailed discussions of theses different approaches are beyond the scope of this chapter, but there are excellent resources available, the most widely used being Bernard (2006).

One such technique is Kleinman's explanatory model (1980). This approach, based on eight questions about an illness episode, provides a framework for clinicians and researchers to assess cultural ideas about illness and its treatment. The questions focus on conception of the illness, perceived causes, severity, and treatment expectations. These questions have been elaborated into a full research tool to use in exploring cultural conceptions of mental health and illness (Weiss et al., 1992).

One of the key challenges in mixed methods research is to create a true team among the quantitative and qualitative researchers. One way to do this is to bring a qualitative researcher onto the team as a full member, rather than typically as a consultant at the beginning of the research. A second is to have all the research team trained in both the qualitative and quantitative methods to be used in the study. A third is to conceptualize the research process as an iterative process of qualitative research to adapt instruments and explore topics, followed by a more structured investigation, followed by more qualitative work to explore unexpected findings and to develop intervention tools, followed by a structured intervention that is evaluated using a mix of qualitative and quantitative approaches. As we continue to improve and expand multicultural mental health research, the creative integration of qualitative and quantitative methods will be an integral part of this process. Unfortunately, there are few models of research programs that have fully achieved this level of integration.

Building Bilingual/Bicultural Research Teams

To achieve the research agenda that follows from the previous sections, it is critical to build diverse teams of researchers. This diversity spans a number of dimensions including discipline, methodological orientation, research training, ethnic background, and language abilities. Minority mental health and wellness research can best be carried out by multidisciplinary teams that have members who come from and/or are expert in the communities to be studied.

Research teams need to be able to design studies that will be effective in minority communities. While this means the team has to have mastery of the key methods and measures in minority mental health and wellness research, this is not sufficient to be successful. The research team must also be able to function effectively in the communities to be studied. This means not only language abilities but also the knowledge of how to relate to the communities, how to gain access to the people to be studied, how to move through the communities in a physical and social sense, and how to bring back the results to have a positive impact on the mental health and wellness of the communities. Community-based participatory research approaches are designed to achieve these goals (Minkler, Wallerstein, & Hall, 2003).

Building such a team requires a commitment to the recruitment and training of a diverse staff. There are now a number of federal programs, particularly through NIH, to facilitate this process. These include training programs for pre- and post-doctoral fellows through NIH and through key social science and health professional associations. The NIH Minority Supplement Program facilitates adding multicultural researchers at different levels of training to research teams. Mechanisms such as the EXPORT grant program and the

Disparities Centers Program provide support for research and training, with a focus on addressing mental health and wellness disparities.

Making diverse teams work requires a level of sensitivity to group process and interpersonal relationships that is not always made explicit in research training. Valuing diverse input into the design and implementation of research programs is an essential skill. Allowing junior researchers to lead when they have more experience in the communities to be studied is often a challenge in research teams. Being able to have everyone contribute from their diverse professional and cultural expertise enriches the research process. One of the first steps is for the research program leaders to think through how the diversity of their team contributes to the research effort and making that explicit at the beginning of and during the research process.

Summary

The methodological challenges of minority mental health and wellness research are myriad. One of the goals of this chapter was to review the substantial progress that has been made in advancing the minority mental health and wellness agenda. Another is to point to new directions for research training, human capacity building, and team development to accelerate the advances in minority mental health and wellness research. Effectively addressing these multiple challenges in minority mental health and wellness research promises not only to improve the research effort for minorities but more importantly to improve their mental health and wellness to reduce existing disparities. When effectively carried out, the minority mental health and wellness agenda will not only impact minorities but the broader society as disparities affect the mental health and wellness of us all.

References

Alegria, M., Vila, D., Woo, M., Canino, G., Takeuchi, D., Vera, M., et al. (2004). Cultural relevance and equivalence in the NLAAS instrument: Integrating etic and emic in the cross-cultural measures for a psychiatric epidemiology and services study. *International Journal of Methods in Psychiatric Research, 13,* 270–288.

Alegria, M., Shrout, P., Sribney, W., Guarnaccia, P., Woo, M., Vila, D., et al. (2007a). Understanding differences in past year mental health disorders for Latinos living in the U.S. *Social Science and Medicine, 65,* 214–230.

Alegria, M., Sribney, W., Woo, M., Guarnaccia, P., & Torres, M. (2007b). Looking beyond nativity: The relation of age of immigration, length of residence, and birth cohorts to the risk of onset of psychiatric disorders for Latinos. *Research in Human Development, 4,* 19–47.

American Anthropological Association. (1997). Response to OMB Directive 15. Last retrieved March 21, 2008; Available at http://www.aaanet.org/gvt/ombdraft.htm

American Anthropological Association. (2007) Project on RACE. Last retrieved March 22, 2008; Available at http://www.understandingrace.org/home.html

Angel, R., & Guarnaccia, P. J, (1989). Mind, Body and Culture: Somatization among Hispanics. *Social Science and Medicine, 28,* 1229–1238.

Bernard, H. R. (2006). *Research methods in anthropology; Qualitative and quantitative approaches* (4th ed.). Lanham, MD: AltaMira Press.

Brislin, R. W. (1970). Back-translation for cross-cultural research. *Journal of Cross-Cultural Psychology, 1,* 187–216.

Brislin, R. W., Lonner, W., & Thorndike, R. (1973). *Cross-cultural research methods.* New York: John Wiley & Sons.

Cabassa, L. J. Lester, R. & Zayas, L. H. (2007). "It's like being in a labyrinth:" Hispanic immigrants' perceptions of depression and attitudes towards treatments. *Journal of Immigrant and Minority Health, 9,* 1–16.

Canino, G., & Bravo, M. (1994). The adaptation and testing of diagnostics and outcome measures for cross cultural research. *International Review of Psychiatry, 6,* 281–286.

Chang, D. F., Myers, H. F., Yeung, A., Zhang, Y., Zhao, J., & Yu, S. (2005). *Shenjing Shuairuo* and the DSM-IV: Diagnosis, distress, and disability in a Chinese primary care setting. *Transcultural Psychiatry, 42,* 204–218.

Chun, K. M., Organista, P. B., & Marin, G. (Eds.). (2003). *Acculturation : Advances in theory, measurement, and applied research.* Washington, DC: The American Psychological Association.

Fetzer Institute. (1999). *Multidimensional measurement of religiousness/ spirituality for use in health research.* Kalamazoo, MI: Fetzer Institute.

Gaboda, D. Tsikiwa, F., Warner, L., & Guarnaccia, P. (2000). *Adjusting for the underreporting of Hispanic ethnicity in New Jersey mortality statistics.* New Brunswick: Rutgers, The State University of New Jersey, Center for State Health Policy, Institute for Health, Health Care Policy and Aging Research.

Good, B. J. (1994). *Medicine, rationality and experience: An anthropological perspective.* Cambridge: Cambridge University Press.

Guarnaccia, P. J., Angel, R., & Worobey, J. L. (1989). The factor structure of the CES-D in the Hispanic Health and Nutrition Examination Survey. *Social Science and Medicine, 29,* 85–94.

Guarnaccia, P. J., Guevara-Ramos, L. M., Gonzales, G., Canino, G. J., & Bird, H. (1992). Cross-cultural aspects of psychotic symptoms in Puerto Rico. *Research in Community and Mental Health, 7,* 99–110.

Guarnaccia, P. J., Canino, G., Rubio-Stipec, M., & Bravo, M. (1993). The prevalence of ataques de nervios in the Puerto Rico Disaster Study: The role of culture in psychiatric epidemiology. *The Journal of Nervous and Mental Disease, 181,* 157–165.

Guarnaccia, P. J., Rivera, M., Franco, F., & Neighbors, C. (1996). The experiences of ataques de nervios: Towards an anthropology of emotion in Puerto Rico. *Culture, Medicine and Psychiatry, 20,* 343–367.

Guarnaccia, P. J. (1996). Anthropological perspectives: The importance of culture in the assessment of quality of life. In B. Spilker (Ed.), *Quality of life and pharmacoeconomics in clinical trials* (2nd ed., pp. 523–528). Philadelphia: Lippincott-Raven Publishers.

Guarnaccia, P. J. (1997). Social and psychological distress among Latinos in the United States. In I. Al-Issa & M. Tousignant, (Eds.), *Ethnicity, immigration and psychopathology* (pp. 71–94). New York: Plenum.

Guarnaccia, P. J., & Rogler, L. H. (1999). Research on culture-bound syndromes: New directions. *American Journal of Psychiatry, 156,* 1322–1327.

Guarnaccia, P. J., Lewis-Fernandez, R., & Rivera Marano, M. (2003). Toward a Puerto Rican popular nosology: *Nervios* and *ataque de nervios. Culture, Medicine and Psychiatry, 27,* 339–366.

Guarnaccia, P. J., Martinez Pincay, I., Alegria, M., Shrout, P. E., Lewis-Fernandez, R., & Canino, G. J. (2007). Assessing diversity among Latinos: Results from the NLAAS. *Hispanic Journal of Behavioral Sciences, 29,* 510–534.

Hahn, R. A., & Mulinare, J. (1992). Inconsistencies in coding race and ethnicity between birth and death in U.S. infants. *Journal of the American Medical Association, 267*, 259–263.

Hayes-Battista, D. E., & Chapa, J. (1987). Latino terminology: Conceptual bases for standardized terminology. *American Journal of Public Health, 77*, 61–68.

Hazuda, H. P., Comeaux, P. J., Stem, M. P., Haffner, S. M., Eifler, C. W., & Rosenthal, M. (1986). A comparison of three indicators for identifying Mexican Americans in epidemiological research. *American Journal of Epidemiology, 123*, 96–112.

Jackson, J. S., Torres, M., Caldwell, C. H., Neighbors, H. W., Neese, R. W., Taylor, R. J., et al. (2004). The National Survey of American Life: A study of racial, ethnic and cultural influences on mental disorder. *International Journal of Methods in Psychiatric Research, 13*, 196–207.

Jenkins, J. & Karno, M. (1992). The meaning of expressed emotion: Theoretical issues raised by cross-cultural research. *American Journal of Psychiatry, 149*, 9–21.

Kessler, R. C., & Ustun, T. B. (2004). The World Mental Health (WMH) Survey Initiative Version of the World Health Organization (WHO) Composite International Diagnostic Interview (CIDI). *International Journal of Methods in Psychiatric Research, 13*, 93–121.

Kleinman, A. (1980). *Patients and healers in the context of culture.* Berkeley: University of California Press.

Kleinman, A. (1982). Neurasthenia and depression: A study of somatization and culture in China. *Culture, Medicine and Psychiatry, 6*, 117–190.

Krieger, N. (1999). Embodying inequality: A review of concepts, measures, and methods for studying health consequences of discrimination. *International Journal of Health Services, 29*, 295–352.

Landrine, H., & Klonoff, E. A. (1996). *African American acculturation: Deconstructing race and reviving culture.* Thousand Oaks, CA: Sage Publications.

Lewis-Fernandez, R. Guarnaccia, P. J., Martinez, I. E., Salman, E, Schmidt, A., & Liebowitz, M. (2002). Comparative phenomenology of *ataques de nervios*, panic attacks, and panic disorder. *Culture, Medicine and Psychiatry, 26*, 199–223.

Lewis-Fernandez, R., Guarnaccia, P., Patel, S., Lizardi, D., & Diaz, N. (2005). *Ataque de nervios*: Anthropological, epidemiological and clinical dimensions of a cultural syndrome. In A. M. Georgiopoulos & J. F. Rosenbaum, (Eds.), *Perspectives in cross-cultural psychiatry* (pp. 63–85.) Philadelphia: Lippincott Williams and Wilkins.

Lewis-Fernandez, R., et al., (in press). Significance of endorsement of psychotic symptoms by U.S. Latinos. *Journal of Nervous and Mental Disease.*

Martinez Pincay, I. E. & Guarnaccia, P. J. (2007). "It's like going through an earthquake": Anthropological perspectives on depression among Latino immigrants. *Journal of Immigrant and Minority Health, 9*, 17–28.

Matias-Carrelo, L. E., Chavez, L. M., Negron, G., Canino, G., Aguilar-Gaxiola, S., & Hoppe, S. (2003). The Spanish translation and cultural adaptation of five mental health outcome measures. *Culture, Medicine and Psychiatry, 27*, 291–313.

Minkler, M., Wallerstein, N., & Hall, B. (2003). *Community-based participatory research for health.* San Francisco, CA: Jossey-Bass.

Morgan, D. L., & Kruger, R. A. (1998). *The focus group kit.* Thousand Oaks, CA: Sage Publications.

Nee, V., & Sanders, J. (1987). On testing the enclave-economy hypothesis. *American Sociological Review, 52*, 771–773.

Office of Management and Budget. (1997). Revisions to the standards for the classification of federal data on race and ethnicity. Last retrieved March 21, 2008; Available at http://www.whitehouse.gov/omb/fedreg/ombdir15.html

Portes, A., & Jensen, L. (1987). What's an enclave: The case for conceptual clarity. *American Sociological Review, 52*, 768–771.

Portes, A., & Rumbaut, R. (2001). *Legacies: The story of the immigrant second generation.* Berkeley, CA: University of California Press.

Reinhard, S. C., Gubman, G. D., Horwitz, A. V., & Minsky, S. (1994). Burden assessment scale for families of the seriously mentally ill. *Evaluation and Program Planning, 1*, 261–269.

Rogler, L. H., Cortes, D. E., & Malgady, R. G. (1991). Acculturation and mental health status among Hispanics: New directions for research. *American Psychologist, 46*, 585–597.

Smedley, B. D., Stith, A. Y., & Nelson, A. R. (Eds.). (2003). *Unequal treatment: Confronting racial and ethnic disparities in health care.* Washington, D.C.: National Academies Press.

Spilker, B. (Ed.). (1996). *Quality of life and pharmacoeconomics in clinical trials* (2nd ed.). Philadelphia, PA: Lippincott-Raven Publishers.

Spradley, J. (1979). *The ethnographic interview.* New York: Holt, Reinhart & Winston.

Stroup, D., & Hahn, R. (1994). Race and ethnicity in public health surveillance. *Public Health Reports, 109*, 7–15.

Suinn, R. M., Rickard-Figueroa, K., Lew, S., & Vigil, P. (1987). The Suinn-Lew Asian Self Identity Acculturation Scale: An initial report. *Educational and Psychological Measurement, 47*, 401–407.

U.S. Bureau of the Census. (2000) Form D-61A. Last retrieved March 21, 2008): Available at http://www.census.gov/dmd/www/pdf/d61a.pdf.

U.S. Bureau of the Census. (2000). State and County QuickFacts. Last retrieved March 21, 2008; Available at http://quickfacts.census.gov/qfd/meta/long_68178.htm

U.S. Bureau of the Census. (2001). Overview of race and Hispanic origin. Last retrieved March 22, 2008; Available at http://www.census.gov/prod/2001pubs/ c2kbr011.pdf

U.S. Department of Health and Human Services. (2001). *Mental health: Culture, race, and ethnicity.* Rockville, MD: U.S. Department of Health and Human Services, Public Health Service, Office of the Surgeon General.

Vazquez-Barquero, J. L., Vazquez Bourgon, E., Herrera Castanedo, S., Saiz, J., Uniarte, M., Morales, F., et al. (2000). Spanish version of the New World Health Organization Disability Assessment Schedule II (WHO-DAS II): Initial phase of development and pilot study. *Actas Española Psychiatrica, 28*, 77–88.

Waters, M. (1990). *Ethnic options: Choosing identities in America.* Berkeley, CA: University of California Press.

Weiss, M., Doongaji, D. R., Siddhartha, S., Wypij, S. Pathare, S., Bhatawdekar, M., et al. (1992). The Explanatory Model Interview Catalogue (EMIC): Contribution to cross-cultural research methods from a study of leprosy and mental health. *British Journal of Psychiatry, 160*, 819–830.

Weller, S. C., Baer, R. D., Garcia de Alba Garcia, J., Glazer, M., Trotter, R., Pachter, L., et al. (2002). Regional variations in Latino descriptions of *susto. Culture, Medicine and Psychiatry, 26*, 449–472.

Williams, D., Lavisso-Mourey, R., & Warren, R. (1994). The concept of race and health status in America. *Public Health Reports, 109*, 26–41.

Zheng, Y. P, Lin, K. M., Takeuchi, D., Kurasaki, K. S., Wang, Y., & Cheung, F. (1997). An epidemiological study of neurasthenia in Chinese-Americans in Los Angeles. *Comprehensive Psychiatry, 38*, 249–259.

Index